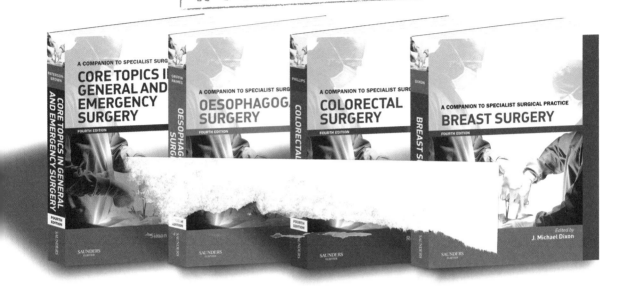

A COMPANION TO SPECIALIST SURGICAL PRACTICE

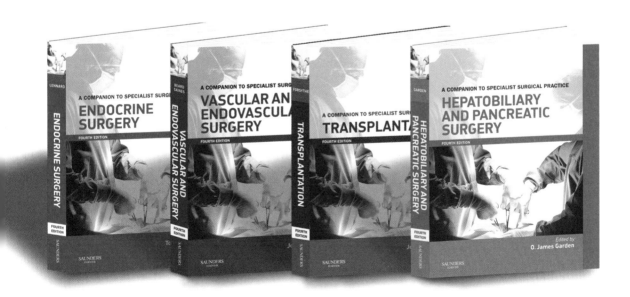

COLORECTAL SURGERY

A Companion to Specialist Surgical Practice

Series Editors
O. James Garden
Simon Paterson-Brown

COLORECTAL SURGERY

FOURTH EDITION

Edited by

Robin K.S. Phillips

MB BS FRCS

Professor of Colorectal Surgery
Imperial College London;
Consultant Surgeon and Clinical Director
St Mark's Hospital
Harrow, Middlesex, UK

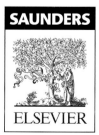

Edinburgh   London   New York   Oxford   Philadelphia   St Louis   Sydney   Toronto   2009

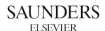

SAUNDERS
ELSEVIER

First edition 1997
Second edition 2001
Third edition 2005
Fourth edition 2009
 Reprinted 2010

ISBN 9780702030109

British Library Cataloguing in Publication Data
A catalogue record for this book is available from the British Library

Library of Congress Cataloging in Publication Data
A catalog record for this book is available from the Library of Congress

Notice
Knowledge and best practice in this field are constantly changing. As new research and experience broaden our knowledge, changes in practice, treatment and drug therapy may become necessary or appropriate. Readers are advised to check the most current information provided (i) on procedures featured or (ii) by the manufacturer of each product to be administered, to verify the recommended dose or formula, the method and duration of administration, and contraindications. It is the responsibility of the practitioner, relying on their own experience and knowledge of the patient, to make diagnoses, to determine dosages and the best treatment for each individual patient, and to take all appropriate safety precautions. To the fullest extent of the law, neither the Publisher nor the Editors assumes any liability for any injury and/or damage to persons or property arising out of or related to any use of the material contained in this book.

The Publisher

 ELSEVIER your source for books, journals and multimedia in the health sciences
www.elsevierhealth.com

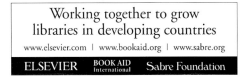

Working together to grow
libraries in developing countries

www.elsevier.com | www.bookaid.org | www.sabre.org

ELSEVIER   BOOK AID International   Sabre Foundation

The Publisher's policy is to use **paper manufactured from sustainable forests**

Printed in China

Commissioning Editor: Laurence Hunter
Development Editor: Elisabeth Lawrence
Project Manager: Andrew Palfreyman
Text Design: Charlotte Murray
Cover Design: Kirsteen Wright
Illustration Manager: Gillian Richards
Illustrators: Martin Woodward and Richard Prime

Contents

Contents

Contributors

David E. Beck, MD, FACS, FASCRS
Chairman, Department of Colon and Rectal Surgery
Ochsner Clinic Foundation
New Orleans, LA, USA

Sue Clark, MD, FRCS(Gen Surg)
Consultant Colorectal Surgeon
St Mark's Hospital
Harrow, UK

Paul Durdey, MS, FRCS
Consultant Colorectal Surgeon
Bristol Royal Infirmary
Bristol, UK

Anton V. Emmanuel, BSc, MD, FRCP
Senior Lecturer and Consultant in
Gastrointestinal Physiology
St Mark's Hospital
Harrow, Middlesex, UK

Nicola S. Fearnhead, MB, BCh, FRCS
Consultant Colorectal Surgeon
Addenbrooke's Hospital
Cambridge, UK

Paul Hatfield, BSc, MB, ChB, MRCP, FRCR, PhD
Consultant Clinical Oncology
St James's Institute of Oncology
St James's University Hospital
Leeds, UK

Adam Haycock, MBBS, MRCP
Specialist Registrar in Gastroenterology
Wolfson Unit for Endoscopy
St Mark's Hospital
Harrow, UK

Ian Jenkins, BSc, MB, FRCS(Ed),
FRCS(Gen Surg)
Laparoscopic Colorectal Fellow
St Mark's Hospital
Harrow, UK

Robin Kennedy, MB, BS, MS, FRCS
Consultant Surgeon
St Mark's Hospital
Harrow, UK

Zygmunt H. Krukowski, MB, ChB, PhD,
FRCS(Ed), Hon FRCS(Glasg), FRCP(Ed)
Professor of Clinical Surgery
University of Aberdeen; Consultant Surgeon
Aberdeen Royal Infirmary Aberdeen, UK

Peter J. Lunniss, BSc, MS, FRCS(Gen Surg)
Senior Lecturer and Honorary
Consultant
Centre for Academic Surgery
Royal London and Homerton
Hospitals
London, UK

Chung Ming Chen, MB, BS, FRCS
Department of General Surgery
Changi General Hospital
Singapore

Neil J.McC. Mortensen, MB, ChB, MD, FRCS
Professor of Colorectal Surgery
John Radcliffe Hospital
Oxford, UK

R. John Nicholls, MA, BChir, FRCS, FRCS(Glasg)
Professor of Colorectal Surgery
Imperial College London; Consultant Surgeon
St Mark's Hospital
Harrow, Middlesex, UK

Robin K.S. Phillips, MB, BS, FRCS
Professor of Colorectal Surgery
Imperial College London;
Consultant Surgeon and Clinical Director
St Mark's Hospital
Harrow, Middlesex, UK

Alexis M.P. Schizas, BSc(Hons), MB, BS(Lond)
Pelvic Floor Unit
St Thomas Hospital
London, UK

John H. Scholefield, MB, ChB, MD, FRCS
Professor of Surgery
Queen's Medical Centre
University Hospital
Nottingham, UK

Contributors

David Sebag-Montefiore, MB, BS, FRCP, FRCR
Consultant Clinical Oncologist
St James's Institute of Oncology
St James's University Hospital
Leeds, UK

Francis Seow-Choen, MB, BS, FRCS(Ed),
FAMS, FRES
Senior Consultant Surgeon
Seow-Choen Colorectal Centre
Singapore

Robert J.C. Steele, MD, FRCS(Ed),
FRCS, FCSHK
Professor of Surgery and Head of Department of
Surgery and Molecular Oncology
University of Dundee Medical School
Ninewells Hospital
Dundee, UK

Paris P. Tekkis, MD, FRCS(Gen Surg)
Senior Lecturer
Imperial College London;
Consultant Colorectal Surgeon
St Mary's Hospital
London, UK

Siwan Thomas-Gibson, MBBS, MRCP, MD
Consultant Gastroenterologist
Wolfson Unit for Endoscopy
St Mark's Hospital
Harrow, UK

Mark W. Thompson-Fawcett, MB, ChB, FRACS
Senior Lecturer and Colorectal Surgeon
University of Otago
Dunedin, New Zealand

Janindra Warusavitarne, BMed, FRACS, PhD
Consultant Surgeon and Clinical Project Leader
GI Cancer Research
Bankstown Hospital and Garvan Institute of
Medical Research
Sydney, Australia

Charles B. Whitlow, MD, FACS, FASCRS
Program Director, Colon and Rectal
Surgery Residency and Staff Colorectal Surgeon
Ochsner Clinic Foundation
New Orleans, LA, USA

Andrew B. Williams, MS, FRCS(Gen Surg)
Consultant Surgeon and Director, Pelvic Floor Unit
St Thomas' Hospital
London, UK

Carolynne Vaizey, MD, MB, ChB,
FRCS(Gen), FCS(SA)
Consultant Surgeon and Chairman of Surgery
St Mark's Hospital
Harrow, UK

Series preface

Since the publication of the first edition in 1997, the *Companion to Specialist Surgical Practice* series has aspired to meet the needs of surgeons in higher training and practising consultants who wish contemporary, evidence-based information on the subspecialist areas relevant to their general surgical practice. We have accepted that the series will not necessarily be as comprehensive as some of the larger reference surgical textbooks which, by their very size, may not always be completely up to date at the time of publication. This Fourth Edition aims to bring relevant state-of-the-art specialist information that we and the individual volume editors consider important for the practising subspecialist general surgeon. Where possible, all contributors have attempted to identify evidence-based references to support key recommendations within each chapter.

We remain grateful to the volume editors and all the contributors of this Fourth Edition. Their enthusiasm, commitment and hard work has ensured that a short turnover has been maintained between each of the editions, thereby ensuring as accurate and up-to-date content as possible. We remain grateful for the support and encouragement of Laurence Hunter and Elisabeth Lawrence at Elsevier Ltd. We trust that our aim of providing up-to-date and affordable surgical texts has been met and that all readers, whether in training or in consultant practice, will find this fourth edition an invaluable resource.

O. James Garden MB, ChB, MD, FRCS(Glas), FRCS(Ed), FRCP(Ed), FRACS(Hon), FRCSC(Hon)
Regius Professor of Clinical Surgery, Clinical and Surgical Sciences (Surgery), University of Edinburgh, and Honorary Consultant Surgeon, Royal Infirmary of Edinburgh

Simon Paterson-Brown MB, BS, MPhil, MS, FRCS(Ed), FRCS
Honorary Senior Lecturer, Clinical and Surgical Sciences (Surgery), University of Edinburgh, and Consultant General and Upper Gastrointestinal Surgeon, Royal Infirmary of Edinburgh

Editor's preface

Colorectal surgery has seen many innovations and changes in the few years since the Third Edition. Multidisciplinary Team Meetings (MDTs) have become embedded in regular UK cancer care, the quality of rectal cancer imaging has gone from strength to strength, and evidence has accrued further with regards to the efficacy of preoperative radiation therapy for all rectal cancer, yet expert opinion remains cautious about its blanket application. As colorectal surgeons increasingly take their part in delivering a colonoscopy service, a fresh chapter on colonoscopy and flexible sigmoidoscopy has been added. Likewise, a myriad of surgical procedures for functional disorders has invited a modern look at less familiar operations, such as the stapled transanal rectal resection (STARR) and external pelvic rectal suspension (EXPRESS) procedures. Enhanced recovery receives its due attention.

The topics are very up to date and the authors are clear and authoritative. Important points are clearly indicated and the references have been reduced to accommodate new chapters and material. Each and every chapter has been thoroughly reviewed and updated. Much is new.

I am confident that readers will enjoy this fourth edition. They will find more than enough to inform, more than enough for examinations worldwide, and more than enough to support them in active consultant practice.

Acknowledgements

I would like to thank Marie Gun, my personal assistant, who has coordinated and chased up the many contributors, followed up on queries and arranged submissions on time.

Robin K.S. Phillips
Harrow

Evidence-based practice in surgery

Critical appraisal for developing evidence-based practice can be obtained from a number of sources, the most reliable being randomised controlled clinical trials, systematic literature reviews, meta-analyses and observational studies. For practical purposes three grades of evidence can be used, analogous to the levels of 'proof' required in a court of law:

1. **Beyond all reasonable doubt.** Such evidence is likely to have arisen from high-quality randomised controlled trials, systematic reviews or high-quality synthesised evidence such as decision analysis, cost-effectiveness analysis or large observational datasets. The studies need to be directly applicable to the population of concern and have clear results. The grade is analogous to burden of proof within a criminal court and may be thought of as corresponding to the usual standard of 'proof' within the medical literature (i.e. $P < 0.05$).

2. **On the balance of probabilities.** In many cases a high-quality review of literature may fail to reach firm conclusions due to conflicting or inconclusive results, trials of poor methodological quality or the lack of evidence in the population to which the guidelines apply. In such cases it may still be possible to make a statement as to the best treatment on the 'balance of probabilities'. This is analogous to the decision in a civil court where all the available evidence will be weighed up and the verdict will depend upon the balance of probabilities.

3. **Not proven.** Insufficient evidence upon which to base a decision, or contradictory evidence.

Depending on the information available, three grades of recommendation can be used:

a. Strong recommendation, which should be followed unless there are compelling reasons to act otherwise.

b. A recommendation based on evidence of effectiveness, but where there may be other factors to take into account in decision-making, for example the user of the guidelines may be expected to take into account patient preferences, local facilities, local audit results or available resources.

c. A recommendation made where there is no adequate evidence as to the most effective practice, although there may be reasons for making a recommendation in order to minimise cost or reduce the chance of error through a locally agreed protocol.

Strong recommendation

Evidence where a conclusion can be reached 'beyond all reasonable doubt' and therefore where a **strong recommendation** can be given.

This will normally be based on evidence levels:

- **Ia.** Meta-analysis of randomised controlled trials
- **Ib.** Evidence from at least one randomised controlled trial
- **IIa.** Evidence from at least one controlled study without randomisation
- **IIb.** Evidence from at least one other type of quasi-experimental study.

Expert opinion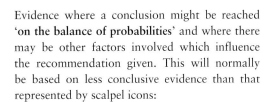

Evidence where a conclusion might be reached 'on the balance of probabilities' and where there may be other factors involved which influence the recommendation given. This will normally be based on less conclusive evidence than that represented by scalpel icons:

- **III.** Evidence from non-experimental descriptive studies, such as comparative studies and case–control studies
- **IV.** Evidence from expert committee reports or opinions or clinical experience of respected authorities, or both.

Evidence in each chapter of this volume which is associated with either a strong recommendation or expert opinion is annotated in the text by either a **scalpel** or **pen-nib** icon as shown above. References associated with **scalpel** evidence will be highlighted in the reference lists, along with a short summary of the paper's conclusions where applicable.

1

Anorectal investigation

Alexis M.P. Schizas
Andrew B. Williams

Introduction

Many tests are available to investigate anorectal disorders, each only providing part of a patient's assessment, so results should be considered together and alongside the clinical picture derived from a careful history and physical examination.

Investigations provide information about structure alone, function alone, or both, and have been directed to five general areas of interest: faecal incontinence, constipation (including Hirschsprung's disease), anorectal sepsis, rectal prolapse (including solitary rectal ulcer syndrome) and anorectal malignancy.

Anatomy and physiology of the anal canal

The adult anal canal is approximately 4 cm long and begins as the rectum narrows, passing backwards between the levator ani muscles. It has an upper limit at the pelvic floor and a lower limit at the anus. The proximal canal is lined by simple columnar epithelium, changing to stratified squamous epithelium lower in the canal via an intermediate transition zone just above the dentate line. Beneath the mucosa is the subepithelial tissue, composed of connective tissue and smooth muscle. This layer increases in thickness throughout life and forms the basis of the vascular cushions thought to aid continence.

Lateral to the subepithelial layer the caudal continuation of the circular smooth muscle of the rectum forms the internal anal sphincter, which terminates caudally with a well-defined border at a variable distance from the anal verge. Continuous with the outer layer of the rectum the longitudinal layer of the anal canal lies between the internal and external anal sphincters in the intersphincteric space. The longitudinal muscle comprises smooth muscle cells from the rectal wall, augmented with striated muscle from a variety of sources, including the levator ani, puborectalis and pubococcygeus muscles. Fibres from this layer traverse the external anal sphincter forming septa that insert into the skin of the lower anal canal and adjacent perineum as the corrugator cutis ani muscle.

The striated muscle of the external sphincter surrounds the longitudinal muscle and forms the outer border of the intersphincteric space. The external sphincter is arranged as a tripartite structure, classically described by Holl and Thompson and later adopted by Gorsch and by Milligan and Morgan. In this system the external sphincter is divided into deep, superficial and subcutaneous portions, with the deep and subcutaneous sphincter forming rings of muscle and, between them, the elliptical fibres of the superficial sphincter running anteriorly from the perineal body to the coccyx posteriorly. Some consider the external sphincter to be a single muscle contiguous with the puborectalis muscle, while others have adopted a two-part model. The latter

1

proposes a deep anal sphincter and a superficial anal sphincter, corresponding to the puborectalis and deep external anal sphincter combined, as well as the fused superficial and subcutaneous sphincter of the tripartite model. Anal endosonography (AES) and magnetic resonance imaging (MRI) have not resolved the dilemma, although most authors report a three-part sphincter where the puborectalis muscle is fused with the deep sphincter.[1]

The external anal sphincter is innervated by the pudendal nerve (S2–S4), which leaves the pelvis via the lower part of the greater sciatic notch, where it passes under the pyriformis muscle. It then crosses the ischial spine and sacrospinous ligament to enter the ischiorectal fossa through the lesser sciatic notch or foramen via the pudendal (or Alcock's) canal.

The pudendal nerve has two branches: the inferior rectal nerve, which supplies the external anal sphincter and sensation to the perianal skin; and the perineal nerve, which innervates the anterior perineal muscles together with the sphincter urethrae and forms the dorsal nerve of the clitoris (penis). Although puborectalis receives its main innervation from a direct branch of the fourth sacral nerve root, it may derive some innervation via the pudendal nerve.

The autonomic supply to the anal canal and pelvic floor comes from two sources. The fifth lumbar nerve root sends sympathetic fibres to the superior and inferior hypogastric plexuses and the parasympathetic supply is from the second to fourth sacral nerve roots via the nervi erigentes. Fibres of both systems pass obliquely across the lateral surface of the lower rectum to reach the region of the perineal body.

The internal anal sphincter has an intrinsic nerve supply from the myenteric plexus together with an additional supply from both the sympathetic and parasympathetic nervous systems. Sympathetic nervous activity is thought to enhance and parasympathetic activity to reduce internal sphincter contraction. Relaxation of the internal anal sphincter may be mediated via non-adrenergic, non-cholinergic nerve activity via the neural transmitter nitric oxide.

Anorectal physiological studies alone cannot separate the different structures of the anal canal; instead, they provide measurements of the resting and squeeze pressures along the canal. Between 60% and 85% of resting anal pressure can be attributed to the action of the internal anal sphincter.[2] The external anal sphincter and the puborectalis muscle generate maximal squeeze pressure.[2] Symptoms of passive anal leakage (where the patient is unaware

that episodes are happening) are attributed to internal sphincter dysfunction, whereas urge symptoms and frank incontinence of faeces are due to external sphincter problems.[3]

Faecal continence is maintained by the complex interaction of many different variables. Stool must be delivered at a suitable rate from the colon into a compliant rectum of adequate volume. The consistency of this stool should be appropriate and accurately sensed by the sampling mechanism. Sphincters should be intact and able to contract adequately to produce pressures sufficient to prevent leakage of flatus, liquid and solid stool. For effective defecation there needs to be coordinated relaxation of the striated muscle components with an increase in intra-abdominal pressure to expel the rectal contents. The structure of the anorectal region should prevent herniation or prolapse of elements of the anal canal and rectum during defecation.

As a result of the complex interplay between the factors involved in continence and faecal evacuation, a wide range of investigations is needed for full assessment. A defect in any one element of the system in isolation is unlikely to have great functional significance and so in most clinical situations there is more than one contributing factor.

Rectoanal inhibitory reflex

Increasing rectal distension is associated with transient reflex relaxation of the internal anal sphincter and contraction of the external anal sphincter, known as the rectoanal inhibitory reflex (**Fig. 1.1**).[4] The exact neurological pathway for this reflex is unknown, although it may be mediated via the myenteric plexus and stretch receptors in the pelvic floor. It is absent in patients with Hirschsprung's disease, progressive systemic sclerosis and Chagas's disease, and initially absent after a coloanal anastomosis, although it rapidly recovers.

The rectoanal inhibitory reflex may enable rectal contents to be sampled by the transition zone mucosa to enable discrimination between solid, liquid and flatus. The rate of recovery of sphincter tone after this relaxation differs for the proximal and distal canal, which may be important in maintaining continence.[5]

Further studies investigating the role of the rectoanal inhibitory reflex in incontinent patients show

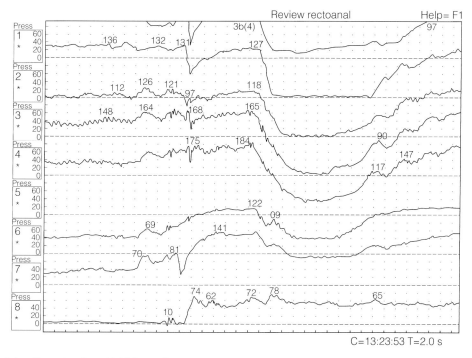

Figure 1.1 • Normal rectoanal inhibitory reflex.

that as rectal volume increases greater sphincter relaxation is seen, whereas constipated patients have a greater recovery velocity of the resting anal pressure in the proximal anal canal.

Manometry

A variety of different catheter systems exist to measure anal pressure and it is important to note that measurements differ depending on the system employed. Systems include microballoons filled with either air or water, microtransducers and water-perfused catheters. These may be hand-held or automated. Hand-held systems are withdrawn in a measured stepwise fashion with recordings made after each step (usually of 0.5–1.0 cm intervals); this is called a station pull-through. Automated withdrawal devices allow continuous data recording (vector manometry).

Water-perfused catheters use hydraulic capillary infusers to perfuse catheter channels, which are arranged either radially or obliquely staggered. Each catheter channel is then linked to a pressure transducer (**Fig. 1.2**). Infusion rates of perfusate (sterile water) vary between 0.25 and 0.5 mL/min per channel. Systems need to be free from air bubbles,

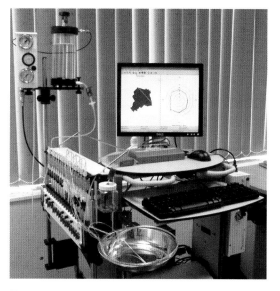

Figure 1.2 • Perfusion system used for anorectal manometry. Standard water perfusion set-up plus computer interface for anorectal manometry. The screen shows a vector volume profile.

which may lead to inaccurate recordings, and must avoid leakage of perfusate onto the perianal skin, which may lead to falsely high resting pressures due to reflex external sphincter action. Perfusion rates should remain constant, because faster rates are associated with higher resting pressures, while larger diameter catheters lead to greater recorded pressure.[6]

Balloon systems may be used to overcome some of these problems and may be more representative of pressure generated within a hollow viscus than recordings using a perfusion system. They are not subject to the same problems as a perfusion system when canal pressures are radially asymmetrical.[6] Balloons can be filled with either air or water. Over the range of balloon sizes used (diameter 2–10 mm), diameter appears to have less of an effect on the pressures recorded than it does with water-perfused catheter systems.

Microtransducers have been developed that can accurately measure canal pressure. However, they are expensive and fragile and more prone to inaccuracies when radial pressure asymmetry is present. They have been validated against water-filled balloon systems and may be useful in the performance of ambulatory studies.

Pressure changes in the anal canal can be measured in a number of ways and each method has been validated for its repeatability and reproducibility, although individual methods are not interchangeable. Although the correlation between measurements made using different systems and catheters is good, the absolute values are different so that when comparing the results of different studies it is essential to consider the method used to obtain the pressure measurements.

Significant variation exists in the results of anorectal manometry in normal asymptomatic subjects. Men have higher mean resting and squeeze pressures.[7] Pressures decline after the age of 60 years, changes most marked in women.[8] These facts must be considered when selecting appropriate control subjects for clinical studies. Normal mean anal canal resting tone in healthy adults is 50–70 mmHg. Resting tone increases in a cranial to caudal direction along the canal such that the maximal resting pressure is found 1–2 cm from the anal verge.[2] The high-pressure zone (the part of the anal canal where the resting pressure is >50% of the maximum resting pressure) is longer in men than women (2.5–3.5 vs. 2.0–3.0 cm).[6,8] In a normal individual the rise in pressure on maximal squeezing should be at least 50–100% of the resting pressure (usually 100–180 mmHg).[9] Reflex contraction of the external sphincter should occur when the rectum is distended, on coughing, or with any rise in intra-abdominal pressure.

In the assessment of patients with faecal incontinence, both resting and maximal squeeze pressures are significantly lower in patients with incontinence than in matched controls,[10] but there is considerable crossover between the pressures recorded in patients and controls.[11]

High-resolution manometry uses closely spaced solid-state sensors simultaneously to measure circumferential pressures in the rectum and throughout the anal canal so there is no need to perform a station pull-through manoeuvre.[12]

Ambulatory manometry

The use of continuous ambulatory manometry to record rectal and anal canal pressures[13] has provided information on the functioning of the sphincter mechanism in a more physiological situation. The generation of giant waves of pressure in the rectum or neorectum may relate to episodes of incontinence in patients after restorative proctocolectomy. Ambulatory manometry has also identified patients in whom episodes of internal sphincter relaxation are not accompanied by reflex external sphincter contraction,[14] a finding that may prove useful in selecting patients likely to benefit from biofeedback treatment.

Vector volume manometry

This technique utilises a radially arranged eight-channel catheter that is automatically withdrawn from the anal canal during rest and squeeze, and computer software that produces a three-dimensional reconstruction of the anal canal (**Fig. 1.3**).[15] This system is able to assess radial symmetry and produces a vector symmetry index (i.e. how far the radial symmetry of the anal canal differs from a perfect circle, which has a vector symmetry index of 1). Sphincter defects are associated with symmetry indices of 0.6 or less.

Vector volume manometry may differentiate between idiopathic and traumatic faecal incontinence by showing global external sphincter weakness rather than a localised area of scarred sphincter indicated by an asymmetrical vectogram.[15] However, there is poor correlation between vectogram and

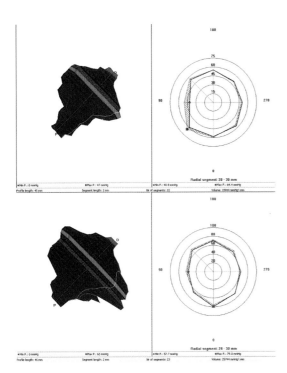

Figure 1.3 • Normal vector volume at squeeze and at rest. Note that asymmetry of the sphincter contour can be normal.

electromyographic or ultrasonic localisation of sphincter defects: the vectogram agrees with electromyographic localisation in only 13% and with ultrasonic localisation in 11%. Vector manometry also consistently records higher pressures than those obtained with conventional manometry.

Anal and rectal sensation

The anal canal is rich in sensory receptors,[16] including those for pain, temperature and movement, with the somatic sensation of the anal transitional mucosa being more sensitive than that of the perianal skin. In contrast, the rectum is relatively insensitive to pain, although crude sensation may be transmitted via the nervi erigentes of the parasympathetic nervous system.[17]

A variety of methods have been used to measure anal sensation. Initial assessment of anal sensation used a stiff bristle to detect light touch in the anal canal and hot and cold metal rods to detect temperature sensation.[16] Thermal sensation has been assessed with water-perfused thermodes;[18] normal subjects can detect a change in temperature of 0.92 °C.[18] The ability of the mucosa to detect a

small electrical current can be assessed by the use of a double platinum electrode and a signal generator providing a square wave impulse at 5 Hz of 100 μs duration. The lowest recorded current of three readings at the point at which the subject feels a tingling or pricking sensation in the anal canal is noted as the sensation threshold. Normal electrical sensation for the most sensitive area of the anal canal (the transition zone) is 4 mA (2–7 mA). Rectal mucosal electrical sensation may also be measured using the same technique as that used for anal mucosal electrical sensation measurement, with slight modification of the stimulus (500 μs duration at a frequency of 10 Hz).[17]

The sensation of rectal filling is measured by progressively inflating a balloon placed within the rectum or by intrarectal saline infusion.[17] Normal perception of rectal filling occurs after inflation of 10–20 mL, the sensation of the urge to defecate occurs after 60 mL, and normally up to 230 mL is tolerated in total before discomfort occurs.[17]

 The clinical use of these measurements may be limited due to the large inter- and intrasubject variation in values and the wide normal range, reducing the discriminatory value of this technique as a clinical investigation.[19]

Temperature sensation may be vital in the discrimination of solid stool from liquid and flatus,[18] and is reduced in patients with faecal incontinence. It is thought that this sensation is important in the sampling reflex, although this is brought into question by the fact that the sensitivity of the anal mucosa to temperature change is not great enough to detect the very slight temperature gradient between the rectum and anal canal.

Anal mucosal electrical sensation threshold increases with age and thickness of the subepithelial layer of the anal canal. Anal canal electrical sensation is reduced in idiopathic faecal incontinence,[20] diabetic neuropathy, descending perineum syndrome and haemorrhoids.[20] There are differing reports on whether there is any correlation between electrical sensation and measurement of motor function of the sphincters (pudendal terminal motor latency and single-fibre electromyography).

The sampling mechanism and maintenance of faecal continence are complex multifactorial processes, as seen by the fact that the application of local anaesthetic to the sensitive anal mucosa does not lead to incontinence and in some individuals actually improves continence.

Rectal compliance

The relation between changes in rectal volume and the associated pressure changes is termed compliance, which is calculated by dividing the change in volume by the change in pressure. Compliance is measured by inflating a rectal balloon with saline or air or by directly infusing saline at physiological temperature into the rectum. In the former method, the filling of the rectal balloon can be either incremental or continuous. When continuous inflation of the rectal balloon is used, the rate of inflation should be 70–240 mL/min.[19] Mean rectal compliance is about 4–14 mL/cmH$_2$O, with pressures of 18–90 cmH$_2$O at the maximum tolerated volume.[21] Reports on the reproducibility of the measurement of rectal compliance are varied and many have found great variation within the same subject;[19,21] the most reproducible measurement is usually the maximum tolerated volume. The use of the barostat to measure rectal compliance has been shown to be reproducible at pressures of between 36 and 48 mmHg. The compliance of the rectum does not differ between men and women up to the age of 60 years, but after this age women have more compliant rectums. It is reduced in Behçet's disease and Crohn's disease and after radiotherapy in a dose-related fashion. It is also reduced in irritable bowel syndrome.

 The association between changes in rectal compliance and faecal incontinence is less clear. Some state that compliance is normal in incontinence whereas others have found a reduction in compliance associated with faecal incontinence,[10] although changes in compliance may be secondary to the incontinence and not causative. Altered compliance may play a role in soiling and constipation associated with megarectum.

Pelvic floor descent

Parks et al. first described the association between excessive descent of the perineum and anorectal dysfunction, and subsequently it has been described in a number of conditions: faecal incontinence, severe constipation, solitary rectal ulcer syndrome, and anterior mucosal and full-thickness rectal prolapse.[22] The presumption in all these conditions is that abnormal perineal descent, especially during straining, causes traction and damage to the pudendal and pelvic floor nerves, leading to progressive neuropathy and muscular atrophy.[22] Irreversible pudendal nerve damage occurs after a stretch of 12% of its length, and often the descent of the perineum in these patients is of the order of 2 cm, which is estimated to cause pudendal nerve stretching of 20%.

Descent of the perineum was initially measured using the St Marks' perineometer. The perineometer is placed on the ischial tuberosities and a movable latex cylinder is positioned on the perineal skin. The distance between the level of the perineum and the ischial tuberosities is measured at rest and during straining.[23] Negative readings indicate that the plane of the perineum is above the tuberosities and a positive value indicates descent below this level. In normal asymptomatic adults the plane of the perineum at rest should be −2.5 ± 0.6 cm, descending to + 0.9 ± 1.0 cm on straining. When measured using dynamic proctography, similar measurements of pelvic floor descent are obtained. The anorectal angle normally lies on a line drawn between the coccyx and the most anterior part of the pubis and descends by 2 ± 0.3 cm on straining.

Excessive perineal descent is found in 75% of subjects who chronically strain during defecation. The degree of descent correlates with age and is greater in women. Although increased perineal descent on straining has been shown to be associated with features of neuropathy, namely decreased anal mucosal electrical sensitivity and increased pudendal nerve terminal motor latency, not all patients with abnormal descent have abnormal neurology.[24] Perineal descent is also associated with faecal incontinence, although the degree of incontinence and the results of anorectal manometry do not correlate with the extent of pelvic floor laxity.[25]

Electrophysiology

Neurophysiological assessment of the anorectum includes assessment of the conduction of the pudendal and spinal nerves, and electromyography (EMG) of the sphincter.

Electromyography

Electromyographic traces can be recorded from the separate components of the sphincter complex both at rest and during active contraction of the striated components. Initially, EMG was used to map sphincter defects before surgery but AES is now so superior in its ability to map defects and is so much better tolerated by patients[26] that EMG has largely become a research tool. Broadly, two techniques of EMG are used: concentric needle studies and single-fibre studies.

Concentric needle EMG records the activity of up to 30 muscle fibres from around the area of the needle both at rest and during voluntary squeeze. The amplitude of the signal recorded correlates with the maximal squeeze pressure,[27] polyphasic long-duration action potentials indicating reinnervation subsequent to denervation injury. The main use of this technique has been in the confirmation and mapping of sphincter defects. Examination of puborectalis EMG may be more sensitive than cinedefecography in the detection of paradoxical puborectalis contraction in obstructed defecation,[28] although paradoxical puborectalis contraction is also present in normal subjects.

The use of an anal plug or sponge can record global electrical activity from the anal sphincters,[27] EMG amplitudes recorded in this way correlating with voluntary squeeze pressure. In the future, sponge electrode EMG may have a role in directing biofeedback retraining for anismus.

When EMG is performed using a needle with a smaller recording area (25 μm diameter) the action potential from individual motor units is recorded. Denervated muscle fibres can regain innervation from branching of adjacent axons, leading to an increase in the number of muscle fibres supplied by a single axon. With multiple readings (an average of 20) using this small-diameter needle, the mean fibre density (MFD) for an area of sphincter can be calculated (i.e. the mean number of muscle action potentials per unit area or axon). Denervation and subsequent reinnervation are also indicated by neuromuscular 'jitter', which is caused by variation in the timing of triggering and non-triggering potentials.[29] An increase in sphincter MFD is often found in cases of idiopathic incontinence and is associated with recognised histological changes in sphincter structure. Atrophic sphincter muscle shows a loss of the characteristic mosaic pattern of distribution of type 1 and type 2 muscle fibres.[30] There is also selective muscle fibre hypertrophy together with fibro-fatty fibre degeneration. These changes predominantly affect the external anal sphincter but the puborectalis and levators are also affected to a lesser extent.[30]

MFD correlates inversely with squeeze pressure and is increased in patients with excessive perineal descent.[31] The correlation with direct assessment of the integrity of sphincter innervation (pudendal nerve terminal motor latency) is less clear.

Pudendal nerve terminal motor latency

Pudendal nerve conduction can be assessed by stimulating as the nerve enters the ischio-rectal fossa at the ischial spines. This investigation only examines the fastest conducting fibres of the pudendal nerve and so can still be normal even in the presence of abnormal sphincter innervation. The normal value for pudendal nerve terminal motor latency (PNTML) is 2.0 ± 0.5 ms.[32]

Prolongation of PNTML is associated with idiopathic faecal incontinence, rectal prolapse, solitary rectal ulcer syndrome, severe constipation and sphincter defects. Nerve latency is delayed with increasing age and is prolonged in 24% of all faecally incontinent patients and 31% of those presenting with constipation.[33]

 PNTML is operator dependent and has a poor correlation with clinical symptoms and histological findings. The American Gastroenterology Association does not recommend the use of this test for the evaluation of patients with faecal incontinence.[34]

Spinal motor latency

Transcutaneous stimulation of the sacral motor nerve roots provides further information on the innervation of the pelvic floor. The motor response from stimulation at the level of the first and fourth lumbar vertebrae can be recorded using standard EMG needles inserted into the puborectalis and external sphincter. By comparing the latency times between the two levels, the latency of the motor component of the cauda equina can be assessed. Up to 23% of patients with idiopathic faecal incontinence will have cauda equina delay.[35]

Defecography/evacuation proctography

Defecography or evacuation proctography involves video fluoroscopy of the patient evacuating barium paste of stool consistency. Barium-soaked gauze may also be inserted into the vagina and barium paste may be applied to the perineum to aid in assessing the anorectal angle and perineal descent.[36] Opacification of the small bowel with an orally ingested contrast medium or injection of contrast into the peritoneum (peritoneography) will reveal enteroceles in 18% of patients with pelvic floor weakness,[37] with only half filling with bowel.[38] Defecography is a dynamic examination; it not only provides information on anorectal structural changes during defecation, but it also assesses function. While anatomical changes during evacuation (namely rectocele, enterocele, rectoanal intussusception, rectal prolapse and changes in anorectal angle) may be evident, the extent and duration of emptying is of more clinical significance.[39]

Anatomical abnormalities demonstrated on proctography are of poor discriminatory value in determining patients from controls.[40] The only measurements that can discriminate between normal subjects and those with severe constipation are the time taken to evacuate and the completeness of evacuation.[41]

During normal evacuation the anorectal angle increases because of relaxation of puborectalis. Normal evacuation should be 90% complete (and 60% complete with a pouch). Rectoceles are significant if they are greater than 3 cm or require digitation to empty.

Dynamic pelvic MRI

Using a modified T2-weighted single-shot fast spin-echo imaging sequence or a T2-weighted fast imaging with steady-state precession MRI sequence, anorectal and pelvic floor motion can be imaged at 1.2- to 2-second intervals.[10] During dynamic MRI, proctography provides pelvic images at rest and when the subject strains. This gives an overview of pelvic floor movement and organ prolapse, and rectal dynamics are assessed during evacuation after

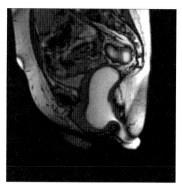

Figure 1.4 • A mid-sagittal image of the anal canal and rectum using MRI proctography, showing an anterior rectocele.

adding 150 mL of ultrasound gel to the rectum[42] (**Fig. 1.4**). There are few differences in the detection of clinically relevant findings between supine MRI and seated MRI, with the exception of detecting rectal intussusceptions, for which seated MRI is superior.[43]

MRI defecography has been shown to alter the surgical approach in 67% of patients who underwent surgery for faecal incontinence.[44] It has also been shown that interobserver agreement for assessing anorectal motion by MRI proctography is better than with barium defecography.

Scintigraphy

Scintigraphy using technetium-labelled sulphur colloid mixed with dilute veegum powder may also be used for defecography.[45] The advantages of this technique are that a quantitative result is obtained and a lower dose of radiation is used. However, the study is not dynamic and does not correlate with patient symptoms or manometric assessment. Radioisotope testing may also be used to assess colonic transit time to diagnose idiopathic slow transit constipation.[46] Colonic transit time is measured more easily by tracking the progress of ingested sets of radio-opaque markers with plain abdominal radiography. Standard protocol takes a single plain abdominal radiograph 5 days after commencing ingestion of the markers (usually different-shaped markers are taken daily over the first 3 days).

Imaging the rectum and anal sphincters

The indications for anorectal imaging may be divided into three broad clinical areas: sepsis and fistula disease, malignancy, and faecal incontinence. The available techniques include surface scanning techniques, namely computed tomography (CT) and body coil MRI, and endoanal imaging, namely anal endosonography (AES), with or without subsequent multiplanar (three-dimensional) reconstruction, and endocoil MRI.

Anal endosonography/endorectal ultrasound

The two-dimensional endoluminal ultrasound of the rectum utilises a transducer that rotates through 360° within a water-filled balloon in order to provide acoustic coupling. The newer three-dimensional endoluminal ultrasound uses a double crystal design with 6–16 MHz frequency range encased in a cylindrical transducer shaft. The transducer is then used with a specially designed restosigmoidoscope and water-filled condom covering the transducer. This allows rectal scanning without moving or replacing the probe. The ultrasonic anatomy has been described in detail as a result of scanning dissected specimens and comprises alternating bands of reflection created by the interfaces between the different anatomical structures present.[47] An alternating bright and dark pattern of rings is seen corresponding to the layers of the rectal wall.

To enable examination of the anal sphincters, the water-filled condom is removed from the three-dimensional transducer and for the two-dimensional endorectal ultrasound (EUS) the water-filled balloon has to be replaced with a water-filled plastic cone (**Fig. 1.5a**). The anal canal mucosa is generally not seen on AES; the subepithelial tissue is highly reflective and surrounded by the low reflection from the internal anal sphincter. The width of the internal sphincter increases with age: the normal width for a patient aged 55 years or younger is 2.4–2.7 mm, whereas in an older patient the normal range is 2.8–3.4 mm. As the width of the sphincter increases it becomes progressively more reflective and more indistinct; this may be due to a relative increase in the fibroelastic content of this muscle as a consequence of ageing. Both the external anal sphincter and the longitudinal muscle are

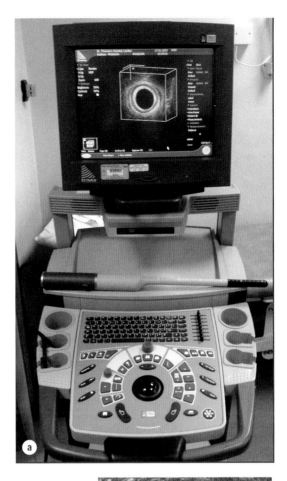

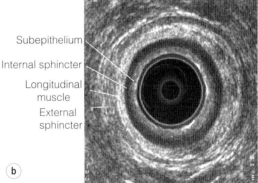

Subepithelium
Internal sphincter
Longitudinal muscle
External sphincter

Figure 1.5 • (a) Bruel–Kjaer three-dimensional endoanal ultrasound machine and 2050 probe. **(b)** The layers of the sphincter are depicted by the three-dimensional endoanal ultrasound probe.

of moderate reflectivity. The intersphincteric space often returns a bright reflection (**Fig. 1.5b**).[48]

The development of high-resolution three-dimensional AES constructed from a synthesis of standard two-dimensional cross-sectional images produces a digital volume that may be reviewed and can be used to perform measurements in any plane, yielding more information on the anal sphincter complex. This provides more reliable measurements, and volume measurements can also be performed.[49] Another development in the use of three-dimensional AES is the volume render mode. This allows analysis of information inside a three-dimensional volume by digitally enhancing individual voxels. The volume-rendered image provides better visualisation performance when there are not large differences in the signal levels of pathological structures compared with surrounding tissues.

Endocoil receiver MRI

MRI provides images with excellent tissue differentiation, although spatial resolution of the anal sphincters using a body coil receiver is poor. When an endoanal receiver coil is used, spatial resolution is vastly improved locally around the coil (within about 4 cm), enabling the acquisition of images of the anal sphincters with both excellent tissue differentiation and spatial resolution. Endocoils have either rectangular or saddle geometry and measure 6–10 cm in length and 7–12 mm in diameter. This increases to 17–19 mm after encasement in an acetal homopolymer (Delrin) former. The coil is inserted in the left lateral position and then secured with sandbags or with a purpose-built holder to avoid movement artefact.[1,48,50]

On T2-weighted images, the external sphincter and longitudinal muscle return a relatively low signal. The internal sphincter returns a relatively high signal and enhances with gadolinium (an intravenous contrast agent used in MRI). The subepithelial tissue has a signal intensity value between that of the internal and external sphincters (**Fig. 1.6**).

Imaging in rectal cancer

CT has an accuracy of 89% in assessing rectal tumours with extensive spread beyond the serosal layer; however, when only cases of moderate tumour spread are assessed, the accuracy is much lower (55%).[51] The accuracy of CT has been improved by the advent of multislice technique CT[52] and further improvement is expected from modern scanners with up to 64 detector rows. CT is also used to assess metastatic disease involving the liver and lungs. The development of positron emission tomography (PET) combined with CT has improved the

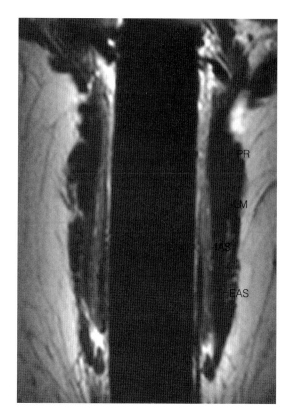

Figure 1.6 • A mid-coronal image of the anal canal using endocoil MRI. EAS, external anal sphincter; IAS, internal anal sphincter; LM, longitudinal muscle; PR, puborectalis.

detection of recurrent rectal carcinoma.[53] PET/CT can also yield additional pretreatment staging information in patients with low rectal cancer.[54] EUS by comparison can correctly detect T-stage rectal cancers in 75–87%[55] of cases, with a trend to over-stage in 22%.[56] Three-dimensional EUS has improved accuracy in T-staging of tumours when compared to two-dimensional EUS (accuracy 87% vs. 82%). Perirectal lymph nodes involved with tumour are seen on EUS as well-defined areas of low reflectivity, although malignant nodal status has also been associated with a degree of inhomogeneity on EUS. EUS is superior to CT and has a positive predictive value for tumour invasion beyond the muscularis propria of 98%. If a lymph node measures greater than 5 mm in diameter on EUS, there is a 45–70% chance that it is involved with tumour.[57]

Body coil MRI has been used to assess the stage of rectal tumours and it would appear to give comparable results to EUS,[58] with an accuracy of 88% at detecting transmural spread, 87% anal sphincter infiltration and over 90% circumferential resection margin involvement.[59] A meta-analysis of 84 studies showed EUS to be slightly superior to MRI in assessing nodal status.[60] Unfortunately, none of the investigations enables reliable detection of nodal spread. Body coil MRI has the advantage over EUS in that it can be performed even in the presence of stenotic tumours. Furthermore, after radiotherapy EUS will tend to over-stage tumours, leading to a marked reduction in its diagnostic accuracy, especially in the differentiation between T2 and T3 tumours. The other area where MRI is superior to EUS is in the assessment of recurrent tumours. The appearances of fibrosis after surgery and recurrent tumour in the pelvis are very similar using either EUS or CT, which makes assessment for recurrent disease very difficult. On MRI the signals from these two tissue types (especially on T2-weighted images) are quite different, allowing greater tissue differentiation.

EUS appears better at estimating the stage of T0, T1, T2 rectal tumours[61] and nodal staging;[60] however, the main determinant of local recurrence is circumferential resection margin and EUS is poor at assessing this, but MRI has been show to be much more accurate.[60]

Imaging in anal sepsis and anal fistulas

Both surface imaging and endoanal imaging have been employed in the assessment of perianal sepsis. CT is unsatisfactory for the assessment of fistulas because of the poor definition of tracks, which is largely due to volume averaging. AES may be used to assess anal fistulas and has been shown to be accurate for the definition of the anatomy of anal sepsis, especially horseshoe collections and the anatomy of complex fistulas.[62] Endosonography is also able to detect and assess sphincter damage caused by chronic sepsis.

Endosonography is less accurate in the assessment of suprasphincteric sepsis and it is often difficult to differentiate between supralevator and infralevator collections, leading to inaccuracy in up to 20% of cases.[63] The internal opening on AES is identified by penetration of the internal anal sphincter by the track because of the lack of definition of the mucosa and is of limited value close to the anal margin.[62] The diagnostic accuracy of AES is increased with the use of hydrogen peroxide injected into fistulous tracks to act as a contrast medium.[64] MRI has the most to offer in the assessment of perianal sepsis. Anal sepsis appears on MRI as areas of very high signal, which enhance with the administration of the intravenous contrast agent gadolinium. Definition is further increased with the use of STIR (short tau inversion recovery) sequences to suppress the signal returned by fat (**Fig. 1.7**).

The use of dynamic contrast-enhanced MRI has been reported to provide better delineation of fistulas than AES, which is better than examination under anaesthetic (EUA). Correct classification with clinical examination has been achieved in 61% of cases using EUA, 81% using AES and 90% using MRI. AES predicts accurately the site of the internal opening in 91% of cases compared with 97% for MRI.[65]

Imaging in faecal incontinence

AES has revealed that many patients who were thought to have idiopathic faecal incontinence in fact have a surgically remediable sphincter defect. It has also been shown that a much higher proportion of women sustain sphincter damage during childbirth than is suspected by clinical assessment alone.[66] While the true incidence of sphincter tears may be lower than initially thought,[67] many women sustain important morphological changes to the sphincter following delivery.[68] The ability of AES to diagnose and correctly assess the extent of external sphincter damage has been validated by comparison with EMG studies and findings at surgery.[69] AES is superior in the differentiation between those patients with idiopathic faecal incontinence and those with a sphincter defect when compared with either simple manometric assessment or vector volume studies.

MRI is also used to assess patients with faecal incontinence and the diagnosis of sphincter defects using endocoil MRI has been validated with surgical confirmation of defect presence and extent.[70] Endocoil MRI may be superior to AES in the detection and assessment of external sphincter defects as a result of better sphincter definition using MRI,[70] although it is more important that the clinician is familiar with the imaging technique used.[71]

MRI has multiplanar capability (i.e. axial, sagittal and coronal images can be acquired), whereas

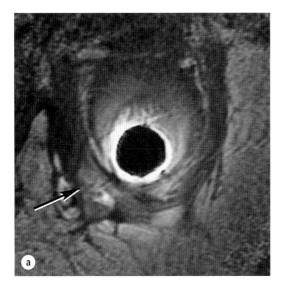

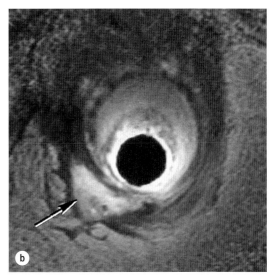

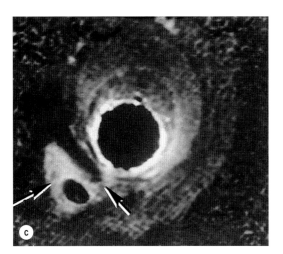

Figure 1.7 • Examples of complex perirectal sepsis as shown by the endoanal magnetic resonance probe. **(a,b)** T1-weighted images of an intersphincteric collection prior to and following gadolinium–DTPA contrast (arrow). **(c)** STIR image of the abscess cavity showing a central gas-containing cavity (long arrow) and a fistula at the 7 o'clock position (short arrow).

standard AES provides only axially oriented images. The acquisition of volume ultrasound data has overcome this problem,[72] and using three-dimensional AES has led to a better understanding of sphincter injury. A direct correlation exists between the length of a defect and the arc of displacement of the two ends of the sphincter.[73]

The use of endocoil MRI has shown that incontinence in the absence of a sphincter defect may be due to atrophy, where the sphincter has been replaced by fat and fibrous tissue.[50,74] The presence of external anal sphincter atrophy on endocoil MRI has been associated with poor results from anterior sphincteroplasty.[75]

Summary

A wide variety of physiological and morphological tests are available for the assessment of the anus and rectum. Although there is no clear correlation between manometric/neurophysiological testing and clinical symptomatology in patients with idiopathic faecal incontinence, there is considerable value in performing these tests before surgery in order to predict long-term outcome. Anorectal investigation has revealed a large group of parous women who have occult sphincter trauma which may have a clinical impact as the women get older.

Anorectal physiological assessment is essential as an objective measure in patients with faecal incontinence and for the diagnosis of Hirschsprung's disease, and may help select those patients who will have acceptable function after colo-anal anastomosis or an ileo-anal pouch.

Endoanal imaging is becoming the gold standard in the preoperative determination of sphincter integrity and defines those patients most likely to benefit from surgical intervention. Endorectal imaging of rectal tumours correlates well with histological assessment of tumour depth and is accurate for the diagnosis of recurrent tumour after anterior resection (especially when using MRI).

In patients with primary evacuatory disorders, neurophysiological testing and defecography assist in the demonstration of unsuspected rectoanal intussusception or rectocele who may benefit from surgery and those who may be suitable candidates for biofeedback therapy.

Anorectal investigation continues to have a major role in clinical research and has helped outline the anatomy of the component parts of the sphincter complex as well as to define the physiology of both defecation and anal continence. The understanding of these processes is vital to the correct management of patients with anorectal disorders.

Key points

- Normal pelvic floor function relies on a complex interplay between various mechanisms.
- Sphincter function may be assessed using anal manometry and electrophysiology.
- Sphincter anatomy may be assessed using AES and MRI, the former being the standard for the diagnosis of sphincter trauma.
- Dynamic MRI and evacuation proctography are useful in the assessment of patients with evacuatory disorders.
- Pelvic MRI is the best imaging modality for anorectal sepsis and can predict recurrence of anal fistulas after surgery, although AES (three-dimensional in particular) provides a useful alternative.
- Preoperative staging of early rectal cancer is superior with EUS. Circumferential resection margin prediction is most accurate when using MRI.

References

1. Desouza NM, Kmiot WA, Puni R et al. High resolution magnetic resonance imaging of the anal sphincter using an internal coil. Gut 1995; 37(2):284–7.

2. Williams AB, Cheetham MJ, Bartram CI et al. Gender differences in the longitudinal pressure profile of the anal canal related to anatomical structure as demonstrated on three-dimensional anal endosonography. Br J Surg 2000; 87:1674–9.

3. Engel AF, Kamm MA, Bartram CI et al. Relationship of symptoms in faecal incontinence to specific sphincter abnormalities. Int J Colorectal Dis 1995; 10(3):152–5.

4. Gowers WR. The automatic action of the sphincter ani. Proc R Soc Lond 1877; 26:77–84.

5. Goes RN, Simons AJ, Masri L et al. Gradient of pressure and time between proximal anal canal and high-pressure zone during internal anal sphincter relaxation. Its role in the fecal continence mechanism. Dis Colon Rectum 1995; 38(10):1043–6.

6. Taylor BM, Beart RW, Phillips SF. Longitudinal and radial variations of pressure in the human anal sphincter. Gastroenterology 1984; 86:693–7.

7. Enck P, Kuhlbusch R, Lubke H et al. Age and sex and anorectal manometry in incontinence. Dis Colon Rectum 1989; 32(12):1026–30.

8. Sun WM, Read NW. Anorectal function in normal subjects: effect of gender. Int J Colorectal Dis 1989; 4:188–96.

9. Jorge JM, Wexner SD. Anorectal manometry: techniques and clinical applications. Southern Med J 1993; 86:924–31.

10. Bharucha AE, Fletcher JG, Harper CM et al. Relationship between symptoms and disordered continence mechanisms in women with idiopathic faecal incontinence. Gut 2005; 54(4):546–55.

    In this study 35% of patients with faecal incontinence had reduced resting pressure and 73% of faecal incontinence patients had reduced squeeze pressures, which was a higher percentage than the control group. This study also found that volume and pressure thresholds for desired defecation were lower in faecal incontinence patients.

 11. McHugh SM, Diamant NE. Effect of age, gender, and parity on anal canal pressures. Contribution of impaired anal sphincter function to fecal incontinence. Dig Dis Sci 1987; 32(7):726–36.

McHugh and Diamant found that in faecally incontinent patients, 39% of women and 44% of men had normal resting and squeeze pressures, and 9% of asymptomatic normal individuals were unable to generate an appreciable pressure on maximal squeeze.

12. Jones MP, Post J, Crowell MD. High-resolution manometry in the evaluation of anorectal disorders: a simultaneous comparison with water-perfused manometry. Am J Gastroenterol 2007; 102(4):850–5.

13. Kumar D, Waldron D, Williams NS et al. Prolonged anorectal manometry and external anal sphincter electromyography in ambulant human subjects. Dig Dis Sci 1990; 35(5):641–8.

14. Sun WM, Read N, Miner PB et al. The role of transient internal anal sphincter relaxation in faecal incontinence. Int J Colorectal Dis 1990; 5:31–6.

15. Braun JC, Treutner KH, Dreuw B et al. Vectormanometry for differential diagnosis of fecal incontinence. Dis Colon Rectum 1994; 37(10):989–96.

16. Duthie HL, Gairns FW. Sensory nerve-endings and sensation in the anal region of man. Br J Surg 1960; 47:585–95.

17. Kamm MA, Lennard-Jones JE. Rectal mucosal electrosensory testing – evidence for a rectal sensory neuropathy in idiopathic constipation. Dis Colon Rectum 1990; 33(5):419–23.

18. Miller R, Bartolo DCC, Cervero F et al. Anorectal temperature sensation: a comparison of normal and incontinence patients. Br J Surg 1987; 74(6):511–5.

19. Kendall GPN, Thompson DG, Day SJ et al. Inter- and intraindividual variation in pressure–volume relations of the rectum in normal subjects and patients with irritable bowel syndrome. Gut 1990; 31:1062–8.

20. Roe AM, Bartolo DC, Mortensen NJ. New method for assessment of anal sensation in various anorectal disorders. Br J Surg 1986; 73(April):310–2.

21. Sorensen M, Rasmussen OO, Tetzschner T et al. Physiological variation in rectal compliance. Br J Surg 1992; 79(10):1106–8.

22. Swash M, Snooks SJ, Henry MM. Unifying concept of pelvic floor disorders and incontinence. J R Soc Med 1985; 78:906–11.

23. Lubowski DZ, Swash M, Nicholls RJ et al. Increase in pudendal nerve terminal motor latency with defaecation straining. Br J Surg 1988; 75(Nov):1095–7.

24. Engel AF, Kamm MA. The acute effect of straining on pelvic floor neurological function. Int J Colorectal Dis 1994; 9(1):8–12.

25. Read NW, Bartolo DC, Read MG et al. Differences in anorectal manometry between patients with haemorrhoids and patients with descending perineum syndrome: implications for management. Br J Surg 1983; 70(11):656–9.

26. Law PJ, Kamm MA, Bartram CI. A comparison between electromyography and anal endosonography in mapping external anal sphincter defects. Dis Colon Rectum 1990; 33(5):370–3.

27. Sorensen M, Tetzschner T, Rasmussen OO et al. Relation between electromyography and anal manometry of the external anal sphincter. Gut 1991; 32(9):1031–4.

28. Karlbom U, Edebol Eeg-Olofsson K, Graf W et al. Paradoxical puborectalis contraction is associated with impaired rectal evacuation. Int J Colorectal Dis 1998; 13(3):141–7.

29. Wexner SD, Marchetti F, Salanga VD et al. Neurophysiologic assessment of the anal sphincters. Dis Colon Rectum 1991; 34(7):606–12.

30. Beersiek F. The pelvic floor: pathophysiology. Ann R Coll Surg 1983; (Sir Alan Parks 1920–1982, Surgeon and Scientist):17–19.

31. Womack NR, Morrison JFB, Williams NS. The role of pelvic floor denervation in the aetiology of idiopathic faecal incontinence. Br J Surg 1986; 73(May):404–7.

32. Kiff ES, Swash M. Slowed conduction in the pudendal nerves in idiopathic (neurogenic) faecal incontinence. Br J Surg 1984; 71(8):614–16.

33. Vaccaro CA, Cheong DM, Wexner SD et al. Pudendal neuropathy in evacuatory disorders. Dis Colon Rectum 1995; 38(2):166–71.

34. Barnett JL, Hasler WL, Camilleri M. American Gastroenterological Association medical position statement on anorectal testing techniques. American Gastroenterological Association. Gastroenterology 1999; 116(3):732–60.

35. Snooks SJ, Swash M, Henry MM. Abnormalities in central and peripheral nerve conduction in patients with anorectal incontinence. J R Soc Med 1985; 78(April):294–300.

36. Delemarre JB, Kruyt RH, Doornbos J et al. Anterior rectocele: assessment with radiographic defecography, dynamic magnetic resonance imaging, and physical examination. Dis Colon Rectum 1994; 37(3):249–59.

37. Kelvin FM, Maglinte DD, Benson JT. Evacuation proctography (defecography): an aid to the investigation of pelvic floor disorders. Obstet Gynecol 1994; 83:307–14.

38. Halligan S, Bartram CI. Evacuation proctography combined with positive contrast peritoneography to demonstrate pelvic floor hernias. Abdom Imaging 1995; 20(5):442–5.

39. Halligan S, Bartram CI. Is barium trapping in rectoceles significant? Dis Colon Rectum 1995; 38(7):764–8.

40. Hiltunen KM, Kolehmainen H, Matikainen M. Does defecography help in diagnosis and clinical decision-making in defecation disorders? Abdom Imaging 1994; 19(4):355–8.

41. Turnbull GK, Bartram CI, Lennard-Jones JE. Radiologic studies of rectal evacuation in adults with idiopathic constipation. Dis Colon Rectum 1988; 31(3):190–7.

42. Bertschinger KM, Hetzer FH, Roos JE et al. Dynamic MR imaging of the pelvic floor performed with patient sitting in an open-magnet unit versus with patient supine in a closed-magnet unit. Radiology 2002; 223(2):501–8.

43. Bharucha AE. Update of tests of colon and rectal structure and function. J Clin Gastroenterol 2006; 40(2):96–103.

44. Hetzer FH, Andreisek G, Tsagari C et al. MR defecography in patients with fecal incontinence: imaging findings and their effect on surgical management. Radiology 2006; 240(2):449–57.

45. McLean RG, King DW, Talley NA et al. The utilization of colon transit scintigraphy in the diagnostic algorithm for patients with chronic constipation. Dig Dis Sci 1999; 44(1):41–7.

46. Gattuso JM, Kamm MA, Morris G et al. Gastrointestinal transit in patients with idiopathic megarectum. Dis Colon Rectum 1996; 39(9):1044–50.

47. Beynon J, Foy DMA, Temple LN et al. The endosonic appearances of normal colon and rectum. Dis Colon Rectum 1986; 29:810–3.

48. Williams AB, Bartram CI, Halligan S et al. Endosonographic anatomy of the normal anal canal compared with endocoil magnetic resonance imaging. Dis Colon Rectum 2002; 45(2):176–83.

49. West RL, Felt-Bersma RJ, Hansen BE et al. Volume measurements of the anal sphincter complex in healthy controls and fecal-incontinent patients with a three-dimensional reconstruction of endoanal ultrasonography images. Dis Colon Rectum 2005; 48(3):540–8.

50. Stoker J, Rociu E, Zwamborn AW et al. Endoluminal MR imaging of the rectum and anus: technique, applications, and pitfalls. Radiographics 1999; 19(2):383–98.

51. Nicholls RJ, York Mason A, Morson BC et al. The clinical staging of rectal cancer. Br J Surg 1982; 69:404–9.

52. Kulinna C, Scheidler J, Strauss T et al. Local staging of rectal cancer: assessment with double-contrast multislice computed tomography and transrectal ultrasound. J Comput Assist Tomogr 2004; 28(1):123–30.

53. Even-Sapir E, Parag Y, Lerman H et al. Detection of recurrence in patients with rectal cancer: PET/CT after abdominoperineal or anterior resection. Radiology 2004; 232(3):815–22.

54. Gearhart SL, Frassica D, Rosen R et al. Improved staging with pretreatment positron emission tomography/computed tomography in low rectal cancer. Ann Surg Oncol 2006; 13(3):397–404.

55. Fuchsjager MH, Maier AG, Schima W et al. Comparison of transrectal sonography and double-contrast MR imaging when staging rectal cancer. Am J Roentgenol 2003; 181(2):421–7.

56. Orrom WJ, Wong WD, Rothenberger DA et al. Endorectal ultrasound in the preoperative staging of rectal tumours. Dis Colon Rectum 1990; 33:654–9.

57. Beynon J, Mortensen NJ, Foy DM et al. Preoperative assessment of mesorectal lymph node involvement in rectal cancer. Br J Surg 1989; 76:276–9.

58. McNicholas MM, Joyce WP, Dolan J et al. Magnetic resonance imaging of rectal carcinoma: a prospective study. Br J Surg 1994; 81(6):911–4.

59. Brown G, Radcliffe AG, Newcombe RG et al. Preoperative assessment of prognostic factors in rectal cancer using high-resolution magnetic resonance imaging. Br J Surg 2003; 90(3): 355–64.

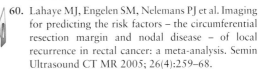

60. Lahaye MJ, Engelen SM, Nelemans PJ et al. Imaging for predicting the risk factors – the circumferential resection margin and nodal disease – of local recurrence in rectal cancer: a meta-analysis. Semin Ultrasound CT MR 2005; 26(4):259–68.

This meta-analysis on the accuracy of preoperative imaging includes studies between 1985 and 2004. It showed that MRI is the only investigation accurate at predicting CRM. EUS is slightly but not significantly superior at predicting nodal status.

61. Bipat S, Glas AS, Slors FJ et al. Rectal cancer: local staging and assessment of lymph node involvement with endoluminal US, CT, and MR imaging – a meta-analysis. Radiology 2004; 232(3):773–83.

A meta-analysis of 90 articles showed that for muscularis propria invasion, EUS and MRI had similar sensitivities but the specificity of EUS (86%) was significantly higher than that of MRI (69%). For perirectal tissue invasion, sensitivity of EUS (90%) was significantly higher than that of CT (79%) and MRI (82%). EUS was more accurate than CT and MRI at diagnosing perirectal tissue invasion and there was no difference in diagnosis of lymph node involvement.

62. Deen KI, Williams JG, Hutchinson R et al. Fistulas in ano: endoanal ultrasonographic assessment assists decision making for surgery. Gut 1994; 35(3):391–4.

63. Choen S, Burnett S, Bartram CI et al. Comparison between anal endosonography and digital examination in the evaluation of anal fistulae. Br J Surg 1991; 78(4):445–7.

64. West RL, Dwarkasing S, Felt-Bersma RJ et al. Hydrogen peroxide-enhanced three-dimensional endoanal ultrasonography and endoanal magnetic resonance imaging in evaluating perianal fistulas: agreement and patient preference. Eur J Gastroenterol Hepatol 2004; 16(12):1319–24.

65. Buchanan GN, Halligan S, Bartram CI et al. Clinical examination, endosonography, and MR imaging in preoperative assessment of fistula in ano: comparison with outcome-based reference standard. Radiology 2004; 233(3):674–81.

This prospective trial of 104 patients with anal fistulas showed that AES with a high-frequency transducer is superior to digital examination but MRI is superior to AES.

66. Donnelly V, Fynes M, Campbell D et al. Obstetric events leading to anal sphincter damage. Obstet Gynecol 1998; 92(6):955–61.

67. Williams AB, Bartram CI, Halligan S et al. Sphincter damage after vaginal delivery – a prospective study. Obstet Gynecol 2000; 97:770–5.

68. Williams AB, Bartram CI, Halligan S et al. Alteration of anal sphincter morphology following vaginal delivery revealed by multiplanar anal endosonography. BJOG 2002; 109(8):942–6.

69. Tjandra JJ, Milsom JW, Schroeder T et al. Endoluminal ultrasound is preferable to electromyography in mapping anal sphincteric defects. Dis Colon Rectum 1993; 36(7):689–92.

70. Stoker J, Hussain SM, Lameris JS. Endoanal magnetic resonance imaging versus endosonography. Radiol Med (Torino) 1996; 92(6):738–41.

71. Malouf AJ, Williams AB, Halligan S et al. Prospective assessment of accuracy of endoanal MR imaging and endosonography in patients with fecal incontinence. Am J Roentgenol 2000; 175(3):741–5.

72. Williams AB, Bartram CI, Halligan S. Review of three-dimensional anal endosonography. RAD 1999; 25(289):47–8.

73. Gold DM, Bartram CI, Halligan S et al. Three-dimensional endoanal sonography in assessing anal canal injury. Br J Surg 1999; 86(3):365–70.

74. Williams AB, Bartram CI, Modhwadia D et al. Endocoil magnetic resonance imaging quantification of external anal sphincter atrophy. Br J Surg 2001; 88(6):853–9.

75. Briel JW, Stoker J, Rociu E et al. External anal sphincter atrophy on endoanal magnetic resonance imaging adversely affects continence after sphincteroplasty. Br J Surg 1999; 86:1322–7.

2

Colonoscopy and flexible sigmoidoscopy

Adam Haycock
Siwan Thomas-Gibson

Introduction

Since flexible endoscopy of the colon was first introduced in 1963 it has become the gold-standard diagnostic test for evaluation of colonic disease. Improvements in technique and technology have also led to advances in therapeutic procedures, and the boundary between endoscopic, laparoscopic and open procedures is becoming increasingly blurred. A good understanding of both the technique and technology is essential for an endoscopist to perform high-quality, safe endoscopy. This chapter gives an insight into how colonoscopy is influencing the practice of colorectal surgery.

Indications and contraindications

Flexible sigmoidoscopy vs. colonoscopy

Indications for colonoscopy or flexible sigmoidoscopy must be weighed against the risk/benefit profile. Colonoscopy has a significantly higher risk of complications relating to sedation, bowel preparation, perforation and bleeding than flexible sigmoidoscopy. Flexible sigmoidoscopy is also quicker, cheaper and easier to perform. However, studies have shown that using a dedicated 60-cm flexible sigmoidoscope, a quarter of cases do not achieve full examinination of the sigmoid colon and the splenic flexure is reached only in the minority of cases, even with 60 cm of scope inserted.[1] The British Society of Gastroenterology (BSG) recommendations are therefore that flexible sigmoidoscopy should be performed with a colonoscope (**Fig. 2.1**).

Contraindications

The only absolute contraindications to endoscopic examination of the colon are a competent patient who is unwilling to give consent, or a known free colonic perforation. Relative contraindications include: acute diverticulitis, immediately postoperative patients, patients with a recent myocardial infarction (within 30 days), pulmonary embolism, severe coagulopathy (particularly for therapeutic procedures) or haemodynamic instability. In fulminant colitis, a limited examination with flexible sigmoidoscopy to ascertain extent of disease and acquire confirmatory biopsies is often helpful. In general, colonoscopy or flexible sigmoidoscopy is considered to be safe in pregnancy, but should probably be deferred in most cases if the indication does not require immediate examination.[2]

Sedation

Sedation during colonoscopy continues to be the subject of much debate and research. A recent large multicentre European audit of current practice[3]

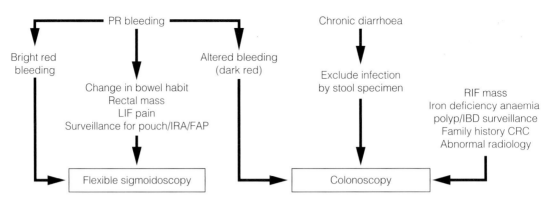

Figure 2.1 • Algorithm for determining colonoscopy or flexible sigmoidoscopy as the initial investigation of choice.

showed that most colonoscopies were done using moderate sedation, and that although deep sedation was associated with shorter procedure times and less difficulties, it was also more resource intensive and required more hospitalisations for complications. Flexible sigmoidoscopy is most often performed unsedated as the use of intravenous sedation would negate many of the potential benefits of the procedure. Unsedated colonoscopy is certainly possible and practical in a subset of patients with few complications and good acceptability.[4]

As the practice and evidence varies widely, current recommendations are to use the minimum amount of drugs within the manufacturers' guidelines to ensure patient comfort and the success of the endoscopy.[5]

Insertion technique

Insertion technique varies greatly even amongst expert colonoscopists. Technique will depend on the local circumstances, sedation practice, endoscopist preference and equipment available. However, there are some basic principles that are recognised to contribute to safe, efficient colonoscopy.

Handling and scope control

Most skilled colonoscopists now adopt the one-person, single-handed approach where the right hand is used to manipulate the shaft and the left hand operates the angulation controls. Tip control is gained by a combination of up/down angulation with the large wheel and clockwise/anticlockwise torque applied with the right hand.

Insertion and steering

A digital rectal examination should be performed to lubricate the anal canal, relax the sphincters and detect any rectal pathology before to insertion. The view is usually initially a 'red-out' due to the lens pressing against the rectal mucosa. Gentle insufflation, slow withdrawal and small amounts of tip angulation are used to gain a view of the lumen.

Tips for insertion and steering

- **Pull back more, push in less.** The first rule of expert colonoscopy is to keep the shaft straight. This allows for accurate tip control, prevents stretching of the mesentery, minimises discomfort and shortens the colon by a 'concertina' effect of telescoping the bowel wall over the shaft. Pulling back often reduces acute angles of bends, disimpacts the tip of the scope and improves the view. In contrast, excessive pushing of the scope often results in formation of large loops, excessive pain, loss of one-to-one tip control and increases the risk of iatrogenic perforation.[6]
- **Insufflate little and suction frequently.** Pain or discomfort during colonoscopy is often due to stretching of the bowel wall due to excessive gas insufflation. Pneumatic perforation of the right colon from over-insufflation has been reported.[7] Frequent suctioning of gas prevents this and may often allow progression of the tip through the colon by the concertina effect.
- **Use torque frequently.** Twisting of the shaft in the right hand clockwise or anticlockwise applies torque to the shaft of the scope. With a straight shaft and bent tip, use of torque will provide lateral movement at the tip and help

to stiffen the scope to prevent looping during advancement. Application of torque is also essential for loop resolution; the majority of sigmoid loops (N loops, 80%; alpha loops, 10%) require clockwise torque and pull-back to resolve; atypical loops (reverse sigmoid N-spiral, 1%; reverse alpha, 5%) require anticlockwise torque.

Patient position change

Moving the patient's position from the left lateral position during both insertion and withdrawal can shift both fluid away from and air into the uppermost segment of bowel, preventing unnecessary suctioning of fluid and insufflation of gas. It can provide mechanical advantage by opening up acute bends, especially at the splenic and hepatic flexures. The effective use of gravity to assist the passage of the endoscope is a simple, cost-neutral, effective technique that is easily learnt. It has been shown to be effective in promoting endoscope tip advancement in two-thirds of cases.[8] However, it does require co-operation from the patient and can be difficult if heavy sedation or general anaesthesia is used (**Fig. 2.2**).

Abdominal hand pressure

The use of abdominal hand pressure aims to prevent the shaft of the endoscope looping by opposing any pressure close to the anterior abdominal wall. Pressure is best used to prevent a loop from forming rather than applying it to an already formed loop, which is unlikely to be successful and may increase the discomfort felt by the patient. Specific pressure on anterior-protruding loops is more likely to be helpful than non-specific pressure.[9] Efficacy in promoting tip advancement is less than for patient position change,[8] as many loops do not protrude anteriorly. However, physicians in a recent audit unanimously advocated use of directed pressure as a technique during colonoscopy.[10]

Three-dimensional imager

A non-invasive magnetic imaging system (ScopeGuide, Olympus Optical Company) has been commercially available since 2002. It uses low-voltage magnetic fields to produce a real-time, three-dimensional image of the entire colonoscope shaft in both anterior–posterior and lateral views, allowing the colonoscopist to visualise the configuration of the scope within the patient, much like with radiological imaging but without the need for X-rays. This can help determine if there is an anterior component to the loop and assist with loop resolution, as well as aiding accurate tip location. A separate hand-pressure sensor can assist with accurate hand-pressure placement.

Two randomised controlled trials have shown improvement in caecal intubation rate and pain scores for both experts and trainees using the imager,[11,12] and one trial showed a benefit in localising lesions[13] with no significant impact on completion rate or length of procedure.

Withdrawal technique

It should be remembered that the aim of colonoscopy is to visualise the whole of the colonic mucosa in order to identify pathology. A systematic review of back-to-back studies[14] has shown a polyp miss rate at colonoscopy of 22% even in expert hands, although most missed polyps were small (<1 cm). All studies investigating miss rates have shown a variation in performance between endoscopists, but this can be wide even with expert examiners (>10 000 procedures), with sensitivities ranging from 17% to 48% in one large study.[15] This implies that there is a link between individual technical skill and outcome measures.

Withdrawal time

Recent publications have stressed the importance of spending sufficient time inspecting the colonic mucosa on withdrawal as a key marker for the adequacy of the examination.

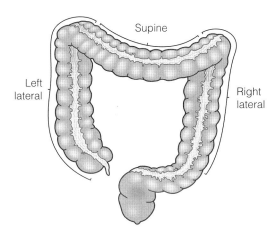

Figure 2.2 • Schema for optimal patient position change.

The current recommendation is that colonoscopists should spend 6–10 minutes during withdrawal inspecting the colonic mucosa.[16] A landmark study[17] looking specifically at withdrawal time found that endoscopists who spent longer on withdrawal had significantly higher adenoma detection rate (ADR) than their quicker colleagues.

Optimal examination technique

Although there is little direct evidence, it seems logical that those colonoscopists who take longer to withdraw also use techniques that increase visualisation of abnormalities. In one study looking at differences in technique between two colonoscopists with different polyp miss rates,[18] a lower miss rate was judged by independent experts to have a superior withdrawal technique for each of the following examination criteria: (1) examining the proximal sides of flexures, folds and valves; (2) cleaning and suctioning; (3) adequacy of distension; and (4) adequacy of time spent viewing. A study looking at the quality of inspection at flexible sigmoidoscopy[19] has included similar criteria: (1) time spent viewing the mucosa; (2) re-examination of poorly viewed areas; (3) suctioning of fluid pools; (4) distension of the lumen; and (5) lower rectal examination.

The following continuous quality improvement targets regarding withdrawal (adapted from Rex et al.[16]) aim to standardise withdrawal technique to maximise detection rates:

1. Mean examination times during withdrawal should average at least 6–10 minutes.
2. Adenoma prevalence rates detected during colonoscopy in persons over 50 years of age undergoing first-time examination should be 25% in men and 15% in women.
3. Documentation of quality of bowel preparation in all cases.

Bowel preparation

It is self-evident that pools of fluid or faeces will obscure good visualisation of the mucosa, and many studies have looked at the effectiveness of various bowel preparations for clearing the colon prior to colonoscopy.

 Evidence-based recommendations on bowel preparation for colonoscopy have been published following an American Task Force review of the literature.[20]

It has been shown that better quality preparation at flexible sigmoidoscopy results in a higher ADR,[21] but crucially important, endoscopists with a higher ADR are more likely to be critical of the quality of bowel preparation.

Position change

The use of position change has been shown in a randomised controlled trial to improve lumenal distension between the hepatic flexure and sigmoid-descending junction during colonoscope withdrawal.[22] The same schema can be used for each segment as previously illustrated for insertion (Fig. 2.2). The interim results of ongoing trials have shown that the improved visualisation that results can also improve polyp detection rates.[22] These data require replication in large multicentre studies as they may have a significant impact on technical performance for those colonoscopists who are used to using moderate or deep sedation for their examinations.

Antispasmodics

Premedication with an antispasmodic such as hyoscine *N*-butyl bromide (Buscopan) has been used for colonoscopy to decrease the amount of muscular spasm caused by peristalsis. Small randomised studies have shown that it can shorten the total procedure time for flexible sigmoidoscopy as compared with placebo,[23] and that it may be beneficial in terms of ease of insertion[24] and the time required for caecal intubation, total procedure time, adequacy of sedation, and scales of patient comfort during colonoscopy.[25] Caution must be taken in patients with a known cardiac history as it can produce a sinus tachycardia. Other antispasmodics such as glucagon and the use of warm water irrigation may be used in patients in whom anticholinergics are contraindicated, although currently there are no data showing any significant benefit.[26]

Rectal retroflexion

Colorectal cancer is most common in the distal colon, and most experts routinely perform retroflexion in the rectum. Although the evidence that this significantly improves detection rates is still being debated,[27,28] it probably allows clearer views of the proximal sides of rectal valves and the top of the anal canal. If the rectal lumen is narrow, a paediatric colonoscope or thin upper gastrointestinal (GI) endoscope can be used.

Endoscopy training in the UK

The largest prospective study of colonoscopy practice in the UK in 2004[29] revealed poor outcomes in terms of completion and perforation rates, as well as deficiencies in almost all aspects of training. Guidelines on training have been published both in the UK and USA.[30,31] Accredited national courses in endoscopy have been developed to provide more readily available and structured training, and have now become essential components of gastroenterology training. Focus has also been placed on ensuring that those endoscopists responsible for training or performing procedures on healthy screening populations are themselves competent to do so. 'Training the Trainers' courses teach experienced endoscopists adult education theory and its application to skills training in endoscopy. Accreditation for colonoscopists wishing to undertake colorectal cancer screening is now mandatory in the UK. Both initiatives are aimed at maximising the provision of high-quality endoscopy and training on a national basis and not just in teaching centres.

The use of endoscopy simulation has now been shown to be of value in the early phase of colonoscopy training with transfer of skills to live patients,[32] and in the management of gastrointestinal bleeding.[33] New computer simulators have been developed (Olympus Colonoscopy Simulator Endo TS-1, Olympus Optical Company) that more accurately model real-life colonoscopy and are currently undergoing evaluation.

 Current European recommendations are that endoscopy simulators, where available, should be used to allow training to occur in a safe, controlled environment.[34]

New optical techniques in endoscopy

There are many new developments in colonoscopic technique that may improve polyp detection and identification of pathology. These range from simple additions to the standard procedure such as the use of dye-spray, through to advanced endoscope technology such as narrow band imaging (NBI) and confocal endomicroscopy.

Chromoendoscopy

Chromoendoscopy is a technique that uses a surface dye such as methylene blue or indigocarmine to make irregularities in the colonic mucosa more readily apparent to the endoscopist (**Fig. 2.3**).

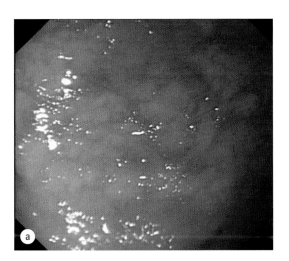
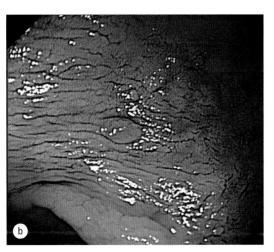

Figure 2.3 • (a) Polyp in white light. **(b)** With indigocarmine dye-spray.

The use of chromoendoscopy has been shown to significantly improve adenoma detection during surveillance of high-risk groups such as ulcerative colitis[35–37] and familial colorectal cancer syndromes.[38,39]

It has also been shown to aid identification of flat or depressed adenomas,[40] which are much more prevalent than was previously thought and have a high risk of malignant transformation. It can, however, be time-consuming and currently there is no substantive evidence for its use during routine colonoscopy.

Narrow band imaging (NBI)

An increased microvascular density is one of the early histological features of colonic adenoma development. NBI uses optical filters to narrow the bandwidth of white light, picking out the central spectrum to enhance the visualisation of the capillary network, thus enabling an adenoma to become more visible against the surrounding mucosa (**Fig. 2.4**). It is activated by a push of a button, which has clear advantages over the use of dye-spray. NBI may have utility in high-risk groups where identifying even diminutive adenomas is important for risk stratification. In ulcerative colitis and hereditary non-polyposis colorectal cancer (HNPCC) patients, the use of NBI has significantly increased the ADR in back-to-back studies.[41,42] Using a classification system of vascular intensity, NBI has good sensitivity and specificity in distinguishing neoplastic and non-neoplastic polyps,[43] and can aid in prediction of histology using pit-pattern recognition (see below). Recent randomised trials have not shown significant benefit in routine endoscopy.[44,45]

High-magnification endoscopy

High-magnification endoscopes can magnify the image up to 100 times, and newer high-definition scopes have a much greater pixel density and ability to improve detail discrimination. In conjunction with dye-spray or NBI their use permits identification of a polyp's surface 'pit pattern' to assist in distinguishing between cancerous, adenomatous and non-adenomatous polyps. A classification system devised by Kudo et al. in 1994[46] has been shown to have a reasonable diagnostic accuracy (overall 86.1%, sensitivity 90.8%, specificity 72.7%) when compared to histological findings[47] (**Fig. 2.5**). There is a learning curve in identification of the patterns, however, so for inexperienced endoscopists it does not significantly reduce the number of biopsies taken. Further work outside of research centres needs to be conducted to confirm its real-world utility.

Retrograde viewing devices

New developments to augment current colonoscopy include the use of an auxiliary imaging device that is inserted into the working channel and extends beyond the colonoscope tip. It then retroflexes, providing a continuous retrograde view during withdrawal to detect lesions missed by the forward-viewing colono-

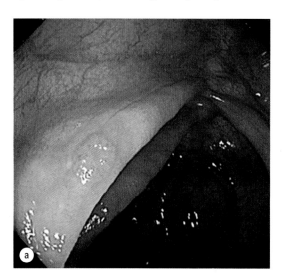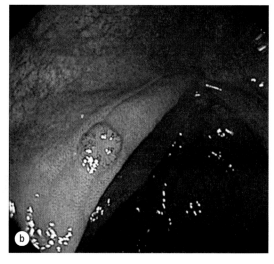

Figure 2.4 • **(a)** Polyp in white light. **(b)** With narrow band imaging.

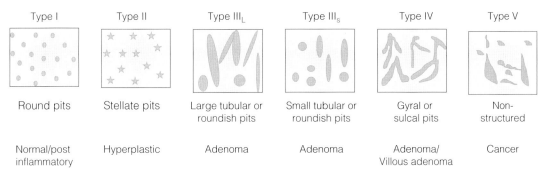

Type I	Type II	Type III$_L$	Type III$_S$	Type IV	Type V
Round pits	Stellate pits	Large tubular or roundish pits	Small tubular or roundish pits	Gyral or sulcal pits	Non-structured
Normal/post inflammatory	Hyperplastic	Adenoma	Adenoma	Adenoma/ Villous adenoma	Cancer

Figure 2.5 • Classification of pit pattern at high-magnification chromoendoscopy (after Kudo).

scope. One such, the Third Eye Retroscope™ (Avantis Medical Systems Inc.), has been shown to significantly improve detection rates of simulated polyps[48] and is currently undergoing further clinical trials.

Confocal laser endomicroscopy

Confocal laser endomicrosopy combines a standard video endoscope with a miniaturised laser microscope. Using intravenous sodium fluorescein as a contrast agent, 'virtual histology' can be created, allowing visualisation of both the surface epithelium and some of the lamina propria, including the microvasculature. Confocal endomicroscopy may have major implications in the future of colonoscopy as it can allow in vivo visualisation of cellular structures, potentially providing accurate identification of colonic intra-epithelial neoplasia and carcinoma. This may enable 'smart' biopsy targeting and increase detection rates and decrease histopathological workload.

Endoscopic therapy

One of the advantages of improving endoscopic skills and technology is the increasingly successful application of novel therapeutic techniques. Therapy that previously required open invasive procedures can now be performed in a minimally invasive way.

Basic therapy

Hot biopsy and snare polypectomy

The ability to remove adenomatous tissue endoscopically forms the basis of all cancer prevention and surveillance programmes. The resectability of a polyp depends on its size, characteristics and accessibility. Polyps that are unlikely to be removable endo-

scopically are those with submucosal invasion, large sessile polyps extending beyond 50% of the bowel wall circumference, large rectal polyps abutting the dentate line, or lesions encircling the appendix.[49]

Small polyps less than 4 mm in size can be removed by hot biopsy in the left colon or cold snare in the right colon. Good hot biopsy technique is essential and involves tenting of the mucosa to concentrate a short burst of current through a pseudostalk, thereby heating directly below the polyp, but not across the bowel wall.[50] Larger stalked polyps are best removed using a conventional large or mini-snare. The stalk should be transected approximately halfway between the polyp and the bowel wall. This ensures a clear resection margin whilst leaving sufficient stalk in situ to facilitate endoscopic treatment should postpolypectomy bleeding occur. Slow transection of the stalk is recommended with low-power coagulating current to allow adequate haemostasis of the blood vessels within the polyp stalk.

Retrieval of the polyp is important to determine the histology and grade of dysplasia. Small polyps can be sucked through the scope into a polyp trap, while larger polyps can be grasped or snared and withdrawn with the scope. Retrieval baskets or Roth nets are particularly useful for retrieving more than one piece of tissue or multiple polyps.

Removal of large (>2 cm), sessile and flat polyps is covered under advanced therapy.

Lower gastrointestinal (GI) bleeding investigation

The lower GI tract accounts for one-quarter to one-third of all hospitalised cases of GI bleeding,[51] with diverticular disease being by far the most common cause. Colitis, cancer, polyps and angiodysplasia account for the majority of the rest. Most lower GI bleeding stops spontaneously and in those cases an elective colonoscopy with standard bowel preparation is appropriate. In the uncommon case of continued bleeding, endoscopic therapy is the treatment of choice as it is currently considered safer, with a greater diagnostic yield, than urgent angiography and embolisation.[52] An urgent therapeutic colonoscopy after rapid purge can decrease both the recurrence of bleeding and the need for surgical intervention.[53] Surgery is reserved for cases of recurrent, uncontrolled or massive bleeding.

Colonic decompression

The three main causes of bowel obstruction are cancer, diverticular disease and a sigmoid volvulus. Flexible sigmoidoscopy with placement of a decompression tube is the initial treatment of choice for a volvulus. It has a high initial success rate (78%) but is only a temporising measure as recurrence is common and elective surgery is therefore still considered the definitive treatment. Emergency surgery is reserved for a volvulus unresponsive to endoscopic therapy or for patients with bowel ischaemia or peritonitis.

Acute colonic pseudo-obstruction (Ogilvie's syndrome) may mimic the signs and symptoms of bowel obstruction. It may be initially treated conservatively with removal of any triggering factor(s), mobilisation, and the use of a parasympathomimetic agent such as neostigmine (if not contraindicated). If this approach fails, then endoscopic placement of a decompression tube is generally accepted as the first invasive therapeutic manoeuvre.[51] Emergency surgery is again only indicated in resistant or complicated cases, such as those with perforation or ischaemia.

Advanced therapy

Endoscopic mucosal resection (EMR)

EMR involves injection of fluid into the submucosal space to lift the mucosa (and the polyp) away from the muscle layer and bowel wall (**Fig. 2.6**). This facilitates removal of sessile or flat lesions, reducing the risk of thermal injury to the bowel wall.[54] The authors found the addition of adrenaline (1:200 000) to improve haemostasis and a few drops of methylene blue to help differentiate the submucosal plane

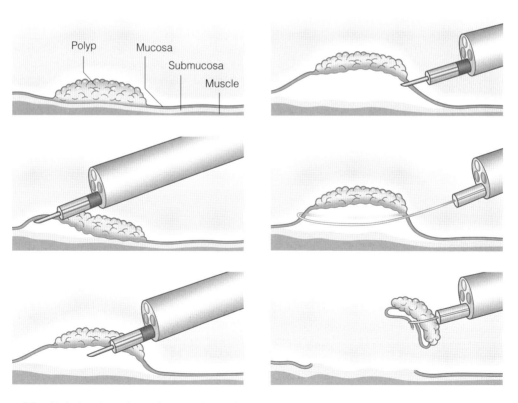

Figure 2.6 • Technique for endoscopic mucosal resection.

helpful. Large lesions (>2 cm) can be safely removed in a piecemeal fashion using a submucosal lift.

 Recurrence may be reduced following piecemeal resection by the use of argon plasma coagulation (APC) to destroy small areas of polyp around the resected margin.[55]

The 'non-lifting' sign, when a polyp fails to lift with a submucosal injection, should raise a suspicion of malignant invasion of the submucosa. Lesions that do not lift should be biopsied, tattooed and referred for surgical resection (see Chapter 17 for tattoo protocol).

Endoscopic submucosal dissection (ESD)

ESD is a technique that has been developed for 'en-bloc' resection of large lesions in the gastrointestinal tract. A deep, submucosal lift is created using a viscous solution such as sodium hyaluronate or 10% glycerine. Mucosal and submucosal incisions are made using a modified needle knife to dissect the mucosa from the submucosa. A transparent hood is attached to the endoscope tip to help retract tissue and maintain the submucosal field of view. The benefit of this technique is that it produces excellent en bloc specimens for histological analysis, but the technique itself is difficult and success depends on excellent endoscopic and haemostatic skills. It is also quite time-consuming, usually taking between 2 and 3 hours in expert hands, and should be performed only when surgical backup is available. It has only recently been applied in the colon, and the current data are limited to small case–control studies.[56–58] Successful en-bloc resection has been reported in 74–98.6% of cases, with a perforation risk in the colon of up to 5%.

Stricture dilatation and stenting

The dilatation of colonic strictures is generally reserved for benign disease, whereas the use of self-expandable metal stents (SEMS) is usually indicated for malignant disease.

Through-the-scope (TTS) balloon dilatators have been used in the management of strictures associated with inflammatory bowel disease, non-steroidal anti-inflammatory drug (NSAID)-induced colonic strictures and diverticular strictures. Success rates vary (around 50%), sometimes requiring multiple attempts,[59] but complication

rates remain high with a risk of perforation or bleeding between 4% and 11%.

SEMS are usually inserted through the scope (TTS) and can be deployed as far as the proximal ascending colon. Preoperative stenting of malignant strictures can allow for one-stage surgical procedures, allowing en-bloc resection of both the stent and tumour in theatre in a fully resuscitated and stable patient.[60] This has a favourable patient outcome and cost compared to surgical intervention alone, and no adverse effect on tumour recurrence rates or survival has been shown.[61] The overall success rate of preoperative stent placement is over 85%. Covered stents can be used for palliation of malignant strictures, with patency established up to a year,[62] although the risk of stent migration is higher than with uncovered stents.

SEMS can also be considered as a potential therapy for selected benign strictures and has been reported with anastomotic strictures unresponsive to dilatation,[63] or Crohn's disease,[64] diverticular disease[60] and radiation-induced strictures.[65]

Natural orifice transluminal endoscopic surgery (NOTES)

As technology and endoscopic skill evolve, the lines between what is possible endoscopically, laparoscopically and traditionally have become increasingly blurred. NOTES involves the intentional puncture of one of the viscera (e.g. stomach, rectum, vagina, urinary bladder) with an endoscope to access the abdominal cavity and perform an intra-abdominal operation. It is currently in its infancy and although the first clinical case series has been published,[66] the debate continues as to the end clinical application.

Competing technologies

Currently, optical colonoscopy remains the gold-standard test for examination of the colon due to its relatively high pathology detection rate and the ability to perform therapy. However, newer techniques are emerging that may be considered as 'disruptive technologies' that will undoubtedly change the current position.

Virtual colonoscopy

Virtual colonoscopy (VC; also frequently termed 'computed tomography (CT) colonography' or 'CT pneumocolon') is a recently established technique for detecting colon cancer and colonic polyps.[67] VC comprises two low-dose CT scans of the abdomen and pelvis, and is less invasive than optical colonoscopy, requires no conscious sedation and is better tolerated by patients. The diagnostic performance characteristics are potentially comparable to expert optical colonoscopy with large polyp (>10 mm in maximal diameter) sensitivity exceeding 90% and cancer sensitivity of 96%,[68] but it lacks the facility for polyp biopsy or removal.

Self-propelling colonoscopes

One disadvantage of traditional optical colonoscopy is the prolonged training required for expertise. There would be significant advantages to providing the same examination and potential for therapy without the need for an experienced operator. A disposable, self-propelling and self-navigating colonoscope (Aer-O-Scope, GI View Ltd., Ramat Gan, Israel) has been developed. It advances through the colon by means of CO_2 introduction between a rectal balloon and a balloon at the tip of the endoscope. It has been shown in porcine models to provide a sensitive inspection of the colonic mucosa without the need for tip manipulation[69] and to be safe in initial human testing.[70] Further evaluation is ongoing.

Colon capsule

Wireless capsule endoscopy (WCE) is a safe, minimally invasive, non-sedation-requiring, patient-friendly modality to visualise the bowel, and is now considered first line for investigation of small bowel disease. The development of the PillCam colon capsule (Given Imaging Ltd., Yoqneam, Israel) aims to widen the application to investigation of colonic disease. It is attractive for similar reasons and, unlike optical colonoscopy, only requires expertise in image interpretation. To date, only two small methodologically flawed pilot studies have been published,[71,72] which found that for patients with positive findings the rates of detection with the PillCam Colon capsule were similar to those obtained with conventional colonoscopy, with no serious adverse events reported.

Conclusions

This chapter has given an overview of the role of flexible sigmoidoscopy and colonoscopy in the diagnosis, treatment and prevention of colorectal disease. Traditional optical endoscopy is becoming more refined and new technologies are emerging that will impact on the need for open or laparoscopic surgery. A focus on training and continual skill development is essential for all those endoscopists wishing to perform high-quality, safe endoscopy.

Key points

- Good technique is vital for high-quality safe endoscopy.
- Sedation practice should be standardised and use the minimum amount of drug required for patient comfort.
- Withdrawal times should be in excess of 6 minutes in normal colonoscopies.
- Advanced imaging techniques are now becoming more widely available and may impact on current practice.
- All endoscopists should be familiar with basic therapeutic techniques (polypectomy, diathermy, decompression) and consider referral for advanced therapy (EMR, ESD, stenting).
- Competing technologies are evolving and need to be evaluated for their utility in clinical practice.

References

1. Painter J, Saunders DB, Bell GD et al. Depth of insertion at flexible sigmoidoscopy: implications for colorectal cancer screening and instrument design. Endoscopy 1999; 31(3):227–31.

2. Siddiqui U, Denise Proctor D. Flexible sigmoidoscopy and colonoscopy during pregnancy. Gastrointest Endosc Clin North Am. 2006; 16(1):59–69.

3. Froehlich F, Harris JK, Wietlisbach V et al. Current sedation and monitoring practice for colonoscopy: an International Observational Study (EPAGE). Endoscopy 2006; 38(5):461–9.

4. Takahashi Y, Tanaka H, Kinjo M et al. Sedation-free colonoscopy. Dis Colon Rectum 2005; 48(4):855–9.

5. Teague R. Safety and sedation during endoscopic procedures. Br Soc Gastroenterol 2003; 000:000.

6. Waye J, Rex D, Williams C. Colonoscopy principles and practice. Blackwell, 2003.

7. Luchette FA, Doerr RJ, Kelly K et al. Colonoscopic impaction in left colon strictures resulting in right colon pneumatic perforation. Surg Endosc 1992; 6(6):273–6.

8. Shah SG, Saunders BP, Brooker JC et al. Magnetic imaging of colonoscopy: an audit of looping, accuracy and ancillary maneuvers. Gastrointest Endosc 2000; 52(1):1–8.

9. Waye JD, Yessayan SA, Lewis BS et al. The technique of abdominal pressure in total colonoscopy. Gastrointest Endosc 1991; 37(2):147–51.

10. Prechel JA, Young CJ, Hucke R et al. The importance of abdominal pressure during colonoscopy: techniques to assist the physician and to minimize injury to the patient and assistant. Gastroenterol Nurs 2005; 28(3):232–6.

11. Hoff G, Bretthauer M, Dahler S et al. Improvement in caecal intubation rate and pain reduction by using 3-dimensional magnetic imaging for unsedated colonoscopy: a randomized trial of patients referred for colonoscopy. Scand J Gastroenterol 2007; 42(7):885–9.

12. Shah SG, Brooker JC, Williams CB et al. Effect of magnetic endoscope imaging on colonoscopy performance: a randomised controlled trial. Lancet 2000; 356(9243):1718–22.

13. Cheung HY, Chung CC, Kwok SY et al. Improvement in colonoscopy performance with adjunctive magnetic endoscope imaging: a randomized controlled trial. Endoscopy 2006; 38(3):214–7.

14. van Rijn JC, Reitsma JB, Stoker J et al. Polyp miss rate determined by tandem colonoscopy: a systematic review. Am J Gastroenterol 2006; 101(2):343–50.

15. Rex DK, Cutler CS, Lemmel GT et al. Colonoscopic miss rates of adenomas determined by back-to-back colonoscopies. Gastroenterology 1997; 112(1):24–8.

16. Rex DK, Bond JH, Winawer S et al. Quality in the technical performance of colonoscopy and the continuous quality improvement process for colonoscopy: recommendations of the U.S. Multi-Society Task Force on Colorectal Cancer. Am J Gastroenterol 2002; 97(6):1296–308.

Guidelines on technical performance and quality improvement for colonoscopy produced by the American Task Force.

17. Barclay RL, Vicari JJ, Doughty AS et al. Colonoscopic withdrawal times and adenoma detection during screening colonoscopy. N Engl J Med 2006; 355(24):2533–41.

Observational study of 12 experienced colonoscopists over 7882 colonoscopies showing a 10-fold difference in ADR between endoscopists and a significant difference in those who spend more or less than 6 minutes during withdrawal in normal colonoscopies.

18. Rex DK. Colonoscopic withdrawal technique is associated with adenoma miss rates. Gastrointest Endosc 2000; 51(1):33–6.

19. Thomas-Gibson S, Rogers PA, Suzuki N et al. Development of a video assessment scoring method to determine the accuracy of endoscopist performance at screening flexible sigmoidoscopy. Endoscopy 2006; 38(3):218–25.

20. Wexner SD, Beck DE, Baron TH et al. A consensus document on bowel preparation before colonoscopy: prepared by a Task Force from The American Society of Colon and Rectal Surgeons (ASCRS), the American Society for Gastrointestinal Endoscopy (ASGE), and the Society of American Gastrointestinal and Endoscopic Surgeons (SAGES). Dis Colon Rectum 2006; 49(6):792–809.

Comprehensive literature review and recommendations from the American Task Force.

21. Thomas-Gibson S, Rogers P, Cooper S et al. Judgment of the quality of bowel preparation at screening flexible sigmoidoscopy is associated with variability in adenoma detection rates. Endoscopy 2006; 38(5):456–60.

22. East JE, Suzuki N, Arebi N et al. Position changes during colonoscope withdrawal improve polyp detection: interim results from a randomised, crossover trial. Endoscopy 2006; 38(Suppl II): A224.

23. Saunders BP, Elsby B, Boswell AM et al. Intravenous antispasmodic and patient-controlled analgesia are of benefit for screening flexible sigmoidoscopy. Gastrointest Endosc 1995; 42(2):123–7.

24. Saunders BP, Williams CB. Premedication with intravenous antispasmodic speeds colonoscope insertion. Gastrointest Endosc 1996; 43(3):209–11.

25. Marshall JB, Patel M, Mahajan RJ et al. Benefit of intravenous antispasmodic (hyoscyamine sulfate) as premedication for colonoscopy. Gastrointest Endosc 1999; 49(6):720–6.

26. Cutler CS, Rex DK, Hawes RH et al. Does routine intravenous glucagon administration facilitate colonoscopy? A randomized trial. Gastrointest Endosc 1995; 42(4):346–50.

27. Chu Q, Petros JG. Extraperitoneal rectal perforation due to retroflexion fiberoptic proctoscopy. Am Surg 1999; 65(1):81–5.

28. Hanson JM, Atkin WS, Cunliffe WJ et al. Rectal retroflexion: an essential part of lower gastrointestinal endoscopic examination. Dis Colon Rectum 2001; 44(11):1706–8.

29. Bowles CJ, Leicester R, Romaya C et al. A prospective study of colonoscopy practice in the UK today: are we adequately prepared for national colorectal cancer screening tomorrow? Gut 2004; 53(2):277–83.

30. ASGE. American Society for Gastrointestinal Endoscopy. Principles of training in gastrointestinal endoscopy. Gastrointest Endosc 1999; 49(6): 845–53.

31. Guidelines for the Training, Appraisal and Assessment of Trainees in Gastrointestinal Endoscopy, 2004 (available from: http://www.thejag.org.uk.

32. Park J, MacRae H, Musselman LJ et al. Randomized controlled trial of virtual reality simulator training: transfer to live patients. Am J Surg 2007; 194(2):205–11.

33. Hochberger J, Matthes K, Maiss J et al. Training with the compactEASIE biologic endoscopy simulator significantly improves hemostatic technical skill of gastroenterology fellows: a randomized controlled comparison with clinical endoscopy training alone. Gastrointest Endosc 2005; 61(2):204–15.

34. Axon AT, Aabakken L, Malfertheiner P et al. Recommendations of the ESGE workshop on ethics in teaching and learning endoscopy. First European Symposium on Ethics in Gastroenterology and Digestive Endoscopy, Kos, Greece, June 2003. Endoscopy 2003; 35(9):761–4.

35. Hurlstone DP, Sanders DS, McAlindon ME et al. High-magnification chromoscopic colonoscopy in ulcerative colitis: a valid tool for in vivo optical biopsy and assessment of disease extent. Endoscopy 2006; 38(12):1213–7.

Biphasic examination with 1800 images from 300 patients obtained via conventional or magnification imaging. Magnification imaging was significantly better than conventional colonoscopy for predicting disease extent in vivo (P < 0.0001).

36. Kiesslich R, Fritsch J, Holtmann M et al. Methylene blue-aided chromoendoscopy for the detection of intraepithelial neoplasia and colon cancer in ulcerative colitis. Gastroenterology 2003; 124(4):880–8.

Randomised controlled trial of 165 patients showing a significantly better correlation between the endoscopic assessment of degree (P = 0.0002) and extent (89% vs. 52%; P < 0.0001) of colonic inflammation and the histopathological findings in the chromoendoscopy group compared with the conventional colonoscopy group. More targeted biopsies were possible, and significantly more neoplasias were detected (32 vs. 10; P = 0.003).

37. Rutter MD, Saunders BP, Schofield G et al. Pancolonic indigo carmine dye spraying for the detection of dysplasia in ulcerative colitis. Gut 2004; 53(2):256–60.

Back-to-back colonoscopies in 100 patients showing significantly more dysplasia detection with chromoendoscopy and targeted biopsies (P=0.02). Chromoendoscopy required fewer biopsies (157 vs. 2904) yet detected nine dysplastic lesions, seven of which were only visible after indigocarmine application.

38. Hurlstone DP, Karajeh M, Cross SS et al. The role of high-magnification-chromoscopic colonoscopy in hereditary nonpolyposis colorectal cancer screening: a prospective "back-to-back" endoscopic study. Am J Gastroenterol. 2005; 100(10):2167–73.

Back-to-back colonoscopies in 25 asymptomatic HNPCC patients. Pan-chromoscopy identified significantly more adenomas than conventional colonoscopy (P = 0.001) and a significantly higher number of flat adenomas (P = 0.004).

39. Lecomte T, Cellier C, Meatchi T et al. Chromoendoscopic colonoscopy for detecting preneoplastic lesions in hereditary nonpolyposis colorectal cancer syndrome. Clin Gastroenterol Hepatol 2005; 3(9):897–902.

Back-to-back colonoscopies in 36 asymptomatic HNPCC patients. The use of chromoendoscopy significantly increased the detection rate of adenomas in the proximal colon, from 3 of 33 patients to 10 of 33 patients (P = 0.045).

40. Hurlstone DP, Cross SS, Adam I et al. Efficacy of high magnification chromoscopic colonoscopy for the diagnosis of neoplasia in flat and depressed lesions of the colorectum: a prospective analysis. Gut 2004; 53(2):284–90.

41. East JE, Suzuki N, von Herbay A et al. Narrow band imaging with magnification for dysplasia detection and pit pattern assessment in ulcerative colitis surveillance: a case with multiple dysplasia associated lesions or masses. Gut 2006; 55(10):1432–5.

42. East JE, Suzuki N, Saunders BP. Comparison of magnified pit pattern interpretation with narrow band imaging versus chromoendoscopy for diminutive colonic polyps: a pilot study. Gastrointest Endosc 2007; 66(2):310–6.

43. Tischendorf JJ, Wasmuth HE, Koch A et al. Value of magnifying chromoendoscopy and narrow band imaging (NBI) in classifying colorectal polyps: a prospective controlled study. Endoscopy 2007; 39(12):1092–6.

44. Adler A, Pohl H, Papanikolaou IS et al. A prospective randomized study on narrow-band imaging versus conventional colonoscopy for adenoma detection: does NBI induce a learning effect? Gut 2007; 57(1):59–64.

45. Rex DK, Helbig CC. High yields of small and flat adenomas with high-definition colonoscopes using either white light or narrow band imaging. Gastroenterology 2007; 133(1):42–7.

46. Kudo S, Hirota S, Nakajima T et al. Colorectal tumours and pit pattern. J Clin Pathol 1994; 47(10):880–5.

47. Liu HH, Kudo SE, Juch JP. Pit pattern analysis by magnifying chromoendoscopy for the diagnosis of colorectal polyps. J Formosan Med Assoc [Taiwan yi zhi] 2003; 102(3):178–82.

48. Triadafilopoulos G, Watts HD, Higgins J et al. A novel nitrograde-viewing auxillary imaging device (Third Eye Retroscope) improves the detection of simulated polyps in anatomic models of the colon. Gastrointest Endosc 2007; 65:139–144.

49. Waye JD. New methods of polypectomy. Gastrointest Endosc Clin North Am 1997; 7(3):413–22.

50. Williams CB. Small polyps: the virtues and the dangers of hot biopsy. Gastrointest Endosc 1991; 37(3):394–5.

51. Peura DA, Lanza FL, Gostout CJ et al. The American College of Gastroenterology Bleeding Registry: preliminary findings. Am J Gastroenterol 1997; 92(6):924–8.

52. Zuckerman GR, Prakash C. Acute lower intestinal bleeding. Part II: Etiology, therapy, and outcomes. Gastrointest Endosc 1999; 49(2):228–38.

53. Jensen DM, Machicado GA, Jutabha R et al. Urgent colonoscopy for the diagnosis and treatment of severe diverticular hemorrhage. N Engl J Med 2000; 342(2):78–82.

54. Waye JD. Endoscopic mucosal resection of colon polyps. Gastrointest Endosc Clin North Am 2001; 11(3):537–48, vii.

55. Brooker JC, Saunders BP, Shah SG et al. Treatment with argon plasma coagulation reduces recurrence after piecemeal resection of large sessile colonic polyps: a randomized trial and recommendations. Gastrointest Endosc 2002; 55(3):371–5.

   Patients with apparent complete excision of adenomatous polyps were randomised to application of APC to the margins or not. Postpolypectomy application of APC reduced recurrence at 3 months (1/10 APC, 7/11 no APC; $P = 0.02$).

56. Hurlstone DP, Atkinson R, Sanders DS et al. Achieving R0 resection in the colorectum using endoscopic submucosal dissection. Br J Surg 2007; 94(12):1536–42.

57. Tamegai Y, Saito Y, Masaki N et al. Endoscopic submucosal dissection: a safe technique for colorectal tumors. Endoscopy 2007; 39(5):418–22.

58. Onozato Y, Kakizaki S, Ishihara H et al. Endoscopic submucosal dissection for rectal tumors. Endoscopy 2007; 39(5):423–7.

59. Saunders BP, Brown GJ, Lemann M et al. Balloon dilation of ileocolonic strictures in Crohn's disease. Endoscopy 2004; 36(11):1001–7.

60. Baron TH, Harewood GC. Enteral self-expandable stents. Gastrointest Endosc 2003; 58(3):421–33.

61. Carne PW, Frye JN, Robertson GM et al. Stents or open operation for palliation of colorectal cancer: a retrospective, cohort study of perioperative outcome and long-term survival. Dis Colon Rectum 2004; 47(9):1455–61.

62. Spinelli P, Mancini A. Use of self-expanding metal stents for palliation of rectosigmoid cancer. Gastrointest Endosc 2001; 53(2):203–6.

63. Guan YS, Sun L, Li X et al. Successful management of a benign anastomotic colonic stricture with self-expanding metallic stents: a case report. World J Gastroenterol 2004; 10(23):3534–6.

64. Matsuhashi N, Nakajima A, Suzuki A et al. Long-term outcome of non-surgical strictureplasty using metallic stents for intestinal strictures in Crohn's disease. Gastrointest Endosc 2000; 51(3):343–5.

65. Yates MR 3rd, Baron TH. Treatment of a radiation-induced sigmoid stricture with an expandable metal stent. Gastrointest Endosc 1999; 50(3):422–6.

66. Hazey JW, Narula VK, Renton DB et al. Natural-orifice transgastric endoscopic peritoneoscopy in humans: initial clinical trial. Surg Endosc 2008; 22(1):16–20.

67. Burling D, Taylor SA, Halligan S. Virtual colonoscopy: current status and future directions. Gastrointest Endosc Clin North Am 2005; 15(4):773–95.

68. Halligan S, Taylor SA. CT colonography: results and limitations. Eur J Radiol 2007; 61(3):400–8.

69. Arber N, Grinshpon R, Pfeffer J et al. Proof-of-concept study of the Aer-O-Scope omnidirectional colonoscopic viewing system in ex vivo and in vivo porcine models. Endoscopy 2007; 39(5):412–7.

70. Vucelic B, Rex D, Pulanic R et al. The aer-o-scope: proof of concept of a pneumatic, skill-independent, self-propelling, self-navigating colonoscope. Gastroenterology 2006; 130(3):672–7.

71. Eliakim R, Fireman Z, Gralnek IM et al. Evaluation of the PillCam Colon capsule in the detection of colonic pathology: results of the first multicenter, prospective, comparative study. Endoscopy 2006; 38(10):963–70.

72. Schoofs N, Deviere J, Van Gossum A. PillCam colon capsule endoscopy compared with colonoscopy for colorectal tumor diagnosis: a prospective pilot study. Endoscopy 2006; 38(10):971–7.

3

Inherited bowel cancer

Sue Clark

Introduction

Individuals develop colorectal cancer as a result of interaction between genotype and the environment to which they are exposed. The lifetime risk of colorectal cancer in the UK population is about 5%. As it is common, many people by chance alone have at least one affected relative;[1] as the number of affected relatives increases, so does the risk of developing the disease.[2] As far as genetic factors are concerned, there is a spectrum of risk: at one end are those with no particular genetic predisposition, and at the other those who will inevitably develop bowel cancer. Between the extremes lie those whose genetic constitution plays some role. While open to error, it is possible to divide the population into three broad categories of risk for colorectal cancer: low, moderate and high risk.

In the high-risk group, the contribution of inheritance (genotype) is overwhelming, though environmental influences may modify disease severity (phenotype). It is this minority (accounting for less than 5% of large bowel cancer) that is traditionally described as being at risk of 'inherited bowel cancer'.

In the low- and moderate-risk groups, genotype may still contribute to risk but less markedly, and is thought to play a part in about 30% of colorectal cancers.[3] This may be due to low penetrance genes that influence dietary carcinogen metabolism.

This chapter deals predominantly with those in the high-risk group. Although these individuals comprise a minority of those at risk overall, there is sufficient knowledge about the specific syndromes that fall within this category to provide important opportunities for cancer prevention.

Assessment of risk

The crucial step in allocating individuals to one of these risk categories is the documentation of an accurate family history which allows an empirical assessment of risk.[2] It should focus on the site and age at diagnosis of all cancers in family members, as well as the presence of related features such as colorectal adenomas. This can be time-consuming, especially when the information needs to be verified. Few surgeons are able to devote the necessary time or skill to do this satisfactorily, and it is here that family cancer clinics or registries for inherited bowel cancer have an important role.[4]

A full personal history should also be taken, with particular attention focused on:

- symptoms (e.g. rectal bleeding, change in bowel habit), which should be investigated as usual;
- previous large bowel polyps;
- previous large bowel cancers;
- cancers at other sites;
- other risk factors for colorectal cancer (inflammatory bowel disease, ureterosigmoidostomy, acromegaly); these

conditions are not discussed further in this chapter, but may warrant surveillance of the large bowel.

The family history has many limitations, particularly in small families. Other difficulties arise because of incorrect information or early death of individuals before they develop cancers. A vast range of complex pedigrees arise, and rather than try to devise guidelines to cover all of them, common sense is needed. If a family seems to fall between risk groups it is safest to manage the family as if in the higher risk group. Despite this, some families will appear to be at high risk simply because of chance clustering of truly sporadic cancer while some, particularly small families with Lynch syndrome, will be assigned to the low- or moderate-risk groups. Even in families affected with an autosomal dominant condition, 50% of family members will not have inherited the causative mutation and will therefore not be at any increased risk of developing cancer.

Family histories evolve, so that the allocation of an individual to a particular risk group may change if further family members develop tumours. It is important that patients are informed of this, particularly if they are in the low- or moderate-risk groups and therefore not undergoing regular surveillance.

Low-risk group

Individuals in this group have:

1. no personal history of bowel cancer; no confirmed family history of bowel cancer; or
2. no first-degree relative (i.e. parent, sibling or child) with bowel cancer; or
3. one first-degree relative with bowel cancer diagnosed at age 45 years or older.

Moderate-risk group

Individuals are allocated to this category if there is:

1. one first-degree relative with bowel cancer diagnosed before the age of 45 years (without the high-risk features outlined below); or
2. two first-degree relatives with bowel cancer diagnosed at any age (without the high-risk features outlined below).

High-risk group

This category encompasses hereditary non-polyposis colorectal cancer (HNPCC) and the various polyposis syndromes. Criteria for inclusion include:

1. member of a family with known familial adenomatous polyposis (FAP) or other polyposis syndrome; or
2. member of a family with known Lynch syndrome; or
3. pedigree suggestive of autosomal dominantly inherited colorectal (or other Lynch syndrome-associated) cancer.

Diagnosis of the polyposis syndromes is comparatively straightforward as there is a recognisable phenotype in each. Lynch syndrome is much more difficult as there is no such characteristic phenotype, other than the occurrence of cancers.

Management

Low-risk group

The risk of bowel cancer even in these individuals may be up to twice the average risk,[2] although this tends to be expressed after the sixth decade of life.

 There is no evidence to support invasive surveillance in this group.[5]

It is important to explain to these individuals that they are at only marginally increased risk of developing colorectal cancer, and that this risk is not sufficient to outweigh the disadvantages of colonoscopy. They should be aware of the symptoms of colorectal cancer, and the importance of reporting if further members of the family develop tumours. Population screening for colorectal cancer has recently been introduced in the UK, and individuals in this risk category should be encouraged to take part.

Moderate-risk group

 There is a three- to sixfold relative risk for individuals in this category,[2] but probably only a marginal benefit from surveillance.[5]

Part of the reason for this is that the incidence of colorectal cancer is very low in the young and rises markedly in the elderly. Even those aged 50 who have a sixfold relative risk by virtue of their family history are less likely to develop colorectal cancer in the following 10 years than are 60-year-olds at average risk.[6]

Current recommendations[5] are that individuals in this risk group should be offered colonoscopy at 35–40 years of age (or at presentation if they are older), and again at the age of 55 years.

If polyps are found, follow-up is modified accordingly. Flexible sigmoidoscopy is not sufficient, as neoplasms in individuals with a strong family history are often proximal; if the caecum is not reached, virtual colonoscopy should be performed.

Again, these individuals should be informed of the symptoms of colorectal cancer, the importance of reporting changes in family history and that they should take part in population screening when they reach the appropriate age.

High-risk group

There is up to a 1 in 2 chance of inheriting a lifetime risk in excess of 50% of developing bowel cancer in this group, and referral to a clinical genetics service is essential. The polyposis syndromes are usually diagnosed from the phenotype, supplemented by genetic testing. Diagnostic confusion can arise, particularly in cases where there are adenomatous polyps insufficient to be diagnostic of FAP. This may occur in MYH-associated polyposis (MAP), FAP with an attenuated phenotype, or Lynch syndrome. A careful search for extracolonic features, mismatch repair immunohistochemistry and microsatellite instability assessment of tumour tissue, and germline mutation detection can sometimes help. Despite this, the diagnosis in some families remains in doubt. In these circumstances the family members should be offered thorough surveillance.

Lynch syndrome

Lynch syndrome is inherited in an autosomal dominant fashion, is responsible for about 2% of colorectal cancers and is the commonest of the inherited bowel cancer syndromes. The terminology in this area is extremely confusing and has recently been revised.[7] Labelled first as the 'cancer family syndrome', the name was changed to hereditary non-polyposis colorectal cancer (HNPCC) to distinguish it from the polyposis syndromes and to highlight the absence of the large numbers of colorectal adenomas found in FAP. However, scanty adenomatous polyps are a feature of Lynch syndrome.

Various different diagnostic criteria have been used, including different definitions based on family history. Mutations in mismatch repair (MMR) genes were identified in some, but not all, families with an apparent dominantly inherited cancer syndrome. It has been suggested that the term Lynch syndrome be used where there is a mismatch repair mutation (irrespective of family history) and 'syndrome X' when there is a strong family history (Amsterdam criteria – see below), but MMR mutation has been excluded. HNPCC can be used to cover both of these groups.

Clinical features

Lynch syndrome is characterised by early onset of colorectal tumours, the average age at diagnosis being 45 years. These tumours have certain distinguishing pathological features. There is a predilection for the proximal colon, and tumours are frequently multiple (synchronous and metachronous). They tend to be mucinous, poorly differentiated and of 'signet-ring' appearance, with marked infiltration by lymphocytes and lymphoid aggregation at their margins. The associated cancers and their frequencies are detailed in Table 3.1.[8] The prognosis of these cancers tends to be better than in the same tumours arising sporadically.

Genetics

Lynch syndrome is due to germline mutations in MMR genes, whose role is to correct errors in base-pair matching during replication of DNA or to initiate apoptosis when DNA damage is beyond repair. The following MMR genes have been identified and mutations in them may be associated with Lynch syndrome: *hMLH1*, *hMSH2*, *hMSH6*, *hPMS1*, *hPMS2*

Table 3.1 • Cancers associated with Lynch syndrome

Site	Frequency (%)
Large bowel	30–75
Endometrium	30–70 (of women)
Stomach	5–10
Ovary	5–10 (of women)
Urothelium (renal pelvis, ureter, bladder)	5
Other (small bowel, pancreas, brain)	<5

and *hMSH3*. The MMR genes are tumour-suppressor genes: patients with Lynch syndrome inherit a defective copy from one parent and tumorigenesis is triggered when the solitary normal gene in a cell becomes mutated or lost, so that DNA mismatches are no longer repaired in that cell. Defective MMR results in the accumulation of mutations in a host of other genes, leading to tumour formation.

A hallmark of tumours with defective MMR is microsatellite instability (MSI). Microsatellites are regions where a short DNA sequence (up to five nucleotides) is repeated. There are large numbers of such sequences in the human genome, the majority in non-coding DNA. Base-pair mismatches occurring during DNA replication are normally repaired by the MMR proteins. In tumours with a deficiency of these proteins this mechanism fails and microsatellites become mutated, resulting in a change in the number of sequence repeats and hence the length of the microsatellite (microsatellite instability). Typically in such a tumour over half of all microsatellites will exhibit this phenomenon.

About 15% of colorectal cancers show MSI. Some of these are from individuals with Lynch syndrome and are due to inherited MMR mutation. The majority, however, occur in older patients and are due to inactivation of MMR genes by promoter methylation, which is not as far as we know related to any inherited factor.

Although predominantly a disorder based on MMR mutations, there is evidence to suggest that other influences affect expression in Lynch syndrome populations. For example, a comparative study between Korean and Dutch families with *hMLH1* mutations found that there were more gastric and pancreatic cancers and fewer endometrial cancers in the Koreans than in the Dutch.[9] This implies either that these Korean families were affected by a modifier gene or genes also prevalent in the general Korean population (which has a high risk for gastric cancer), or that environmental influences exist to which the Korean population are exposed and which interact with the mutations responsible for Lynch syndrome-related cancers.

Diagnosis

Pedigree

Over the years a confusing range of 'criteria' have emerged. The International Collaborative Group on HNPCC (ICG-HNPCC) proposed the Amsterdam criteria in 1990 (Box 3.1). These were not intended as a diagnostic definition but rather as a means to identify families very likely to have a dominantly inherited cancer predisposition. The aim was to target genetic research on a well-defined group that was likely to yield positive results. While families fulfilling these criteria very likely have Lynch syndrome, many affected families will not meet the stringent conditions.[10] The Amsterdam criteria were modified by the ICG-HNPCC in 1999 (Box 3.2) to include Lynch syndrome-associated cancers other than colorectal cancer (Amsterdam II criteria).[11] Subsequent studies have shown that approximately half the families which meet these criteria have Lynch syndrome (i.e. an MMR mutation is identified), and a similar proportion of individuals with Lynch syndrome come from families meeting these criteria (i.e. 50% of Lynch syndrome families do not meet the Amsterdam criteria).

Genetic testing is expensive and time-consuming. The circumstances under which it is offered vary from centre to centre, but generally an affected individual (i.e. with a Lynch syndrome-related cancer) from a family fulfilling the Amsterdam I or II criteria would be offered testing. In families where the

Box 3.1 • Amsterdam criteria I

- At least three relatives with colorectal cancer, one of whom should be a first-degree relative of the other two
- At least two successive generations should be affected
- At least one colorectal cancer should be diagnosed before age 50 years
- FAP should be excluded
- Tumours should be verified by pathological examination

Box 3.2 • Amsterdam criteria II

- At least three relatives with a Lynch syndrome-associated cancer (colorectal, endometrial, small bowel, ureter, renal pelvis), one of whom should be a first-degree relative of the other two
- At least two successive generations should be affected
- At least one colorectal cancer should be diagnosed before age 50 years
- FAP should be excluded
- Tumours should be verified by pathological examination

Amsterdam criteria are not met, but where clinical suspicion remains, analysis of tumour tissue can provide further useful information.

Analysis of tumour tissue

A reference panel of five microsatellite markers is used to detect MSI; if two of the markers show instability, the tumour is designated 'MSI-high'. About 15% of colorectal cancers are MSI-high, but only 5–10% of these will be from patients with Lynch syndrome. The value of MSI testing is that Lynch syndrome is due to MMR mutation and therefore virtually all tumours arising as a result of Lynch syndrome will be MSI-high. The Bethesda guidelines[12] (Box 3.3) were proposed to determine whether tumour tissue from an individual should be tested for MSI. The aim was to provide a sensitive set of guidelines that would encompass nearly all Lynch syndrome-associated colorectal cancers but also many 'sporadic cancers', and to use MSI testing to exclude those individuals lacking MSI-high, whose cancers are extremely unlikely to be caused by Lynch syndrome. Those designated MSI-high can then be further investigated using immunohisto-chemistry and genetic testing. Using this approach, approximately 90% of individuals with colorectal cancer due to Lynch syndrome can be identified.

MSI testing is expensive and requires DNA extraction. A simpler approach is to use standard immunohistochemical techniques to identify MMR proteins,[13] although care is needed in interpreting the results.

Box 3.3 • Bethesda criteria for determining whether the tumour tissue from an individual with colorectal cancer should be tested for microsatellite instability

- Colorectal cancer diagnosed at age <50 years
- Multiple colorectal or other Lynch syndrome-associated tumours, either at the same time (synchronous) or occurring over a period of time (metachronous)
- Individuals diagnosed with colorectal cancer at <60 years, in whom the tumour has microscopic characteristics indicative of microsatellite instability
- Individuals with colorectal cancer who have one or more first-degree relatives diagnosed with a Lynch syndrome-related tumour at age 50 years or younger
- Individuals with colorectal cancer who have two or more first- or second-degree relatives diagnosed with a Lynch syndrome-related tumour at any age

Genetic testing

The decision whether to perform germline genetic testing on a blood sample from an at-risk or affected person takes the features of the patient, family and tumour into account. This cautious approach is currently justified on the grounds of cost, since genetic testing for MMR genes in the first member of the family (mutation detection) costs around £1000. Once a mutation has been detected in a family, testing other at-risk family members to determine whether they too carry the abnormal gene (predictive testing) is much more straightforward, and allows those without the mutation to be discharged from further surveillance.

As with the other syndromes described in this chapter, testing should be undertaken only after the patient has been counselled appropriately and given informed consent. The consent process should include an offer to provide written information, including a frank discussion of the benefits and risks (e.g. to employment, insurance) of genetic testing. A multidisciplinary clinic where counselling is available is ideal.[14] However, not every individual will accept an offer of genetic testing. Significant predictors of test uptake by individuals include an increased perception of risk, greater confidence in the ability to cope with unfavourable genetic news, more frequent thoughts of cancer and having had at least one colonoscopy.[15]

Germline gene testing may have several outcomes (Box 3.4) and the results should be relayed via the multidisciplinary clinic, where counselling is available.[16] There are also complexities of interpretation of results that mandate this (missense mutations, genetic heterogeneity).[17] Unregulated genetic testing for cancer risk has led to errors and adverse outcomes for individuals.[18] Failure to detect a mutation may be due to a variety of factors: some cases may be due to mutation in regulatory genes rather than the MMR genes themselves; there may be other genes involved that have not yet been identified;

Box 3.4 • Outcomes of genetic testing

Mutation detected
Test at-risk family members (predictive testing): if positive, surveillance and/or other management (e.g. surgery); if negative, no surveillance required

Mutation not detected
Keep all at-risk members under surveillance

there may be a technical failure to identify a mutation which is present; or the family history may be a cluster of sporadic tumours. When this happens, the at-risk family members should continue to be screened.

 Families meeting the Amsterdam criteria but with MSI-negative tumours are at lower risk, so that 3- to 5-yearly colonoscopy is sufficient.[19]

Surveillance

 There is good evidence that regular colonoscopy significantly reduces the 80% risk of colorectal cancer in Lynch syndrome patients.[20]

Colonoscopy must be meticulous, because tiny cancers may be present[21] and frequent as interval cancers are common.

 Thus, colonoscopy every 1–2 years from age 25 years (or 5 years younger than the youngest affected relative, whichever is the earlier)[13] is recommended for at-risk individuals. Surveillance should continue until about 75 years or until the causative mutation in that family has been excluded.[13]

Screening for extracolonic cancers is available, but there is currently little evidence of benefit. Recommendations vary from centre to centre, but surveillance is generally advised where there is a family history of cancers at a particular site. Box 3.5 shows the options for extracolonic surveillance.[13]

Box 3.5 • Extracolonic surveillance in Lynch syndrome

- Annual transvaginal ultrasound ± colour flow Doppler imaging ± endometrial sampling
- Annual CA125 level and clinical examination (pelvic and abdominal)
- Upper gastrointestinal endoscopy every 2 years
- Annual urinalysis/cytology
- Annual abdominal ultrasound of renal tracts, pelvis, pancreas
- Annual liver function tests, CA19-9, CEA

Intervention

Surgery
Prophylactic

The option of prophylactic colectomy rather than colonoscopic surveillance should be discussed with mutation carriers, because of the high risk of colorectal cancer. A similar situation pertains to prophylactic hysterectomy and bilateral salpingo-oophorectomy in women who have completed their families.

Colectomy might be subtotal, with an ileorectal anastomosis, or might take the form of a restorative proctocolectomy. The risk of metachronous cancer in the retained rectum after ileorectal anastomosis has been estimated to be about 12% at 12 years.[22] Regular endoscopy via the anus should be carried out postoperatively, at intervals no greater than 12 months.

 Use of a decision analysis model indicates large gains in life expectancy for carriers of MMR mutation when offered some intervention. Benefits were quantified as 13.5 years from surveillance, 15.6 years from proctocolectomy and 15.3 years from subtotal colectomy compared with no intervention.[23]

Adjusting for quality of life showed that surveillance led to the greatest quality-adjusted life expectancy benefit. This study provides a mathematically based indication of benefit only: individual circumstances need to be incorporated into the decision-making process when making recommendations.

Treatment

 There is a risk of metachronous bowel tumour of 16% after 10 years of follow-up.[24]

For those with colonic tumours, colectomy with ileorectal anastomosis has a prophylactic element in that the entire colon is removed, but without the additional morbidity of proctectomy. Proctocolectomy (with or without ileo-anal pouch reconstruction) is the option of choice in patients who present with rectal cancer.

Medical
Studies of colorectal cancer cells lines deficient in MMR genes have shown that MSI is reduced in cells

exposed to non-steroidal anti-inflammatory drugs (NSAIDs).[25] This provides some theoretical support for the CAPP2 (Colorectal Adenoma/Carcinoma Prevention Programme 2) study, recently completed in Lynch syndrome patients, using aspirin and resistant starch as chemopreventive agents. As yet, however, there is no evidence to support the use of any medical therapy in Lynch syndrome.

The benefit of cytotoxic chemotherapy (notably 5-fluorouracil) for cancers in the setting of Lynch syndrome has been questioned.[13] This may be because some agents act by damaging DNA, which results in apoptosis. MMR proteins are thought to play a part in signalling the presence of irreversible DNA damage and initiating apoptosis, a pathway absent in these tumours.

Familial adenomatous polyposis

Less common than Lynch syndrome, the risk of colorectal cancer in patients with FAP is nearly 100%. FAP is usually characterised by:

- hundreds of colorectal adenomatous polyps at a young age (second or third decade of life) (**Fig. 3.1**);
- duodenal adenomatous polyps;
- multiple extraintestinal manifestations (Box 3.6);
- mutation in the tumour-suppressor adenomatous polyposis coli (*APC*) gene on chromosome 5q;

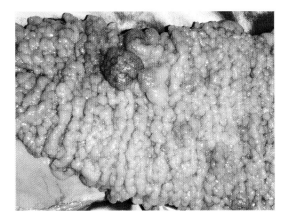

Figure 3.1 • Colectomy specimen from a patient with FAP.

Box 3.6 • Extracolonic manifestations in FAP

Ectodermal origin

- Epidermoid cysts
- Pilomatrixoma
- Tumours of central nervous system
- Congenital hypertrophy of the retinal pigment epithelium

Mesodermal origin

- Connective tissue: desmoid tumours, excessive adhesions
- Bone: osteoma, exostosis, sclerosis
- Dental: dentigerous cyst, odontoma, supernumerary teeth, unerupted teeth

Endodermal origin

- Adenomas and carcinomas of duodenum, stomach, small intestine, biliary tract, thyroid, adrenal cortex
- Fundic gland polyps
- Hepatoblastoma

- autosomal dominant inheritance (offspring of affected individuals have a 1 in 2 chance of inheriting FAP).

Diagnosis

FAP was originally defined by the presence of over 100 colorectal adenomas. This clinical definition is still useful, as a mutation in the *APC* gene can only be identified in up to 80% of affected individuals. The majority of new cases come from families with a known history of the disease, but confusion can arise as approximately 20% are due to a new mutation.[26] In these circumstances there will be no family history of colorectal cancers at a young age or of multiple polyps. Further potential sources of confusion are the recent discovery of MAP (see later) and the well-documented existence of a milder form of the condition, known as attenuated FAP.[27]

Inadequate colonoscopy may lead to a false diagnosis of attenuation, an error that can be avoided by the use of dye-spray (chromoendoscopy).[28] A further point that should be borne in mind is that some individuals with Lynch syndrome have a number of adenomatous polyps. Where the diagnosis requires confirmation, the use of dye-spray and random biopsies looking for microadenomas (a hallmark of FAP and MAP, but not seen in Lynch syndrome) are helpful, as is upper gastrointestinal (GI) endoscopy (50% of FAP patients and some

MAP patients have gastric fundic gland polyps and around 90% duodenal adenomas), as are testing for MSI and immunohistochemistry of tumours.

Genetic testing

 The issue of genetic testing is a useful paradigm highlighting the fundamental role played by registries. Identification of at-risk family members who might be offered gene testing is critical and is usually made possible by the comprehensive collation of family pedigrees that such registries are uniquely positioned to obtain and update.[29]

An uncontrolled approach to testing and the release of results can lead to inadequate counselling and the provision of incorrect information to patients.[30]

An affected family member should be tested first. The mutation can be located in approximately 80% of affected individuals. Once the mutation has been identified, at-risk members of the family can be offered simple blood testing. Should the known family mutation not be found in the at-risk individual, that person can be discharged from further surveillance[31] but should be informed that he or she remains at the same risk of sporadic colorectal cancer as any member of the general population. Such an approach eliminates unnecessary colonic examination and costs less than conventional clinical screening.[32]

Genotype–phenotype correlation

The site of the mutation in the *APC* gene can influence the expression of FAP.[33] Genotype–phenotype correlation is seen in the association between certain mutations and severe FAP (dense colorectal polyposis with relatively early colorectal cancer development), and between other mutations and less severe FAP ('attenuated' polyposis).[34] However, individuals with identical mutations can display differences in phenotypic expression, suggesting that other modifier genes and the environment play a role in disease expression.[35]

Some of the multiple extracolonic manifestations of FAP (see Box 3.6),[36] such as desmoid disease, also show some correlation with the mutation site; others, notably duodenal polyposis and malignancy, do not.

These genotype–phenotype correlations have led to suggestions that the findings of molecular analysis might guide both surveillance and treatment.[34,37,38] At present, however, it is important to emphasise that

prophylactic colectomy or proctocolectomy (almost always with a pouch) remain the management options of choice for all patients with proven FAP.

Surveillance

If the family mutation is known, at-risk family members are usually offered predictive genetic testing in their early teens. If this is not possible, then clinical surveillance is required. It is very unusual for significant colorectal polyps to develop before the teenage years and while cancers have been described in children, they are exceptionally rare. If an individual has symptoms attributable to the large bowel (anaemia, rectal bleeding or change in bowel habit), colonoscopy should be performed. Otherwise annual flexible sigmoidoscopy starting at 13–15 years of age is recommended. If no polyps are detected, 5-yearly colonoscopy should be started at the age of about 20 years, with annual flexible sigmoidoscopy in the intervening years.

The large bowel

Surgery
Prophylactic

Once the diagnosis has been made, either by predictive genetic testing or by the detection of adenomatous polyposis during surveillance of an at-risk family member, the aim is to offer prophylactic surgery before a cancer develops. If the diagnosis has been made on the basis of flexible sigmoidoscopy, colonoscopy should be performed to assess the colonic polyp burden. If the individual is symptomatic or the polyps are dense or large, surgery should be undertaken as soon as is practical. In other cases it is usual to defer surgery until a time when its social and educational impact will be minimised, usually a long summer vacation or 'gap' after leaving school.

As the surgical options have increased, so has the controversy surrounding the choice between them. Increasingly, laparoscopically assisted surgery is becoming available and has great attractions in this group, where a good cosmetic result makes surgery more acceptable. The available operations are:

- colectomy and ileorectal anastomosis (IRA);
- restorative proctocolectomy (RPC) with an ileal pouch–anal anastomosis;
- total proctocolectomy and end ileostomy (almost exclusively for those with very low rectal cancer).

Most young people facing prophylactic colectomy want to avoid a permanent ileostomy, so the choice really lies between the first two options. The biggest attraction of RPC is that the entire large bowel is removed, so that there is no risk of polyps or cancer developing in a retained rectum. However, a cuff of rectal mucosa is retained when a stapled anastomosis is performed, and cancers at this site have been reported.[39] A mucosectomy can be done to remove this area and a handsewn pouch anal anastomosis created, but this is a more technically demanding technique, which probably also results in poorer functional outcome. Furthermore, follow-up studies have shown adenoma formation within ileo-anal pouches, so there is concern that over time these may develop into invasive cancers.[40]

The advantages of IRA are that it is a one-stage procedure (whereas RPC often involves a temporary defunctioning ileostomy) with lower morbidity and mortality.

The functional results in terms of stool frequency and leakage are generally slightly better than after RPC.[41]

Sexual and reproductive function can both be compromised by proctectomy. There is a small but definite risk of erectile and ejaculatory dysfunction in men undergoing proctectomy. In addition there is a pouch failure rate of about 10%, resulting in the need for a permanent ileostomy. These potential complications are particularly difficult to accept for essentially healthy young people undergoing surgery for prophylaxis rather than treatment.

Recent studies have shown that RPC for both FAP[42] and ulcerative colitis adversely affects fertility in women.

It is known that some groups are at particular risk of developing rectal cancer after IRA. These are individuals with numerous rectal polyps, carriers of certain mutations (such as at codon 1309) and those presenting over the age of 25–30 years. Historical data show a cumulative rectal cancer risk of up to 30% by 60 years of age, but at the time many of these patients underwent IRA, RPC was not available. IRA was the only option to avoid a permanent ileostomy, and thus was done in circumstances when it would not now be recommended.

In selected cases the risk of rectal cancer is low and IRA is a reasonable option.[43]

Many patients will have experience of one or both operations from other family members who have undergone them, which may affect their choice. Ultimately, they need to be informed about the advantages and disadvantages of both procedures, as well as the implications of their genotype (if identified) so that their decision can be as informed as possible.

Treatment

In the presence of a colonic cancer, the surgical decision-making is essentially the same as in prophylactic surgery. In individuals with severe rectal polyposis, in those carrying a mutation at codon 1309 of the *APC* gene or in those aged over 25–30 years, the risk of subsequent uncontrollable rectal polyposis requiring completion proctectomy, or of rectal cancer itself, are high and outweigh the disadvantages of RPC. In younger patients, those with few rectal polyps, mutations at other sites and the few older patients with a genuine attenuated phenotype, IRA may represent a better option. Ultimately, it remains for the informed patient to make a choice.

When rectal cancer is present, the choice is between RPC and proctocolectomy and ileostomy. As in any case of rectal cancer, a very low tumour precludes sphincter preservation. Careful local staging and multidisciplinary management are crucial in these cases.

Surveillance after surgery

Follow-up is required after all procedures. After IRA or RPC, peranal digital and flexible endoscopic examination are mandatory at intervals of up to 12 months, depending on findings. The NSAID sulindac has been used to control rectal adenomas[44] and pouch adenomas.[45]

A recent trial using the selective cyclo-oxygenase (COX)-2 inhibitor celecoxib (marketed in Europe as Onsenal) has shown a moderate reduction in large bowel polyps in treated patients.[46]

These drugs must be used with caution in view of earlier reports of cancer despite chemoprevention (with sulindac) and surveillance in this setting and also because of a threefold increase in adverse cardiovascular events (admittedly anyway rare in most younger FAP patients) when Onsenal is used. Following colectomy, the major causes of mortality and morbidity are duodenal cancers and desmoid tumours. This knowledge guides postoperative management.[29]

Upper gastrointestinal tract polyps

Non-adenomatous gastric polyps (fundic gland polyps) occur in approximately 50% of patients with FAP. Their malignant potential is extremely low but not non-existent.[47]

 Duodenal adenomas occur in nearly all patients with FAP but are severe in only 10%, with malignant change occurring in 5%.[48]

Surveillance of the upper gastrointestinal tract

Surveillance usually begins in the third decade of life (in the asymptomatic patient), with endoscopies at intervals of between 6 months and 5 years depending on the severity of duodenal polyposis.[49] A staging system for duodenal polyposis has been developed (Table 3.2) to allow surveillance to be

tailored to disease severity and to identify individuals at high risk of developing malignancy.[50]

 Upper gastroduodenal endoscopy leads to a moderate gain in life expectancy.[51]

The periampullary area must be examined, being at particularly high risk, so a side-viewing as well as end-viewing scope should be used in the examination.[52]

Management of duodenal polyposis

 Management of severe duodenal polyposis is difficult. Chemopreventive options have some benefit.[53]

Interventions such as endoscopic removal or open duodenotomy are associated with high recurrence rates.[54] The risk of endoscopic-induced duodenal perforation may be obviated by using argon plasma coagulation.[55] Advanced endoscopic techniques, often under general anaesthesia, are currently being investigated in patients with Spigelman stage III disease.

While prophylactic pancreatico-duodenectomy or pylorus-preserving pancreatico-duodenectomy has been described with good outcomes,[48,54] associated morbidity and mortality are substantial. However, the poor prognosis once invasive disease is present and the high rate of progression to

Table 3.2 • Spigelman staging of severity of duodenal polyposis in FAP

	Points allocated		
	1	**2**	**3**
Number of polyps	1–4	5–20	>20
Polyp size (mm)	1–4	5–10	>10
Histological type	Tubular	Tubulovillous	Villous
Degree of dysplasia	Mild	Moderate	Severe
Total points	**Spigelman stage**	**Recommended follow-up interval**	
0	0	5 years	
1–4	I	5 years	
5–6	II	3 years	
7–8	III	1 year and consider endoscopic therapy	
9–12	IV	Consider prophylactic duodenectomy	

cancer of advanced polyposis (36% over 10 years in one series) means that this aggressive approach can be justified in some cases with Spigelman stage IV disease. Cancer risk and hence the need for intervention is minimal in patients with stage 0–II disease.

Desmoid tumours

Desmoid tumours are fibromatous lesions consisting of clonal proliferations of myofibroblasts (**Fig. 3.2**). They occur in approximately 15% of individuals with FAP, with a mortality rate of about 10%.[56,57] Most exhibit cycles of growth and resolution and, while causing discomfort and being unsightly, may not cause significant problems. Most desmoids associated with FAP arise either intra-abdominally (usually within the small bowel mesentery) or on the abdominal wall, although they can appear in the extremities and trunk. They are histologically benign, but within the abdomen can cause small bowel and ureteric obstruction, intestinal ischaemia or perforation, all of which can be fatal. A model of desmoid tumour development, based on the appearance of a precursor plaque-like lesion, has been proposed, offering a possibility for prevention or early treatment.[58]

The aetiology of desmoid tumours is multifactorial, with contributions from trauma (e.g. operative), oestrogens, specific *APC* gene mutations and modifier genes.

Management

The challenge in the management of these bizarre tumours is to identify the minority which are rapidly and relentlessly progressive and to avoid harming patients with unnecessarily aggressive attempts to treat the rest. Ureteric obstruction is not infrequent, and as the consequences can be obviated by ureteric stenting it is wise to perform regular renal tract imaging in patients otherwise being managed non-operatively every 6 months.

Computed tomography (CT) provides the best imaging with respect to size and relationship to surrounding structures, but T2-weighted magnetic resonance imaging (MRI) sequences may provide useful information about cellularity and growth potential. Ultrasound can be used to monitor the ureters.

Treatment options include NSAIDs, antioestrogens, surgical excision and cytotoxic chemotherapy.[59]

Anecdotal successes with a variety of NSAIDs and antioestrogens abound (e.g. sulindac 150–200 mg twice daily alone or in combination with very-high-dose tamoxifen 80–120 mg daily), although good evidence of efficacy is lacking. Evaluation of these treatments is further hampered by the natural history of desmoids, which have been documented to regress spontaneously and exhibit relentless growth in only a small minority of patients.

Evidence[56] supports the use of surgery as first-line treatment for abdominal wall and body wall desmoids, although the recurrence rate is high.

There is no evidence to support the concern that this might be increased by the use of prosthetic materials to repair any resulting defect. Surgery should usually be avoided where possible for intra-abdominal desmoids, being associated with high mortality, morbidity and recurrence rates. However, perforation with peritonitis, complete intestinal obstruction or erosion through the body wall may force the surgeon's hand.

MYH-associated polyposis (MAP)

Recent study of patients with the phenotype of FAP but no identifiable *APC* mutation has led to the discovery of this form of adenomatous polyposis,

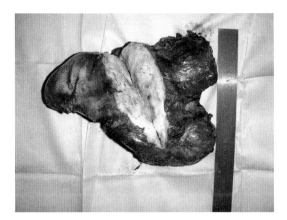

Figure 3.2 • A desmoid tumour excised from the abdominal wall.

which has considerable clinical overlap with FAP, but is genetically distinct.[60]

Clinical features

The large bowel

As in FAP, the most consistent feature of MAP is the development of colonic adenomas and carcinomas. The number of polyps is very variable,[61] with about half the patients in one series having a phenotype consistent with classical FAP (hundreds of polyps) and half having an attenuated phenotype with fewer than 100 polyps. Some cases of cancer have been reported in individuals with a definite genetic diagnosis of MAP, but very few polyps indeed, and the lifetime risk of colorectal cancer is almost 100% by the age of 60. The distribution differs from FAP in that there is a greater proportion of right-sided cancers, which also develop slightly later, at an average of 47 years.

The upper gastrointestinal tract

Gastric fundic gland polyps and duodenal adenomas occur in MAP, but less commonly, with 20–30% having duodenal polyps.[62]

Other manifestations

It has been suggested that there is an increased frequency of breast cancer in MAP, up to 18% in one series.[63] Osteomas and dental cysts have also been documented. To date no MAP patient with desmoid has been reported.

Genetics

This condition is due to biallelic mutation of the mutY human homologue (MYH) gene on chromosome 1p. Thus, for the first time, autosomal recessive inheritance has been described in the context of inherited bowel cancer. The frequency of mutation carriage (heterozygosity) in the general population may be as high as 1 in 200, but individuals who are heterozygotes appear to be at most only at minimally increased risk of colorectal cancer.

Genetic testing is available, and should be considered in individuals with a clinical diagnosis of FAP, but no detectable APC mutation, as well as patients presenting with fewer adenomas. The recessive inheritance means that there will often be no family history of colorectal cancer or polyps. This mode of inheritance also poses challenges in terms of genetic counselling and family testing strategies.

Management

The management of an affected individual is essentially the same as for FAP, although as a higher proportion has an attenuated phenotype, and the age of onset may be a little later, it may be that more patients can be managed, at least initially, by annual colonoscopy and polypectomy. Upper gastrointestinal tract surveillance is started at around the age of 25.

There is insufficient evidence currently to support breast screening, but female patients should be informed of the potentially increased risk. Breast self-examination and participation in population-based breast cancer screening should be encouraged.

The lifetime risk of a heterozygote carrier developing colorectal cancer has not yet been fully clarified, but studies to date indicate that any increase in risk is modest (in the range 1.5–2 times). Thus surveillance is not currently recommended.

Peutz–Jeghers syndrome

Peutz–Jeghers syndrome is an autosomal dominant condition characterised by mucocutaneous pigmentation (**Fig. 3.3**) together with multiple gastrointestinal hamartomatous polyps. The gene responsible in some patients is STK11 (LKB1) on chromosome 19p13, although there is evidence of genetic heterogeneity as mutation at this site has been excluded in some families.

A 78-year follow-up of the original family described by Peutz is instructive.[64] Survival of affected family members was found to be reduced as a result of bowel obstruction and the development of a range of cancers.

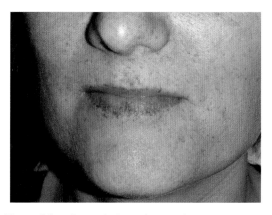

Figure 3.3 • Peutz–Jeghers pigmentation.

Bowel obstruction

The commonest polyp-related complication is bowel obstruction, often caused by intussusception with a polyp at the apex. Repeated episodes result in increasingly difficult laparotomies and loss of bowel length.

Cancer risk

 The incidence of subsequent bowel obstruction can be reduced by adequate intraoperative small bowel enteroscopy, allowing identification and removal of all polyps at the time of initial laparotomy.[65]

Individuals with Peutz–Jeghers syndrome are at increased risk particularly of gastrointestinal malignancy, with a lifetime risk of colorectal cancer of about 20% and of gastric cancer of about 5%. Other areas at increased risk include the breasts (female), ovaries, cervix, pancreas and testes.[66]

Surveillance and management

Up-to-date surveillance protocols are best obtained from local registries. Most involve annual review with physical examination and measurement of haemoglobin. Upper and lower gastrointestinal endoscopies (with polypectomy) and capsule endoscopy or barium follow-through are performed every 2–3 years to detect premalignant polyps or early cancers. If large polyps are seen in the small bowel or symptoms suggesting intermittent small bowel obstruction occur, or if there are small bowel polyps with anaemia, a double-balloon enteroscopy or laparotomy with on-table enteroscopy and polypectomy is recommended to clear the small bowel of polyps and prevent frank obstruction.

As far as malignancy at other sites is concerned, where surveillance programmes have been shown to be useful in the general population they should be used. Breast and testicular self-examination can be advised, and it is important to stress that females should remain up to date with cervical smears and standard breast screening. However, ovarian and pancreatic ultrasound are much more controversial as benefit is not likely.

Juvenile polyposis

Not to be confused with the finding of an isolated juvenile polyp (which has very low, if any, malignant potential), juvenile polyposis is an autosomal dominant condition where multiple characteristic hamartomatous juvenile polyps occur, mostly in the colon but also in the upper gastrointestinal tract and small bowel. Other features sometimes associated are macrocephaly and congenital heart disease. Some affected individuals harbour germline mutations in the *SMAD4* gene,[67] while others have germline mutations in the *BMPR1A* gene.

There is a risk of gastrointestinal cancer in excess of 50%, warranting regular endoscopic screening.[68] Regular oesophago-gastroduodenoscopy and colonoscopy, with polypectomy for large polyps, is mandatory. Occasionally prophylactic colectomy is required.

Cowden disease

The *PTEN* gene on chromosome 10q22 is associated with this syndrome, which consists of gastrointestinal hamartomas and cancers, plus a high risk of cancer of the female breast, thyroid, uterus and cervix, benign fibrocystic breast disease, non-toxic goitre and varied benign mucocutaneous lesions, particularly trichilemmomas. Targeted screening seems sensible, but there is little evidence to support it.

Other inherited colorectal cancer syndromes

Multiple hyperplastic polyps that have adenomatous features (mixed polyposis syndromes) are associated with a high risk for colorectal cancer,[69] as is hyperplastic polyposis. Both conditions can be inherited. Endoscopy and even timely colectomy may be necessary. Large (>1 cm) multiple and right-sided hyperplastic polyps (as opposed to the much more common, though frequently multiple, diminutive rectal and sigmoid ones) should alert the surgeon to potential future risk.

A variant mutation of the *APC* gene on chromosome 5q (E1317Q) has been associated with an increased risk of colorectal cancer without any of the syndromes described above, particularly in the Ashkenazi Jewish population.[70] Research into the same population has provided evidence for the existence of another colorectal cancer susceptibility gene on chromosome 15q.[71] Caution should therefore be exercised in discharging Ashkenazi Jewish kindred on the basis of a negative gene test, as mutations in the other colorectal cancer genes found in this population may be present.[72]

Summary

The emerging complexity of inherited bowel cancer, coupled with rapid advances in knowledge, reinforce the need for the availability of experienced, informed and up-to-date opinion in the areas of diagnosis and management. Individual surgeons will rarely be able to meet all of these needs. Patients and their families are best served by the existence of good working relationships between managing clinicians, family cancer clinics and registries based in expert centres.

Key points

- Genetic factors make a significant contribution to colorectal cancer.
- High-risk families should be referred to special interest registries, genetics units or clinical groups.
- HNPCC and FAP are the main autosomal dominant conditions involved.
- An understanding of these conditions is required to recognise and diagnose them.
- Individuals with these conditions are at risk of a range of extracolonic tumours, so need specialised follow-up.

References

1. Fuchs CS, Giovannucci EL, Colditz GA et al. A prospective study of family history and the risk of colorectal cancer. N Engl J Med 1994; 331:1669–74.

2. Houlston RS, Murday V, Harocopos C et al. Screening and genetic counselling for relatives of patients with colorectal cancer in a family cancer clinic. Br Med J 1990; 301:366–8.

3. Lichtenstein P, Holm NV, Verkasalo PK et al. Environmental and heritable factors in the causation of cancer: analyses of cohorts of twins from Sweden, Denmark and Finland. N Engl J Med 2000; 343:78–85.

4. Lips CJM. Registers for patients with familial tumours: from controversial areas to common guidelines. Br J Surg 1998; 85:1316–18.

5. Dunlop MG. Guidance on large bowel surveillance for people with two first degree relatives with colorectal cancer or one first degree relative diagnosed with colorectal cancer under 45 years. Gut 2002; 51(Suppl V):17–20.

6. Dunlop MG, Campbell H. Screening for people with a family history of colorectal cancer. Br Med J 1997; 314:1779–80.

7. Jass JR. Hereditary non-polyposis colorectal cancer: the rise and fall of a confusing term. World J Gastroenterol 2006; 12:4943–50.

8. Aarnio M, Sankila R, Pukkala E et al. Cancer risk in mutation carriers of DNA-mismatch repair genes. Int J Cancer 1999; 81:214–18.

9. Park JG, Park YJ, Wijnen JT et al. Gene–environment interaction in hereditary nonpolyposis colorectal cancer with implications for diagnosis and genetic testing. Int J Cancer 1999; 82:516–19.

10. Simmang CL et al. and the Standards Committee of the American Society of Colon and Rectal Surgeons. Practice parameters for detection of colorectal neoplasms. Dis Colon Rectum 1999; 42:1123–9.

11. Vasen HFA, Watson P, Mecklin J-P et al. New clinical criteria for hereditary nonpolyposis colorectal cancer (HNPCC, Lynch syndrome) proposed by the International Collaborative Group on HNPCC. Gastroenterology 1999; 116:1453–6.

12. Umar A, Boland CR, Terdiman JP et al. Revised Bethesda Guidelines for hereditary nonpolyposis colorectal cancer (Lynch syndrome) and microsatellite instability. J Natl Cancer Inst 2004; 96:261–8.

13. Vasen HFA, Moslein G, Alonso A et al. Guidelines for the clinical management of Lynch syndrome (hereditary non-polyposis colorectal cancer). J Med Genet 2007; 44:353–62.

14. Scholefield JH, Johnson AG, Shorthouse AJ. Current surgical practice in screening for colorectal cancer based on family history criteria. Br J Surg 1998; 85:1543–6.

15. Esplen MJ, Madlensky L, Butler K et al. Motivations and psychosocial impact of genetic testing for HNPCC. Am J Med Genet 2001; 103:9–15.

16. Burke W, Petersen G, Lynch P et al. Recommendations for follow-up care of individuals with an inherited predisposition to cancer: I. Hereditary nonpolyposis colon cancer. JAMA 1997; 277:915–19.

17. Syngal S, Fox EA, Li C et al. Interpretation of genetic test results for hereditary nonpolyposis colorectal cancer: implications for clinical predisposition testing. JAMA 1999; 282:247–53.

18 Neergaard L. Unregulated gene tests can cause life altering errors. Associated Press, 20 September 1999. Available at http://www.nandotimes.com.

19. Dove-Edwin I, de Jong AE, Adams J et al. Prospective results of surveillance colonoscopy in dominant familial colorectal cancer with and without Lynch syndrome. Gastroenterology 2006; 130:1995–2000.

20. Jarvinen HJ, Aarnio M, Mustonen H et al. Controlled 15-year trial on screening for colorectal cancer in families with hereditary nonpolyposis colorectal cancer. Gastroenterology 2000; 118:829–34.

A prospective controlled trial showing that colonoscopic surveillance in Lynch syndrome led to a 63% reduction in colorectal cancer and a significant decrease in mortality.

21. Church J Hereditary colon cancers can be tiny: a cautionary case report of the results of colonoscopic surveillance. Am J Gastroenterol 1998; 93:2289–90.

22. Rodriguez-Bigas MA, Vasen HF, Mecklin J-P et al. Rectal cancer risk in hereditary nonpolyposis colorectal cancer after abdominal colectomy. Ann Surg 1997; 225:202–7.

23. Syngal S, Weeks JC, Schrag D et al. Benefits of colonoscopic surveillance and prophylactic colectomy in patients with hereditary nonpolyposis colorectal cancer mutations. Ann Intern Med 1998; 129:787–96.

24. de Vos tot Nederveen Cappel WH, Nanengast FM, Griffioen G et al. Surveillance for hereditary non-polyposis colorectal cancer: a long-term study on 114 families. Dis Colon Rectum 2002; 45:1588–94.

25. Ruschoff J, Wallinger S, Dietmaier W et al. Aspirin suppresses the mutator phenotype associated with hereditary nonpolyposis colorectal cancer by genetic selection. Proc Natl Acad Sci USA 1998; 95:11301–6.

26. Bisgaard ML, Fenger K, Bulow S et al. Familial adenomatous polyposis (FAP): frequency, penetrance and mutation rate. Hum Mutat 1994; 3:121–5.

27. Hernegger GS, Moore HG, Guillem JG. Attenuated familial adenomatous polyposis: an evolving and poorly understood entity. Dis Colon Rectum 2002; 45:127–34.

28. Wallace MH, Frayling IM, Clark SK et al. Attenuated adenomatous polyposis coli: the role of ascertainment bias through failure to dye-spray at colonoscopy. Dis Colon Rectum 1999; 42: 1078–80.

29. Vasen HFA, Bülow S and the Leeds Castle Polyposis Group. Guidelines for the surveillance and management of familial adenomatous polyposis (FAP): a world wide survey among 41 registries. Colorectal Dis 1999; 1:214–21.

30. Giardiello FM, Brensinger JD, Petersen GM et al. The use and interpretation of commercial APC gene testing for familial adenomatous polyposis. N Engl J Med 1997; 336:823–7.

31. Berk T, Cohen Z, Bapat B et al. Negative genetic test results in familial adenomatous polyposis: clinical screening implications. Dis Colon Rectum 1999; 42:307–10.

32. Bapat B, Noorani H, Cohen Z et al. Cost comparison of predictive genetic testing versus conventional clinical screening for familial adenomatous polyposis. Gut 1999; 44:698–703.

33. Wu JS, Paul P, McGannon EA et al. APC genotype, polyp number, and surgical options in familial adenomatous polyposis. Ann Surg 1998; 227:57–62.

34. Vasen HFA, van der Luijt RB, Slors JFM et al. Molecular genetic tests as a guide to surgical management of familial adenomatous polyposis. Lancet 1996; 348:433–5.

35. Crabtree MD, Tomlinson IPM, Hodgson SV et al. Explaining variation in familial adenomatous polyposis: relationship between genotype and phenotype and evidence for modifier genes. Gut 2002; 51:420–3.

36. Brett MCA, Hershman MJ, Glazer G. Other manifestations of familial adenomatous polyposis. In: Phillips RKS, Spigelman AD, Thomson JPS (eds) Familial adenomatous polyposis and other polyposis syndromes. London: Edward Arnold, 1994; pp. 142–58.

37. Soravia C, Berk T, Madlensky L et al. Genotype–phenotype correlations in attenuated adenomatous polyposis coli. Am J Hum Genet 1998; 62: 1290–301.

38. Bertario L, Russo A, Radice P et al. Genotype and phenotype factors as determinants for rectal stump cancer in patients with familial adenomatous polyposis. Ann Surg 2000; 231:538–43.

39. Van Duijvendijk P, Vasen HA, Bertario L et al. Cumulative risk of developing polyps or malignancy at the ileal pouch–anal anastomosis in patients with familial adenomatous polyposis. J Gastrointest Surg 1999; 3:325–30.

40. Parc YR, Olschwang S, Desaint B et al. Familial adenomatous polyposis: prevalence of adenomas in the ileal pouch after restorative proctocolectomy. Ann Surg 2001; 233:360–4.

41. Aziz O, Athanasiou T, Fazio VW et al. Meta-analysis of observational studies of ileorectal versus ileal pouch-anal anastomosis for familial adenomatous polyposis. Br J Surg 2006; 93:407–17.

42. Olsen KO, Juul S, Bulow S et al. Female fecundity before and after operation for familial adenomatous polyposis. Br J Surg 2003; 90:227–31.

43. Church J, Burke C, McGannon E et al. Risk of rectal cancer after colectomy and ileorectal anastomosis for familial adenomatous polyposis: a function of available options. Dis Colon Rectum 2003; 46:1175–81.

44. Giardiello FM, Offerhaus JA, Tersmette AC et al. Sulindac induced regression of colorectal adenomas in familial adenomatous polyposis: evaluation of predictive factors. Gut 1996; 38:578–81.

45. Ho JWC, Yuen ST, Chung LP et al. The role of sulindac in familial adenomatous polyposis patients with ileal pouch polyposis. Aust NZ J Surg 1999; 69:756–8.

46. Steinbach LT, Lynch P, Phillips RKS et al. The effect of celecoxib, a cyclo-oxygenase inhibitor, in familial adenomatous polyposis. N Engl J Med 2000; 342:1946–58.

A randomised controlled trial of celecoxib in patients with FAP who had previously undergone colectomy and ileorectal anastomosis. A reduction in adenoma size and number was seen with celecoxib.

47. Hofgartner WT, Thorp M, Ramus MC et al. Gastric adenocarcinoma associated with fundic gland polyps in a patient with attenuated familial adenomatous polyposis. Am J Gastroenterol 1999; 94:2275–81.

48. Groves CJ, Saunders BP, Spigelman AD et al. Duodenal cancer in patients with familial adenomatous polyposis (FAP): results of a 10 year prospective study. Gut 2002; 50:636–41.

49. Burke CA, Beck GJ, Church JM et al. The natural history of untreated duodenal and ampullary adenomas in patients with familial adenomatous polyposis followed in an endoscopic surveillance program. Gastrointest Endosc 1999; 49:358–64.

50. Spigelman AD, Williams CB, Talbot IC et al. Upper gastrointestinal cancer in patients with familial adenomatous polyposis. Lancet 1989; ii:783–5.

51. Vasen HFA, Bülow S, Nyrhøj T et al. Decision analysis in the management of duodenal adenomatosis in familial adenomatous polyposis. Gut 1997; 40:716–19.

52. Wallace MH, Phillips RKS. Upper gastrointestinal disease in patients with familial adenomatous polyposis. Br J Surg 1998; 85:742–50.

53. Phillips RKS, Wallace MH, Lynch PM et al. A randomised, double blind, placebo controlled study of celecoxib, a selective cyclooxygenase 2 inhibitor, on duodenal polyposis in familial adenomatous polyposis. Gut 2002; 50:857–60.

54. Penna C, Bataille N, Balladur P et al. Surgical treatment of severe duodenal polyposis in familial adenomatous polyposis. Br J Surg 1998; 85:665–8.

55. Grund KE, Storek D, Farin G. Endoscopic argon plasma coagulation (APC). First clinical experiences in flexible endoscopy. Endosc Surg Allied Technol 1994; 2:42–6.

56. Clark SK, Neale KF, Landgrebe JC et al. Desmoid tumours complicating familial adenomatous polyposis. Br J Surg 1999; 86:1185–9.

57. Church JM, McGannon E, Ozuner G. The clinical course of intra-abdominal desmoid tumours in patients with familial adenomatous polyposis. Colorectal Dis 1999; 1:168–73.

58. Clark SK, Smith TG, Katz DE et al. Identification and progression of a desmoid precursor lesion in patients with familial adenomatous polyposis. Br J Surg 1998; 85:970–3.

59. Sturt NJ, Clark SK. Current ideas in desmoid tumours. Fam Cancer 2006; 5:275–85.

60. Al Tassan N, Chmiel NH, Maynard J et al. Inherited variants of MYH associated with somatic G:C–T:A mutations in colorectal tumours. Nat Genet 2002; 30:227–32.

61. Sieber OM, Lipton L, Crabtree M et al. Multiple colorectal adenomas, classic adenomatous polyposis and germ-line mutations in MYH. N Engl J Med 2003; 348:791–9.

62. Kanter-Smoler G, Bjork J, Fritzell K et al. Novel findings in Swedish patients with MYH-associated polyposis: mutation detection and clinical characterization. Clin Gastroenterol Hepatol 2006; 4:499–506.

63. Nielsen M, Franken PF, Reinards TH et al. Multiplicity in polyp count and extracolonic manifestations in 40 Dutch patients with MYH associated polyposis coli (MAP). J Med Genet 2005; 42:e54.

64. Westerman AM, Entius MM, de Baar E et al. Peutz–Jeghers syndrome: 78-year follow-up of the original family. Lancet 1999; 353:1211–15.

65. Edwards DP, Khosraviani K, Stafferton R et al. Long-term results of polyp clearance by intraoperative enteroscopy in the Peutz–Jeghers syndrome. Dis Colon Rectum 2003; 46:48–50.

66. Hearle N, Schumacher V, Menko FH et al. Frequency and spectrum of cancers in the Peutz–Jeghers syndrome. Clin Cancer Res. 2006; 12:3209–15.

67. Friedl W, Kruse R, Uhlhaas S et al. Frequent 4-bp deletion in exon 9 of the SMAD4/MADH4 gene in familial juvenile polyposis patients. Genes Chrom Cancer 1999; 25:403–6.

68. Howe JR, Mitros FA, Summers RW. The risk of gastrointestinal carcinoma in familial juvenile polyposis. Ann Surg Oncol 1998; 5:751–6.

69. Ilyas M, Straub J, Tomlinson IPM et al. Genetic pathways in colorectal and other cancers. Eur J Cancer 1999; 35:335–51.

70. Lamlum H, Al Tassan N, Jaeger E et al. Germline APC variants in patients with multiple colorectal adenomas, with evidence for the particular importance of E1317Q. Hum Molec Genet 2000; 9:2215–21.

71. Tomlinson I, Rahman N, Frayling I et al. Inherited susceptibility to colorectal adenomas and carcinomas: evidence for a new predisposition gene on 15q14–q22. Gastroenterology 1999; 116:789–95.

72. Yuan ZQ, Wong N, Foulkes WD et al. A missense mutation in both hMSH2 and APC in an Ashkenazi Jewish HNPCC kindred: implications for clinical screening. J Med Genet 1999; 36:793–4.

4

Colonic cancer

Robert J.C. Steele

Introduction

Colorectal cancer is a major health problem. In the UK, it is the second most common cause of cancer death, accounting for some 16 000 deaths in 2004. In 2002 there were approximately 35 000 new cases, of which about 13 000 were rectal and 22 000 colonic.[1] Although the overall numbers in men and women are similar, the incidence of rectal cancer is higher in men and that of colonic cancer is higher in women. The 5-year relative survival rate is currently in the region of 50% and has improved over the last 30 years from a figure of around 20% in 1971–75.[1]

Surprisingly, there is no precise definition of colonic cancer. Although the colon comprises the large bowel proximal to the rectum, the definition of the rectum is unclear. Anatomical texts describe the top of the rectum as the point where the sigmoid mesocolon ends or that part of the large bowel level with the third sacral vertebra.[2] Surgeons, on the other hand, prefer to think of the rectum as the segment of large bowel lying within the true pelvis. As far as rectal cancer is concerned, the UK definition is a tumour within 15 cm of the anal verge on rigid sigmoidoscopy,[3] whereas authorities from the USA have preferrred 11 or 12 cm.[4] Perhaps the simplest definition is the intraoperative identification of the fusion of the two antemesenteric taenia into an amorphous area where the true rectum begins.

These distinctions are important for two reasons. First, adjuvant radiotherapy is not appropriate for colonic tumours and, secondly, comparisons between outcomes for colorectal cancer surgery are impossible unless uniform definitions are adopted. This problem has yet to be addressed by international consensus.

Natural history

Within the colon, about 50% of cancers arise in the left side and 25% in the right (**Fig. 4.1**); in 4–5% of cases there are synchronous lesions. It is now widely accepted that the majority of colonic cancers arise from pre-existing adenomatous polyps, the supporting evidence being as follows:[5]

1. The prevalence of adenomas correlates well with that of carcinomas, the average age of adenoma patients being around 5 years younger than patients with carcinomas.
2. Adenomatous tissue often accompanies cancer, and it is unusual to find small cancers with no contiguous adenomatous tissue.
3. Sporadic adenomas are identical histologically to the adenomas of familial adenomatous polyposis (FAP), and this condition is unequivocally premalignant.
4. Large adenomas are more likely to display cellular atypia and genetic abnormalities than small lesions.
5. The distribution of adenomas throughout the colon is similar to that for carcinomas.
6. Adenomas are found in up to one-third of all surgical specimens resected for colorectal cancer.

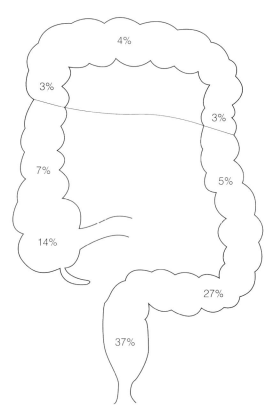

Figure 4.1 • Frequency of anatomical locations of colorectal cancer. Based on data from the Royal College of Surgeons audit in Trent Region and Wales.

7. The incidence of colorectal cancer has been shown to fall with a long-term screening programme involving colonoscopy and polypectomy.

 It should be recognised that, although the majority of adenomas diagnosed in the West are polypoid or exophytic, the flat adenoma, defined as an adenoma where the depth of the dysplastic tissue is no more than twice that of the mucosa, is now a recognised entity.[6] There is good evidence that these lesions are premalignant, and may indeed have a greater tendency towards malignant transformation than polypoid adenomas. They are difficult to find, but may account for up to 40% of all adenomas.[6] Reliable diagnosis requires a skilful, experienced colonoscopist and the use of dye sprayed on to the colonic mucosa to highlight the contours of the abnormal tissue.

When invasion has taken place, colonic cancer can spread directly and via the lymphatic, blood and transcoelomic routes.

Direct spread

Direct spread occurs longitudinally, transversely and radially, but as adequate proximal and distal clearance is technically feasible in the majority of colonic cancers, it is radial spread which is of most importance. In a retroperitoneal colonic cancer, radial spread may involve the ureter, duodenum and muscles of the posterior abdominal wall; the intraperitoneal tumour may involve small intestine, stomach, pelvic organs or the anterior abdominal wall.

Lymphatic spread

In general, the lymphatic spread of colonic cancer progresses from the paracolic nodes along the main colonic vessels to the nodes associated with either cephalad or caudal vessels, eventually reaching the para-aortic glands in advanced disease. This orderly process does not always occur, however, and in about 30% of cases nodal involvement can skip a tier of glands.[7] In contrast to rectal disease, it is rare for a colonic cancer which has not breached the muscle wall to exhibit lymph node metastases[7] (overall, about 15% of cases confined to the bowel wall will be found to have lymph node metastases).

Blood-borne spread

The most common site for blood-borne spread of colorectal cancer is the liver, presumably arriving by the portal venous system. Up to 37% of patients may have detectable liver metastases at the time of operation, and around 50% of patients may be expected to develop overt disease at some time. The lung is the next most common site, with around 10% of patients developing lung metastases at some stage; other reported sites include ovary, adrenal, bone, brain and kidney.

Transcoelomic spread

Colonic cancer may spread throughout the peritoneum, either via the subperitoneal lymphatics or by virtue of viable cells being shed from the serosal surface of a tumour, giving rise to malignant ascites, which is relatively rare.

Aetiology

Knowledge of molecular genetics in sporadic colorectal cancer has increased rapidly in recent years, but the stimuli which lead to these carcinogenic changes are still obscure. In this section, a brief consideration of the genetic basis of colorectal cancer is followed by discussion of aetiological factors.

Genetic factors

The genetic changes associated with colorectal cancer have been widely studied, and the molecular background to inherited colorectal cancer is dealt with in Chapter 3. However, the genetic events in sporadic colorectal cancer are also quite well understood. Mutations of the adenomatous polyposis coli (APC) gene, which is central to ordered cell motility, are thought to occur early as they are found in 60% of all adenomas and carcinomas.[8] K-ras mutations, which induce cell growth by activating growth factor signal transduction, similarly occur in both adenomas and carcinomas. However, as they are more common in large adenomas than in small adenomas they are thought to represent a later event.[9] Mutation of the p53 gene is common in invasive colonic cancers but rare in adenomas and is therefore deemed to be a late event which accompanies the development of invasion.[10] This is thought to be important as the p53 protein has roles in the repair of DNA and the induction of programmed cell death.[11]

The sequence of events described above is depicted in **Fig. 4.2**, but it must be stressed that this merely illustrates one possible multistep process; indeed, there is now good evidence that K-ras and p53 mutations very rarely occur in the same tumour, suggesting alternative pathways to carcinogenesis.[12] Many other genetic events have been observed in sporadic colorectal cancer, and no single event has been seen in all cancers. Thus the range of mutations, inactivations and deletions is wide, and it is likely that no single pattern will be applicable to every tumour. Nevertheless, knowledge of specific genetic events which take place in colorectal carcinogenesis may well have implications for diagnosis, prognosis and ultimately for gene therapy. For example, there is now evidence that K-ras mutations are not only associated with advanced stage at presentation, but also with poor prognosis in node-negative disease.[13]

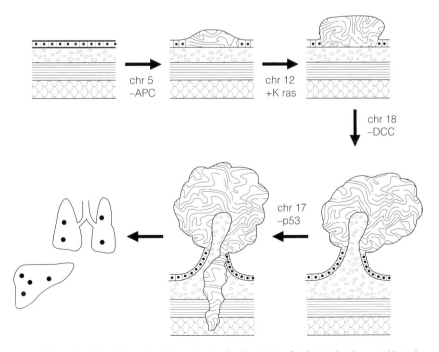

Figure 4.2 • A possible sequence of genetic changes in the development of colorectal polyps and invasive cancer.

Diet and lifestyle

 In 2007, the World Cancer Research Fund (WCRF) published its report on Food, Nutrition, Physical Acitivity and the Prevention of Cancer based on a systematic review of the world literature.[14] With respect to colon cancer, evidence for decreased risk was found for physical exercise, dietary fibre, calcium, garlic, non-starchy vegetables and pulses. Evidence for increased risk was uncovered for obesity, red meat, processed meat, alcohol, animal fat and sugar. It is clear that being overweight and underactive stand out as major risk factors, and governments worldwide have recognised this as an area for action. Smoking is also important and long-term smoking is associated with relative risks of between 1.5 and 3.0.[15]

Predisposing conditions

Long-standing inflammatory bowel disease, both ulcerative colitis and Crohn's disease, increases the risk of colorectal cancer, and this is discussed elsewhere. Previous gastric surgery has also been implicated, and although the association is controversial, the risk may be about twofold. Altered bile acid metabolism may play a role in this process, both after gastrectomy and after vagotomy. The risk after ureterosigmoidostomy is well established, although this operation has now been largely superseded by the use of an isolated ileal conduit for urinary diversion.

Presentation

Colon cancer can present as an emergency or with chronic symptoms which are well recognised. Right-sided cancer typically presents with anaemia, as the liquid nature of the faeces and the wider diameter of the colon make obstructive symptoms unusual. When the tumour is situated in the descending or sigmoid colon, change of bowel habit, colicky abdominal pain and blood in the stool are the commonest symptoms. Occasionally, the patient may notice the primary tumour as a mass and even more rarely a sigmoid cancer may cause pneumaturia and urinary infection by fistulation into the bladder, and a gastrocolic fistula may cause faecal vomiting or severe diarrhoea.

Unfortunately, many of the symptoms of colon cancer are common and non-specific, and there has been a good deal of recent work attempting to refine the indications for investigation. Guidelines have been developed to classify those at high risk warranting urgent investigation based on change in bowel habit, rectal bleeding in the absence of anal symptoms, palpable abdominal or rectal masses and anaemia (Box 4.1).[16] These guidelines are not particularly discriminatory, however, and weighted scoring systems may be more accurate.

Investigation

Currently, investigative techniques include barium enema, sigmoidoscopy, colonoscopy and computed tomography (CT) colography.

A barium enema usually demonstrates a colonic cancer as an irregular polypoid lesion or as an 'apple core' stricture with destruction of the mucosal

Box 4.1 • UK Department of Health criteria for high and low risk of colorectal cancer

Higher risk

- Rectal bleeding with a change in bowel habit to looser stools or increased frequency of defecation persisting for 6 weeks (all ages)
- Change in bowel habit as above without rectal bleeding and persisting for 6 weeks (>60 years)
- Persistent rectal bleeding without anal symptoms* (>60 years)
- Palpable right-sided abdominal mass (all ages)
- Palpable rectal mass (not pelvic) (all ages)
- Unexplained iron deficiency anaemia (all ages)

Low risk

Patients with no iron deficiency anaemia, no palpable rectal or abdominal mass

- Rectal bleeding with anal symptoms and no persistent change in bowel habit (all ages)
- Rectal bleeding with an obvious external cause, e.g. anal fissure (all ages)
- Change in bowel habit without rectal bleeding (<60 years)
- Transient changes in bowel habit, particularly to harder or decreased frequency of defecation (all ages)
- Abdominal pain as a single symptom without signs and symptoms of intestinal obstruction (all ages)

* Soreness, discomfort, itching, lumps, prolapse or pain.
Reproduced from Thompson MR, Heath I, Ellis BG et al. Identifying and managing patients at low risk of bowel cancer in general practice. Br Med J 2003; 327:263–5. With permission from BMJ Publishing Group Ltd.

pattern; benign polyps may also be seen as typical filling defects. It must be stressed, however, that false-positive and false-negative results may occur in up to 1% and 7% of cases respectively, with errors usually occurring in the sigmoid colon and caecum.[17]

Although rigid sigmoidoscopy may provide satisfactory rectal visualisation, it has been largely superseded by flexible sigmoidoscopy. This provides useful supplementary information, and neoplasia may be detected in the sigmoid colon in 25% of cases with 'normal' barium enemas, especially if there is coexisting diverticular disease. It may therefore be argued that colonoscopy should be the investigation of choice, but it carries a risk of perforation (much greater than barium enema), and even in good hands failure to achieve caecal intubation can be expected in 10% of cases. In addition, precise localisation of a tumour seen at colonoscopy is difficult as the only reliable landmarks are the anus and the terminal ileum.

Preoperative histological confirmation of a colonic cancer is ideal, but this can be achieved only by performing endoscopy in every case. If a barium enema demonstrates an unequivocal carcinoma, then biopsy may be deemed unnecessary, but where there is any reasonable doubt regarding the nature of a stricture or other lesion, then endoscopic visualisation and biopsy are mandatory.

 CT as a primary investigative modality is now coming to the fore with the development of CT colography or 'virtual colonoscopy', which is effective in detecting polypoid lesions down to 6 mm in diameter. This is fast becoming a standard investigation and is replacing the barium enema as the radiological investigation of choice.

When the diagnosis has been made, staging of the primary tumour, liver and lungs is now considered mandatory in the majority of cases. A fit patient with metastatic disease may be suitable for active treatment, whereas an elderly patient with a relatively asymptomatic primary and evidence of widespread dissemination may escape resection. Multislice CT of the chest and abdomen is now regarded as the staging modality of choice, supplanting chest X-ray and ultrasound.[18] Until recently, magnetic resonance imaging (MRI) scanning was considered to be less useful because of the long image acquisition time, but with ultrafast scanning MRI may become the investigation of choice for both distant and local disease.

Screening

Colon cancer is a suitable candidate for screening. Prognosis after treatment is much better in early stage disease and the polyp–carcinoma sequence (see above) offers an opportunity to prevent cancer by treating premalignant disease. The ideal screening test should detect the majority of tumours without a large number of false positives, i.e. it should have high sensitivity and specificity. In addition, it must be safe and acceptable to the population offered screening. In colorectal cancer, the most widely studied test is Haemoccult, a guaiac-based test which detects the peroxidase-like activity of haematin in faeces. Because this activity is diminished as haemoglobin travels through the gastrointestinal tract,[19] upper gastrointestinal bleeding is less likely to be detected than colonic bleeding. On the other hand, false-positive results may be produced by ingestion of animal haemoglobin or vegetables containing peroxidase, and because of the intermittent nature of bleeding from tumours, the sensitivity of Haemoccult is only about 50–70%.[20]

Screen-detected tumours are much more likely to be at an early stage than symptomatic disease, but this does not prove that screening is beneficial. Even improved survival in patients whose tumours are detected by screening is not conclusive because of the biases inherent in screening. These biases are threefold, and comprise selection bias, length bias and lead-time bias.

Selection bias arises from the tendency of people who accept screening to be particularly health conscious and therefore atypical of the population as a whole. Length bias indicates the tendency for screening to detect a disproportionate number of cancers which are slow growing, and which thereby have a good prognosis. Lead-time bias results from the time between the date of detection of a cancer by screening and the date when it would have been diagnosed had the subject not been screened. As survival is measured from the time of diagnosis, screening advances the date at which diagnosis is made, thus lengthening the survival time without necessarily altering the date of death.

Because of these biases, effectiveness can be assessed only by comparing disease-specific mortality in a population offered screening with that in an identical population not offered screening. This has to be done in the context of a well-designed randomised controlled trial, and for colorectal cancer three trials using faecal occult blood (FOB) have reported mortality data.[21–23] The first of these was carried out in Minnesota,[21] and showed a significant 33% reduction in colorectal cancer-specific mortality with annual FOB testing and a significant 21% reduction in a group offered biennial screening. In Nottingham, a trial of biennial FOB testing demonstrated a 15% reduction in cumulative mortality[22] and an almost identical study carried out in Funen, Denmark, showed an 18% reduction in mortality.[23]

There seems little doubt that FOB screening can reduce mortality from colorectal cancer, when applied to unselected populations, and the challenges for the future are to increase uptake and to improve the sensitivity and specificity of the screening test. Worldwide there is increasing interest in using faecal immunological testing (FIT) for blood, which appears to be more accurate than the indirect guaiac test.[24]

Another approach is to use endoscopy as a primary screening test. As 70% of cancers and large adenomas are found in the distal 60 cm of the large bowel, flexible sigmoidoscopy has been proposed as a screening test, and there is good evidence that it is more sensitive than FOB testing, Once-only flexible sigmoidoscopy has been investigated as a screening modality in a multicentre randomised study,[25] but the effect on mortality is not yet known. Sophisticated stool tests utilising polymerase chain reaction (PCR) to detect abnormal DNA and proteomic technology have yet to bear fruit.

Surveillance of high-risk groups

Individuals at high risk of colon cancer are not suitable for the population screening strategies described above, as the tests employed are not sufficiently sensitive. Surveillance strategies for patients with inflammatory bowel disease and for individuals with a family history of colon cancer are dealt with elsewhere. However, another important group is made up of those with adenomatous polyps and, particularly where screening is available, this group poses a significant challenge in terms of the use of colonoscopy resources. For this reason, guidelines have been developed that classify patients as being at low, intermediate or high risk for adenoma recurrence.[26] The low-risk category includes those with one or two adenomas less than 1 cm in diameter, and either no follow-up or a repeat colonoscopy at 5 years is recommended. For those at intermediate risk, defined as three to four adenomas or at least one adenoma greater than 1 cm in diameter, colonoscopy at 3 years is recommended. High-risk patients, those with five of more small adenomas or three or more where at least one is greater than 1 cm in diameter, should have another colonoscopy at 1 year. While the evidence upon which these guidelines is based is not very strong, they represent a very sensible approach, and one that has been adopted widely in the UK.

Elective surgery

Given that a patient is fit for surgery, and does not have advanced disseminated disease, resection of a colonic cancer is the only advisable primary treatment. There is also good evidence that adjuvant chemotherapy is of value in certain patient groups; this is dealt with elsewhere.

Preparation for surgery

 The first priority is to obtain informed consent, and the surgeon must be prepared to discuss the risks of death, complications such as anastomotic dehiscence, venous thromboembolism and wound infection, and disease recurrence. The patient must also be assessed for fitness for operation. This implies obtaining a full history and examination, full blood count, urea and electrolyte examination, and electrocardiogram (ECG) where indicated. In addition, investigations for disseminated disease should be performed as outlined above.

Blood transfusion

The patient must have blood taken for crossmatch, but the amount of blood requested will depend on the individual procedure. Group and save alone will be suitable for most right hemicolectomies, whereas for other types of colectomy and depending on the operating technique it is prudent to have at least two units of blood available.

There is still some debate as to the effects of blood transfusion on prognosis in colorectal cancer. Since the report by Burrows and Tartter[27] that blood transfusion may be associated with an increased likelihood of recurrence, there have been many reports, some making allowance for case mix, which have reached conflicting conclusions.

A randomised trial comparing the use of predeposited autologous and allogenic blood in patients undergoing resection for colorectal cancer has shown no difference in prognosis.[28] For this reason, observed effects of blood transfusion on recurrence must be treated with caution.

Bowel preparation

Immediately before surgery, many surgeons require the patient to undergo some form of mechanical bowel preparation.

A wide variety of washouts, enemas and purgatives have been used, and one of the most popular regimens uses Picolax®. This combines a senna compound (10 mg sodium picosulphate), which is activated by colonic bacteria and causes vigorous mass contraction, with magnesium citrate, which reduces water and sodium reabsorption, so that a large hyperosmolar fluid load reaches the caecum.

A popular alternative is polyethylene glycol salt solution, which can achieve preparation within 3 hours. It does, however, necessitate 4–5 L of oral intake, and many elderly patients find this difficult. Nasogastric whole-gut irrigation with an electrolyte solution obtains excellent results, but patients find it very unpleasant.

Whatever approach is taken, care must be taken not to attempt preoperative preparation in the presence of obstruction. If a patient experiences excessive pain or abdominal distension during preparation, it should be stopped. In such cases, the use of intraoperative preparation should be considered (see below).

It is by no means certain that bowel preparation is essential to prevent anastomotic leakage or its consequences. Most anastomotic leaks are caused by technical error (such as poor knotting/ suturing or too much tension) or biological failure (usually from ischaemia), neither of which will

be influenced by bowel preparation. The effects of an early leak (usually due to poor technique) would probably be obviated by bowel preparation, but most leaks occur late after the patient has recommenced oral feeding so that any value of preoperative bowel preparation will have been lost. For this reason there is an increasing tendency for surgeons to omit bowel preparation altogether and, indeed, the results of several randomised trials support this view.[29] It remains sensible to prepare the bowel if a proximal stoma is likely in order to prevent a column of stool feeding an anastomotic leak, should one occur.

Thromboembolism prophylaxis

Although there have been no studies confined to patients with colorectal cancer, a meta-analysis of appropriate randomised trials has shown that rates of deep vein thrombosis (DVT), pulmonary embolism and death from pulmonary embolism can all be significantly reduced by the use of subcutaneous heparin in general surgical patients.[30]

Offset against the advantages are the problems of increased bleeding, particularly when performing pelvic surgery, so that there still remains room for surgeons to choose. Low-molecular-weight heparin has received attention recently, and a large randomised trial of patients undergoing abdominal surgery has shown that it is less likely to cause bleeding-related complications than standard heparin.[31]

Other measures include graduated compression stockings, intravenous dextran and intermittent pneumatic calf compression. Stockings alone are less effective than other methods, and dextran is not as effective as heparin, but there is at least one trial indicating that intermittent compression is equivalent to heparin in reducing the incidence of DVT.

Antibiotic prophylaxis

All patients should receive antibiotic prophylaxis, as there is good evidence from several randomised trials that systemic antibiotics reduce the risk of sepsis after colorectal surgery.[32]

The choice of antibiotic and the route of administration are still open to debate, but in the UK the intravenous use of metronidazole for *Bacteroides fragilis* combined with broad-spectrum cover against gut anaerobes is favoured.

 A single dose of cephalosporin plus metronidazole is just as effective as a three-dose regimen in preventing wound infection.[33]

If there is significant contamination at the time of surgery, then prolonging antibiotic therapy for 3–5 days may be appropriate. Whatever regimen is used, it is important that the antibiotics are given immediately before the inoculation of bacteria into the wound, and the ideal timing is immediately after induction of anaesthesia.

Bladder catheterisation

This is usually done after the patient has been anaesthetised to monitor urine output per- and postoperatively. The urethral route is most commonly used, although there is evidence that suprapubic catheterisation may be preferable.[34]

Resection

Radical excision of a colonic tumour along with the appropriate vascular pedicle and accompanying lymphatic drainage is the most appropriate operation to obtain local control. Occasionally, a very limited resection may be appropriate in an unfit patient or one with widespread disease.

Classical resection removes the lymphatic drainage that lies along the named arterial blood supply, thereby rendering the associated colon ischaemic; thus right hemicolectomy removes the ileocolic and right colic arteries, transverse colectomy removes the middle colic artery and left hemicolectomy removes the left colic artery. However, transverse colectomy has fallen out of favour owing to a perception that anastomotic leakage is unacceptably high, and the distinction between left hemicolectomy and sigmoid colectomy is irrelevant if the principle of radical excision of the vascular pedicle is accepted. Thus, many surgeons would now hold that the decision as to type of operation lies between right hemicolectomy and left hemicolectomy, with the extent of bowel resection dependent on site of tumour.

A standard right hemicolectomy involves division of the ileocolic and right colic arteries at their origins from the superior mesenteric artery (**Fig. 4.3**). The marginal artery or the right branch of the middle

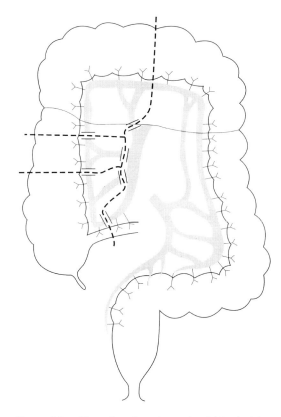

Figure 4.3 • Alternative sites of vascular division in right hemicolectomy.

colic artery will also need division to complete vascular isolation. For tumours of the descending colon and sigmoid colon, a formal left hemicolectomy involves division of the inferior mesenteric artery at its origin from the aorta (**Fig. 4.4**).

Splenic flexure carcinoma

The main controversy arises with tumours in the region of the splenic flexure, and here there are two options. One is to regard the tumour as left sided, and to carry out a left hemicolectomy, dividing the inferior mesenteric artery at its origin and dividing the left branch of the middle colic artery. A more conservative approach to this operation is to preserve the inferior mesenteric trunk, but this is essentially a segmental resection. The other approach is to carry out an extended right hemicolectomy, dividing the middle colic artery and the ascending branch of the left colic artery.

Expert opinion is divided as to which approach to take, but left hemicolectomy will necessitate anastomosis between right colon and rectum,

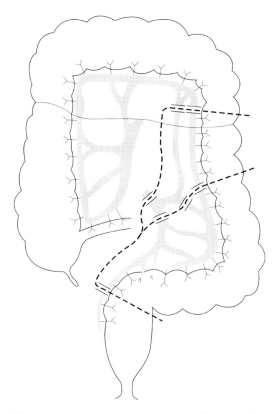

Figure 4.4 • Alternative sites of vascular division in left hemicolectomy.

which may be difficult to achieve without tension in some patients. Furthermore, the blood supply of the colon is inconstant. In 6% of cases there is no left colic artery and the blood supply of the splenic flexure is from the middle colic artery. In 22% of cases the middle colic artery is absent and the blood supply of the splenic flexure comes from both the left and right colic arteries. A cancer operation involves removing the tumour with its associated lymphatic drainage, and as the lymphatic drainage follows the arterial blood supply, it would seem sensible to ligate the right colic, middle colic and left colic arteries, making extended right hemicolectomy necessary.

For these reasons, I prefer extended right hemicolectomy, with an anastomosis between sigmoid colon and mobile well-vascularised ileum. It must be stressed, however, that the ideal operation will be dictated by individual anatomy, the most important criteria being lack of tension and good blood supply as evidenced by brisk bleeding and good colour at the cut bowel ends.

The Large Bowel Cancer Project found a high local recurrence rate and poor survival for patients with splenic flexure carcinoma, regardless of stage and presentation, which may reflect surgical inadequacy of primary treatment.[35]

Advanced tumours

When a tumour is locally advanced, it may still be possible to achieve a curative resection if the surgeon is prepared to resect adjacent involved organs, such as ureter, duodenum, stomach, spleen, small bowel, bladder and uterus (Rupert Turnbull at the Cleveland Clinic classified tumours that involved other organs as Dukes' D, for which he achieved a number of cures). In addition, about 5% of women will have macroscopic ovarian metastases and a further 2% will have microscopic disease. For this reason, a few surgeons carry out routine oophorectomy in all women with colorectal cancer.

In a patient with a truly inoperable tumour of the colon an ileocolonic bypass may be appropriate for lesions of the right side, whereas for tumours of the distal colon a defunctioning colostomy may be preferable. With multiple colonic tumours, a subtotal or total colectomy should be considered.

Operative technique

 The descriptions of operative technique given here refer to open surgery only, as the laparoscopic approach is dealt with elsewhere. For all colonic resections, it is my preference to have the patient in the legs apart position using a split-leg table, even if access to the anus or pelvis is not required, as this facilitates distribution of surgeon, scrub nurse and assistants around the table. The use of a multicomponent self-retaining retractor such as the 'Omnitract®' is also advised.

Right hemicolectomy

I prefer midline incisions for all colonic resections, as there is no muscle damage and access is gained to all parts of the abdomen and pelvis. For a right hemicolectomy it is useful to have two-thirds of the incision above the umbilicus to facilitate mobilisation of the hepatic flexure.

With the surgeon standing on the patient's right, the right colon is retracted towards the midline by the assistant, and the peritoneum in the right paracolic gutter is divided. This extends from the caecal pole to the hepatic flexure, and cephalad to this point the lesser sac is entered and the greater omentum divided below the gastroepiploic arcade up to the point of intended division of the transverse colon. The right colon is then retracted firmly towards the midline, and the plane between the colonic mesentery and the posterior abdominal wall is carefully developed with diathermy, taking care not to damage the duodenum. As this is done, the ureter and gonadal vessels will fall away safely. This is done until the superior mesenteric vessels are clearly identified so that the right colic and ileocolic vessels can be ligated and divided very close to their origins. The bowel wall is then cleared at the sites of transection and single crushing clamps are applied. Soft clamps may be applied on proximal small bowel and distal large bowel, and the bowel is divided on the crushing clamps, leaving them on the specimen.

Left hemicolectomy

A long midline incision is employed, extending from above the umbilicus to the symphysis pubis. The operator stands on the patient's left side, and the assistant retracts the sigmoid colon medially. The peritoneum lateral to the sigmoid and descending colon is divided close to the 'white line' of fusion using diathermy. It should then be possible to see the plane between the mesentery and the retroperitoneal structures, which can be further developed using a combination of firm medial traction of the bowel by the assistant and countertraction applied by the operator on the retroperitoneum using a swab or forceps.

This manoeuvre will ensure that ureter and gonadal vessels are swept away. Care must be taken to identify the hypogastric nerves, and these should be separated from the mesentery or they may be damaged as the upper rectum is prepared for anastomosis. The splenic flexure should then be mobilised, and this is best done by dissecting the greater omentum off the transverse colon and continuing laterally towards the flexure. If the tumour is in the region of the splenic flexure, however, it is advisable to divide the gastrocolic ligament and take the omentum with the specimen. In either event, the spleen is at risk from tears caused by traction on its peritoneal attachments and, despite extreme care, splenectomy is sometimes necessary. For minor tears, however, application of a haemostatic agent such as oxycellulose is sufficient.

Once the left colon has been mobilised, the origin of the inferior mesenteric artery is identified by

dividing the peritoneum over the aorta close to the fourth part of the duodenum, ligated and divided. To obtain full mobility it is then necessary to divide the inferior mesenteric vein just below the inferior border of the pancreas. The colon is then divided as described for right hemicolectomy at a convenient point in the transverse colon and at the rectosigmoid junction.

Anastomosis

For anastomosis after resection of a colonic cancer, I prefer to use hand suturing, although it is appreciated that stapling may produce excellent results.

Appositional serosubmucosal anastomosis

This method, initially described by Matheson et al.,[36] utilises a single layer of interrupted 3/0 braided polyamide. For mobile anastomoses (usually ileocolic) the first step is to ensure that the ends to be anastomosed are roughly equal in circumference. This is usually achieved by making an incision on the antemesenteric aspect of the small bowel, although some surgeons prefer to use an end-to-side technique. One side of the anastomosis is performed on the serosal aspect of the bowel between the mesenteric and antemesenteric borders, placing the sutures 4 mm apart and 4 mm deep, ensuring that the muscle layer and the submucosa but not the mucosa have been included (**Fig. 4.5**). The sutures are left untied until they have all been inserted (**Fig. 4.6**), and each knot is then tied by hand to ensure a snug but non-constrictive result. The half-completed anastomosis is then turned over and the process repeated. Mesenteric defects are not closed.

For colorectal or ileorectal anastomoses, the posterior row of sutures is inserted first, holding each suture with a specially designed suture clamp or individual artery forceps. If artery forceps are used, they should be threaded on to a forceps holder to avoid tangling. Again, the sutures are tied by hand after insertion of the whole row, the knots being tied on the luminal side of the anastomosis after the proximal bowel has been 'parachuted' down the sutures to the upper rectum (**Fig. 4.7**). The knot tails

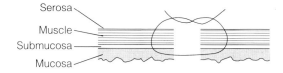

Figure 4.5 • Placement of the appositional serosubmucosal suture.

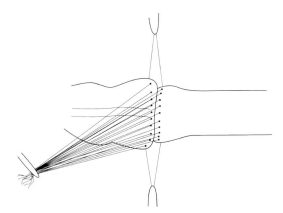

Figure 4.6 • Ileocolic anastomosis. The sutures are left untied until they have all been inserted.

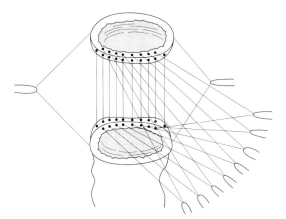

Figure 4.7 • Colorectal anastomosis. The sutures are held in individual forceps and the colon slid down to the rectum before tying.

are then cut so that they are covered by the cut edges of the undisturbed mucosal layers. On completion of the posterior aspect of the anastomosis, the anterior part is performed in a similar fashion, but with the knots tied on the extraluminal side. This type of anastomosis is greatly facilitated by the use of curved 'Heaney' needle holders, with the needle mounted facing out from the convex side of the tip.

Stapled anastomoses

After right hemicolectomy the most widely employed stapled anastomosis is the 'functional end-to-end'. Here, the ends of the colon and ileum are stapled closed at the time of specimen excision, and two small enterotomies are made to permit insertion of the limbs of a linear cutting stapler. The anastomosis is then performed by firing the stapler, taking care not to include mesentery (**Fig. 4.8**), and after

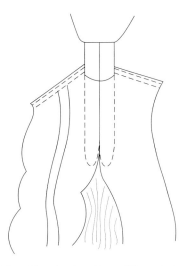

Figure 4.8 • 'Functional end-to-end' ileocolonic stapled anastomosis.

checking the staple line for bleeding the remaining defect is closed with a linear stapler. After left hemicolectomy, a true end-to-end anastomosis can be performed using a circular anastomosing stapler introduced per anum (**Fig. 4.9**), but in some male patients the intact rectum can be difficult to negotiate.

Results of anastomotic techniques

The interrupted serosubmucosal technique is recommended for its adaptability to any anastomosis involving the colon, but it is also associated with the best results in the literature, with leak rates of 0.5–3% in sizeable series.[37,38]

 Stapling has been compared with hand suturing in several randomised trials and, although the results vary, there seems to be no consistent difference in colonic anastomotic dehiscence between the two approaches. In one trial there was evidence that tumour recurrence was less in the stapled group, but no distinction between rectal and colonic resections was made.[39]

Drains

 After the anastomosis is complete, many surgeons will leave a drain in the peritoneal cavity either to minimise the consequences of an anastomotic leak or to prevent the accumulation of fluid which might be infected. There is no evidence to support this practice, however, and three randomised trials have shown there to be no advantage associated with drainage of colonic or colorectal anastomoses.[40–42]

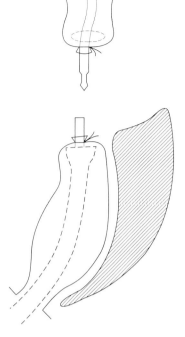

Figure 4.9 • End-to-end colorectal anastomosis using a circular stapling device.

Postoperative care/complications

After colectomy, postoperative care is similar to that of any patient undergoing major abdominal surgery, and there is now increasing interest in 'fast-track' or enhanced recovery. This involves a multimodal approach to postoperative recovery that is based on early feeding, early mobilisation, i.v. fluid and sodium restriction, and avoidance of both drains and nasogastric intubation; initial epidural analgesia with avoidance of parenteral opiates may also be employed. A median hospital stay (including readmissions) after open colonic surgery of 3 days can be achieved if this policy is pursued, but it involves considerable commitment, not only from the patient, but also from anaesthetic staff, nursing staff and community healthcare.[43]

Anastomotic dehiscence

Although patients undergoing colectomy may suffer any of the complications associated with major abdominal surgery, anastomotic breakdown is the major source of morbidity specific to this type of operation. Subclinical leaks occur more frequently than clinically obvious leaks, but after resection of a colonic tumour the overall significant leak rate should currently be no more than 4%.[18]

A leak may present in a variety of ways, and the onset of symptoms may be quite insidious. Warning signs are pyrexia, increasing pulse rate and abdominal distension due to paralytic ileus, as well as unexplained cardiorespiratory disturbance. The patient may then go on to develop localised or generalised peritonitis, or a faecal fistula, usually through the wound. Occasionally a patient will develop sudden generalised peritonitis and septicaemic shock as a result of rapid faecal contamination of the peritoneal cavity.

Because of the heterogeneous nature of the symptoms, a leak should be suspected in any patient with an anastomosis who is not progressing as well as expected. Investigations which may prove useful in a doubtful case include a full blood count, abdominal and chest radiographs, and a water-soluble contrast enema (increasingly CT is employed). The white cell count is usually raised, although not inevitably. Plain radiographs will frequently demonstrate distended loops of bowel and gas may be seen under the diaphragm, although both of these may be seen after any laparotomy in the absence of a leak. The most useful investigation is a water-soluble contrast enema (often now CT), and in the patient with clinical signs consistent with a leak, extravasation of contrast at the anastomosis secures the diagnosis.

The treatment of an anastomotic dehiscence depends on the specific mode of presentation. The patient with general peritonitis requires laparotomy after appropriate resuscitation. With a major disruption, the anastomosis should be taken down and the two ends exteriorised if possible; primary repair of the anastomotic dehiscence should not be attempted. After dealing with the anastomosis, careful peritoneal toilet must be performed using copious quantities of warm saline with or without antibiotic, and the patient will require at least 5 days of intravenous antibiotic therapy.

In the patient with localised peritonitis who remains otherwise well, a conservative approach with systemic antibiotics may be appropriate, but laparotomy should not be delayed if there is any deterioration. A faecal fistula can also be treated in this way, but care must be taken with the surrounding skin, and nutritional support may be required if drainage is prolonged.

Emergency management

In the UK, about 20% of patients with colonic cancer will present as an emergency and 16% will present with obstruction. Bleeding and perforation are less common modes of emergency presentation; when perforation occurs, it is often in the caecum as a result of distal obstruction in the face of a competent ileocaecal valve. Obstruction is thus the most likely reason for emergency or urgent operation.

Investigation

The patient with obstruction will usually present with colicky abdominal pain and abdominal distension, with a variable degree of vomiting and change of bowel habit. Paradoxically, the obstructed patient may complain of diarrhoea rather than constipation, owing to overflow. The first specific investigation in this case will be a plain abdominal radiograph, which will demonstrate the typical features of large or, in the case of an obstructing caecal cancer, small bowel obstruction.

Particular attention should be paid to the size of the caecum on the radiograph, and whether or not gas is present in small bowel loops. If the caecum is 12 cm or more in diameter and there is no evidence of decompression into the small bowel, then there is significant risk of caecal perforation and urgent intervention is required. The same applies when the caecum is tender to palpation.

Before committing the patient to laparotomy, however, it is important to identify the site of obstruction, as colonic pseudo-obstruction can mimic the clinical and radiological signs of mechanical obstruction. Increasingly, the water-soluble contrast enema is being replaced by an abdominal CT with contrast. Barium should not be used as it can become inspissated in the segment of colon distal to the obstruction, and if there is a perforation barium can enter the peritoneal cavity with disastrous consequences.

Management of obstruction

Once mechanical obstruction is diagnosed and the patient resuscitated, laparotomy should proceed with experienced surgical and anaesthetic staff in attendance, preferably during daylight hours. The first task

at laparotomy is usually to decompress the gaseous distension of the large bowel, and this can be achieved by inserting a 19-gauge (white) needle attached to suction into the lumen through a convenient taenia. If a larger tube is required to evacuate large amounts of liquid faeces, this should be inserted into the caecum via an enterotomy in the terminal ileum.

When the bowel can be safely handled, a decision must be made as to the type of operation required. If the obstruction is due to a right-sided lesion, it is usually easy and safe to carry out a standard right hemicolectomy. If, however, the cancer is on the left side, several options are available.

Traditionally, obstructing left-sided cancers were treated by a three-stage approach, starting with a defunctioning loop colostomy, followed by resection and anastomosis, and then by closure of the defunctioning stoma. This gradually gave way to a two-stage procedure, with primary resection of the tumour in the form of a Hartmann operation, where the proximal colon is brought out as an end colostomy and the distal segment either closed off or brought out as a mucous fistula.[44]

Recently, however, there has been a move towards one-stage procedures, and here the choice lies between a subtotal colectomy with ileocolic or ileorectal anastomosis and a left hemicolectomy after on-table colonic irrigation.[45] For tumours in the region of the splenic flexure, the former approach is often sensible, especially if there is doubt about the viability of the caecum.

There is also an argument for subtotal colectomy for tumours in the more distal colon, but a randomised trial comparing both strategies found that patients treated by left hemicolectomy had more acceptable postoperative bowel function.[46]

If a decision is made to perform a left hemicolectomy, then many surgeons will wish to irrigate the colon proximal to the site of obstruction using the technique described by Dudley et al.[47] This is illustrated in **Fig. 4.10**, and although anaesthetic scavenging tubing inserted proximal to the tumour and a large Foley catheter inserted into the caecum by means of an enterotomy in the appendix or the terminal ileum were originally described, a number of dedicated devices are now available.

Clearly the choice of operation will depend on individual circumstances, and few surgeons would

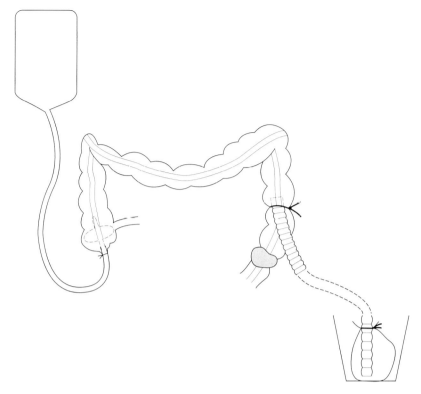

Figure 4.10 • On-table colonic irrigation.

attempt an anastomosis in the presence of severe intra-abdominal sepsis or in a severely ill patient. In these cases, a Hartmann resection is acceptable, and in some situations a defunctioning stoma may be the best option. Increasingly, expanding metal stents are being used in obstructing left-sided colonic tumours. Although most experience has been palliative in intent, more lesions are now being treated in this way to allow decompression followed by bowel preparation and elective resection of the tumour.[48]

Management of perforation

In the patient who is found to have a perforated caecum as a result of an obstructing distal cancer, an extended right hemicolectomy or subtotal colectomy is the treatment of choice. Whether or not an anastomosis is fashioned will depend on the degree of peritoneal contamination. For the cancer which has perforated primarily, it is important to resect the lesion itself to eliminate not only the malignancy but also the source of sepsis. This

can be technically demanding, and for left-sided lesions will almost always necessitate a Hartmann procedure.

Management of advanced disease

The surgical management of the advanced primary tumour is covered in the section on elective surgery. In colonic cancer, local recurrence usually occurs at the suture line and, in the absence of disseminated disease, re-resection should be attempted, although palliative bypass may be all that can be achieved. The patient with distant metastases poses different challenges.

Operable metastases

Hepatic resection for colorectal cancer metastases is now widely practised, but there is still debate as to its value. It has never been tested by a randomised trial, and all comparative studies have used retrospective data from historical controls.[49]

With careful patient selection, hepatectomy for colorectal metastases can be associated with a 5-year survival of around 33%,[49] and although the most widely accepted criterion for resection is one to three resectable metastases in one lobe of the liver, many surgeons are now extending their indications.

The role of preoperative chemotherapy in these patients is currently unclear, and the reults of a phase III multicentre international trial are awaited. There is, however, some non-randomised evidence that preoperative treatment with 5-fluorouracil plus folinic acid (FUFA) and oxaliplatin may improve both resectability and long-term survival.

In a proportion of patients with liver disease that is not amenable to resection, in situ ablation using cryotherapy or radiofrequency energy may be employed.[50] This may prolong survival, but as yet must be regarded as palliative.

Pulmonary metastases may also be amenable to resection, but as only 10% of patients develop such metastases and only 10% of these have disease confined to the lung, very few patients will be suitable. Nonetheless, segmental resection of the lung may be associated with 5-year survival rates of 20–40%.[51]

Inoperable disseminated disease

In the patient with widespread disease, chemotherapy containing 5-fluorouracil (5-FU) is the only established therapeutic option, but this can only be regarded as palliative. Few studies have compared chemotherapy with supportive treatment only, and the survival benefits, although significant, are not great. Based on a recent meta-analysis, patients with ECOG scores of 2, 1 and 0 treated with this type of chemotherapy have median survival times or 4, 10 and 14 months respectively.[52]

Recently, the oral 5-FU prodrugs UFT and capecitabine have come into use, and as they have been found to offer equivalent survival with the advantage of increased ease of delivery they are now regarded as suitable single agents for first-line use. Even more recently, combination chemotherapy with intravenous 5-FU and either irinotecan or oxaliplatin has been demonstrated to enhance survival as both first- and second-line therapy. Both of these strategies have been approved in the UK by the National Institute for Clinical Excellence (NICE).[54]

Looking to the future, monclonal antibody treatment either in the form of bevacizumab (an antibody against vascular endothelial growth factor)[55] or cetuximab (an antibody against epidermal growth factor receptor)[56] has been shown to confer survival advantages in combination with conventional chemotherapy. These agents are awaiting NICE approval.

Pathological staging

Accurate, detailed and consistent pathology reporting for colorectal cancer is important for estimating prognosis and planning further treatment in terms of adjuvant therapy (see Chapter 6). Both macroscopic and histological appearances must be described in some detail, and the following information should be available.

Microscopic description

1. Size of the tumour (greatest dimension).
2. Site of the tumour in relation to the resection margins.
3. Any abnormalities of the background bowel.

Microscopic description

1. Histological type.
2. Differentiation of the tumour, based on the predominant grade within the tumour.[57]
3. Maximum extent of invasion into/through the bowel wall (submucosa, muscularis propria, extramural).
4. Serosal involvement by tumour, if present.[58]
5. A statement on the completeness of excision at the cut ends (including the 'doughnuts' from stapling devices) and at any radial margin.
6. The number of lymph nodes examined, the number containing metastases, and whether or not the apical node is involved.
7. Extramural vascular invasion if present.[59]
8. Pathological staging of the tumour according to Dukes' classification.[60,61]

Dukes' staging is simple, reproducible and widely recognised, but TNM staging is becoming increasingly recognised as the international standard; the two systems are described in Table 4.1. Some pathologists use the Jass classification,[62] although its usefulness may be limited by observer variation in the degree of lymphocytic infiltration at the advancing margin of the tumour (one of the four parameters that contribute to the classification) and the fact that its prognostic value appears to be confined to rectal tumours.

After curative resection, cancer registry data indicate that age-adjusted 5-year survival for Dukes' stage A colonic cancer is 85%, for stage B 67% and for stage C 37%. These results can be improved on as evidenced by individual series,[64] and the 'Will Rogers' effect (stage migration owing to variable quality of pathology reporting) may play a role in this respect.

Recommendations for best practice

The recommendations given here represent a summary of the evidence-based guidelines from the Association of Coloproctology and the Scottish Intercollegiate Guidelines Network for the management of colorectal cancer as they apply to colonic tumours.[18,64]

Investigation

1. Patients with suspicious symptoms or a proven colorectal cancer should be investigated with either endoscopic visualisation of the whole rectum plus a high-quality double-contrast barium enema or a total colonoscopy or CT colography.

Table 4.1 • Clinicopathological staging of colorectal cancer

Dukes' staging* (based on histological examination of the resection specimen)	
A	Invasive carcinoma not breaching the muscularis propria
B	Invasive carcinoma breaching the muscularis propria, but not involving regional lymph nodes
C1	Invasive carcinoma involving the regional lymph nodes (apical node negative)
C2	Invasive carcinoma involving the regional lymph nodes (apical node positive)
TNM staging†	
T	Primary tumour
TX	Primary tumour cannot be assessed
T0	No evidence of primary tumour
Tis	Carcinoma in situ
T1	Tumour invades submucosa
T2	Tumour invades muscularis propria
T3	Tumour invades through muscularis propria into subserosa or into non-peritonealised pericolic or perirectal tissues
T4	Tumour perforates the visceral peritoneum or directly invades other organs or structures‡
N	Regional lymph nodes
NX	Regional lymph nodes cannot be assessed
N0	No regional lymph node metastasis
N1	Metastasis in 1–3 pericolic or perirectal lymph nodes
N2	Metastasis in 4 or more pericolic or perirectal lymph nodes
N3	Metastasis in any lymph node along the course of a named vascular trunk
M	Distant metastasis
M0	No distant metastases
M1	Distant metastases

* Dukes' stage D has come to mean the presence of distant metastases.
† UT, ultrasound depth; yT, following neoadjuvant therapy.
‡ Direct invasion in T4 includes invasion of other segments of the colorectum by way of the serosa, e.g. invasion of the sigmoid colon by a carcinoma of the caecum.

2. Unless it cannot alter management, all patients should have screening (preoperative where possible) for lung and liver metastases by means of CT scanning.

Preparation for surgery

1. All patients undergoing surgery for colon cancer should give informed consent. This implies being given information about the likely benefits and risks of the proposed treatment and details of any alternatives.
2. Mechanical bowel preparation before surgery is no longer recommended (except where an upstream stoma is planned – rare with colonic tumours and more applicable to total mesorectal excision surgery).
3. Subcutaneous heparin or intermittent compression should be employed as thromboembolism prophylaxis in surgery for colorectal cancer unless there is a specific contraindication.
4. All patients undergoing surgery for colorectal cancer should have antibiotic prophylaxis. It is impossible to be dogmatic as regards the precise regimen, but a single dose of appropriate intravenous antibiotics appears to be effective.

Elective surgical treatment

1. Any tumour with a distal margin at 15 cm or less from the anal verge using a rigid sigmoidoscope should be classified as rectal.
2. Although no definite recommendations can be made regarding anastomotic technique, the interrupted serosubmucosal method is adaptable to all colonic anastomoses and has the lowest reported leak rate in the literature.
3. Laparoscopic surgery for colorectal cancer should be performed only by experienced laparoscopic surgeons who have been properly trained in colorectal surgery, and who are prepared to audit their results very carefully.

Emergency treatment

1. Emergency surgery should be carried out during daytime hours as far as possible by experienced surgeons and anaesthetists.
2. In patients presenting with obstruction, steps should be taken to exclude pseudo-obstruction before operation.

3. Stoma formation should be carried out in the patient's interests only, and not as a result of lack of experienced surgical staff or appropraite stenting facilities.
4. The overall mortality for emergency/urgent surgery should be 20% or less.

Treatment of advanced disease

1. It is recommended that effective palliation with optimal quality of remaining life should be the main aim of therapy in advanced disease.
2. Consideration should be given to palliative chemotherapy in patients with local advanced and metastatic disease. Thus, patients with advanced disease who remain in good general condition should have the opportunity to discuss the possible benefits of palliative therapy with an oncologist.
3. Consideration should also be given to surgical treatment in selected patients with locally advanced and metastatic disease. In particular, the patient with limited hepatic involvement should be considered for partial hepatectomy by an experienced liver surgeon.

Outcomes

Surgeons should carefully audit the outcome of their colorectal cancer surgery.

1. They should expect to achieve an operative mortality of less than 20% for emergency surgery and 5% for elective surgery for colorectal cancer.
2. Wound infection rates after surgery for colorectal cancer should be less than 10%.
3. Surgeons should expect to achieve an overall leak rate below 4% for colonic resection.
4. Surgeons should examine carefully their practice with a view to meeting or improving on targets set by national long-term mortality statistics.

Pathology

All resected colorectal tumours should be submitted for histological examination. For this to be useful, the report should reach an acceptable standard, providing information which will be useful in assessing prognosis, planning treatment and carrying out audit.

References

1. Cancer Research UK Statistics on Colorectal Cancer; http://www.cancerresearchuk.org/aboutcancer/statistics/statstables/colorectalcancer.

2. Williams PL, Warwick R. Gray's anatomy. Edinburgh: Churchill Livingstone, 1980, p. 1356.

3. UKCCCR. Handbook for the clinicopathological assessment and staging of colorectal cancer. UKCCCR, 1989.

4. Bass BL, Enker WE, Lightdale CJ. Advances in colorectal carcinoma surgery. New York: World Medical Press, 1993, p. 37.

5. Leslie A, Carey FA, Pratt NR et al. The colorectal adenoma–carcinoma sequence. Br J Surg 2002; 89:845–60.

6. Rembacken BJ, Fujii T, Cairns A et al. Flat and depressed colonic neoplasms: a prospective study of 1000 colonoscopies in the UK. Lancet 2000; 355:1211–4.

7. Jinnai D. In: Goligher JC (ed.) Surgery of the anus, rectum and colon, 4th edn. London: Baillière Tindall, 1982, p. 447.

8. Powell SM, Zilz N, Beazer-Barclay Y et al. APC mutations occur early during colorectal tumorigenesis. Nature 1992; 359:235–7.

9. Scott N, Bell SM, Sagar P et al. p53 expression and K-ras mutation in colorectal adenomas. Gut 1993; 34:621–4.

10. Kikuchi-Yanoshita R, Konishi M, Ito S et al. Genetic changes of both p53 alleles associated with the conversion from colorectal adenoma to early carcinoma in familial adenomatous polyposis and non-familial adenomatous polyposis patients. Cancer Res 1992; 52:3965–71.

11. Kastan MB, Onyekwere O, Sidransky D et al. Participation of p53 protein in the cellular response to DNA damage. Cancer Res 1991; 51:6304–11.

12. Smith G, Carey FA, Beattie J et al. Mutations in APC, Kirsten-ras, and p53 – alternative genetic pathways to colorectal cancer. Proc Natl Acad Sci USA 2002; 99:9433–8.

13. Conlin A, Smith G, Carey FA et al. The prognostic significance of K-ras, p53, and APC mutations in colorectal cancer. Gut 2005; 54:1283–6.

14. World Cancer Research Fund. Food, nutrition, physical activity and the prevention of cancer; a global perspective. Washington, DC: AICR, 2007.

15. Giovannucci E. An updated review of the epidemiological evidence that cigarette smoking increases risk of colorectal cancer. Cancer Epidemiol Biomarkers Prev 2001; 10:725–31.

16. Thompson MR, Heath I, Ellis BG et al. Identifying and managing patients at low risk of bowel cancer in general practice. Br Med J 2003; 327:263–5.

17. Anderson N, Cook HB, Coates R. Colonoscopically detected colorectal cancer missed on barium enema. Gastrointest Radiol 1991; 16:123–7.

18. Association of Coloproctology of Great Britain and Ireland. Guidelines for the management of colorectal cancer, 3rd edn. Association of Coloproctology of Great Britain and Ireland, 2007.

19. Burton RM, Landreth KS, Barrows GH et al. Appearance, properties and origin of altered human haemoglobin in faeces. Lab Invest 1976; 35:111–5.

20. Bennett DH, Hardcastle JD. Early diagnosis and screening. In: Williams NS (ed.) Colorectal cancer

(Clinical Surgery International, Vol. 20). Edinburgh: Churchill Livingstone, 1996; pp. 21–37.

21. Mandel JS, Church TR, Ederer F et al. Colorectal cancer mortality: effectiveness of biennial screening for fecal occult blood. J Natl Cancer Inst 1999; 91:434–7.

22. Hardcastle JD, Robinson MHE, Moss SM et al. Randomised controlled trial of faecal occult blood screening for colorectal cancer. Lancet 1996; 348:1472–7.

23. Kronborg O, Fenger C, Olsen J et al. A randomized study of screening for colorectal cancer with fecal occult blood test at Funen in Denmark. Lancet 1996; 348:1467–71.

    These three randomised trials (Refs 21–23) provide evidence that disease-specific mortality can be reduced by faecal-occult blood screening for colorectal cancer, and form the basis for current debates regarding the introduction of national screening programmes in several countries.

24. Allison JE, Sakoda LC, Levin TR et al. Screening for colorectal neoplasms with new fecal occult blood tests: update on performance characteristics. J Natl Cancer Inst 2007; 99:1462–70.

25. UK Flexible Sigmoidoscopy Screening Trial Investigators. Single flexible sigmoidoscopy screening to prevent colorectal cancer: baseline findings of a UK multicentre randomised trial. Lancet 2002; 359:1291–300.

26. Atkin WS, Saunders BP. Surveillance guidelines after removal of colorectal adenomatous polyps. Gut 2002; 51(Suppl v):v6–vv979.

27. Burrows L, Tartter P. Effect of blood transfusions on colonic malignancy recurrence rate. Lancet 1982; ii:662.

28. Busch ORC, Hop WCJ, Hoynck van Papendrecht MAW et al. Blood transfusions and prognosis in colorectal cancer. N Engl J Med 1993; 328:1372–6.

29. Guanega K, Attallah AN, Castro AA et al. Mechanical bowel preparation for elective colorectal surgery. The Cochrane Database of Systematic Reviews 2006; issue 2. John Wiley and Sons Ltd.

30. Collins R, Scrimgeour A, Yusuf S et al. Reduction in fatal pulmonary embolism and venous thrombosis by perioperative administration of subcutaneous heparin. N Engl J Med 1988; 318:1162–73.

    This important meta-analysis established the use of low-dose subcutaneous heparin as a prophylactic measure in abdominal surgery.

31. Kakkar VV, Cohen AT, Edmonson RA et al. Low molecular weight versus standard heparin for prevention of venous thromboembolism after major abdominal surgery. Lancet 1993; 341:259–65.

32. Keighley MRB, Williams NS. Perioperative care. In: Keighley MRB, Williams NS (eds) Surgery of the anus, rectum and colon, 3rd edn. Elsevier Saunders, 2008.

33. Rowe-Jones DC, Peel ALG, Kingston RD et al. Single dose cefotaxime plus metronidazole versus three dose cefotaxime plus metronidazole as prophylaxis against wound infection in colorectal surgery: multicentre prospective randomised study. Br Med J 1990; 300:18–22.

    As a result of several trials, the place of prophylactic antibiotics in colorectal surgery is now firmly established, and a single dose is as effective as multiple doses

34. O'Kelly TJ, Mathew A, Ross S et al. Optimum method for urinary drainage in major abdominal surgery: a prospective randomised trial of suprapubic versus urethral catheterisation. Br J Surg 1995; 82:1367–8.

35. Aldridge MC, Phillips RKS, Hittinger R et al. Influence of tumour site on presentation, management and subsequent outcome in large bowel cancer. Br J Surg 1986; 73:663–70.

36. Matheson NA, McIntosh CA, Krukowski ZH. Continuing experience with single layer appositional anastomosis in the large bowel. Br J Surg 1985; 72:S104–6.

    These results have yet to be bettered, and form a persuasive argument for the use of the serosubmucosal anastomotic technique.

37. Carty NJ, Keating J, Campbell J et al. Prospective audit of an extramucosal technique for intestinal anastomosis. Br J Surg 1991; 78:1439–41.

38. Leslie A, Steele RJC. The interrupted serosubmucosal anastomosis – still the gold standard. Colorectal Dis 2003; 5:362–6.

39. Docherty JG, McGregor JR, Akyol AM et al. Comparison of manually constructed and stapled anastomoses in colorectal surgery. Ann Surg 1995; 221:176–84.

40. Hoffmann J, Shoukouh-Amiri MH, Damm P et al. A prospective, controlled study of prophylactic drainage after colonic anastomoses. Dis Colon Rectum 1987; 30:449–52.

41. Johnson CD, Lamont PM, Orr N et al. Is a drain necessary after colonic anastomosis? J R Soc Med 1989; 82:661–4.

42. Sagar PM, Couse N, Kerin M et al. Randomised trial of drainage of colorectal anastomosis. Br J Surg 1993; 80:769–71.

43. Wind J, Polle SW, Fung Kon Jin PH et al. Systematic review of enhanced recovery programmes in colonic surgery. Br J Surg 2006; 93:800–9.

44. Rothenberger DA, Mayoral J, Deen K. Obstruction and perforation. In: Williams NS (ed.) Colorectal cancer (Clinical Surgery International, Vol. 20). Edinburgh: Churchill Livingstone, 1996; pp. 123–33.

45. Koruth NM, Krukowski ZH, Youngson GG et al. Intra-operative colonic irrigation in the management of left-sided large bowel emergencies. Br J Surg 1985; 72:708–11.

46. SCOTIA Study Group. Single-state treatment for malignant left-sided colonic obstruction: a prospective randomised trial comparing subtotal colectomy with segmental resection following intraoperative irrigation. Br J Surg 1996; 82:1622–7.

    One of the few randomised trials of surgical technique in emergency colonic surgery, this study indicates that segmental resection of obstructed colon cancer provides better long-term results than subtotal colectomy.

47. Dudley HAF, Radcliffe AG, McGeehan D. Intraoperative irrigation of the colon to permit primary anastomosis. Br J Surg 1980; 67:80.

48. Watson AJ, Shanmugam V, Mackay I et al. Outcomes after placements of colorectal stents. Colorectal Dis 2005; 7:70–3.

49. Garden OJ, Rees M, Poston GJ et al. Guidelines for resection of colorectal liver metastases. Gut 2006; 55(Suppl III):iii1–8.

50. Seifert JK, Junginger T, Morris DL. A collective review of the world literature on hepatic cryotherapy. J R Coll Surg Edinb 1998; 43:141–54.

51. Shirouzu K, Isomoto H, Hayashi A et al. Surgical treatment for patients with pulmonary metastases after resection of primary colorectal carcinoma. Cancer 1995; 76:393–8.

52. Thirion P, Wolmark N, Haddad E et al. Impact of chemotherapy in patients with colorectal metastases confined to the liver: a re-analysis of 1,458 non-operable patients randomised in 22 trials and 4 meta-analyses. Proc Am Soc Clin Oncol 1999; 10:1317–20.

53. Grothley A, Sarjent D. Overall survival of patients with advanced colorectal cancer correlates with availability of fluorouracil, irinotecan and oxaliplatin regardless of whether doublet or singlet agent therapy is used first line. J Clin Oncol 2005; 23:9441–2.

54. National Institute for Clinical Excellence (NICE) Guidance on Cancer Services. Improving outcomes in colorectal cancer. Manual update. NICE, 2004.

55. Hurwitz H, Fechrenbacher L, Novotny W et al. Bevacizumab plus irinotecan, florouracil and leucovorin for metastatic colorectal cancer. N Engl J Med 2004; 350:2335–42.

56. Cunningham D, Humblet Y, Siena S et al. Cetuximab monotherapy and cetuximab plus irinotecan in irinotecan refractory metastatic colorectal cancer. N Engl J Med 2004; 351:337–45.

57. Halvorsen TB, Seim E. Degree of differentiation in colorectal adenocarcinomas: a multivariate analysis of the influence on survival. J Clin Pathol 1988; 41:532–7.

58. Shepherd NA, Baxter KJ, Love SB. Influence of local peritoneal involvement on pelvic recurrence and prognosis in rectal cancer. J Clin Pathol 1995; 48:849–55.

59. Talbot IC, Ritchie S, Leighton M et al. Invasion of veins by carcinoma of the rectum: method of detection, histological features and significance. Histopathology 1981; 5:141–63.

60. Dukes CE, Bussey HJR. The spread of rectal cancer and its effect on prognosis. Br J Cancer 1958; 12:309–20.

61. UICC TNM classification of malignant tumours, 5th edn. Wiley-Liss, 1997.

62. Jass JR, Love SB, Northover JMA. A new prognostic classification of rectal cancer. Lancet 1987; i:1303–6.

63. Hawley PR. In: Goligher JC (ed.) Surgery of the anus, rectum and colon, 4th edn. London: Baillière Tindall, 1984; p. 549.

64. Scottish Intercollegiate Guidelines Network. Guidelines for the management of colorectal cancer. SIGN, 2003.

5

Rectal cancer

Robin K.S. Phillips

Introduction

From a surgeon's perspective, the rectum begins where the two antemesenteric taenia on the sigmoid colon fuse together. This is roughly at the level of the sacral promontory, 15 cm from the anus.

Rectal cancer at presentation is either truly local (or locoregional) or has spread elsewhere, usually to the liver. Preoperative scanning and intraoperative palpation may not always demonstrate small occult metastases within the liver substance but, if present, they will be responsible for death over the next 5 years.[1]

Role of pathology

Histopathological examination of the resected specimen simply allows an estimate of any occult hepatic metastases already present in the liver at the time of apparently curative resection, the chance increasing with depth of primary tumour penetration, grade and lymph node status.

The depth of primary tumour penetration can be gauged very accurately by endoanal ultrasound,[2] but intra- and interobserver variation[3] and variation within the tumour[4] make estimation of grade inexact. Thus a preoperative biopsy may reveal a rectal cancer that is not obviously poorly differentiated and yet examination of the subsequently resected whole specimen may show unsuspected areas of poor differentiation within the tumour.

It is not possible to combine the information on depth of primary tumour penetration and on grade and thereby make the information on lymph node status redundant. This is important, as depth and grade (subject to the caveat raised above) can be assessed preoperatively much more accurately than lymph node status. Nevertheless, lymph node status remains central to all rectal cancer staging systems (TNM,[5] Dukes,[6] Jass[7]).

Objectives of rectal cancer surgery

A tumour that is truly local will be cured by adequate locoregional therapy; inadequate locoregional therapy will lead to local recurrence. A tumour that has already spread widely to the liver will be incurable by surgical means alone. It does not matter whether abdominoperineal excision of the rectum is performed, or indeed an anterior resection, the occult hepatic metastases will still kill the patient. Similarly, in the presence of many occult hepatic metastases, it does not matter whether preoperative or postoperative radiotherapy is used, or no radiotherapy, the patient will still die.

From time to time it is stated that preoperative radiotherapy can 'downstage' the primary tumour, but one must be very careful in interpreting this downstaging. The original histology provides an estimate of the likelihood of occult hepatic metastases already present in the liver at the time of resection; the application of radiotherapy makes no difference to this original estimate, even if it makes the primary tumour smaller (or makes it go away completely) and lymph nodes disappear. Thus one must be very cautious about estimating likely outcome based on the histopathological examination of a resected pre-irradiated rectal cancer. This is because there is no useful yardstick by which to measure the likelihood of occult hepatic metastases based on the pathology of irradiated rectal cancer specimens.

From the above discussion, it can be seen that longer-term survival is in many ways outside the control of the rectal cancer surgeon, being dependent on the presence or absence of occult hepatic metastases at the time of presentation. However, the surgeon can control (i) death in hospital, (ii) local recurrence and (iii) quality of life.

Death in hospital

Death in hospital involves patient factors, tumour factors and surgeon-related factors. Clearly, in an elderly patient with an obstructing tumour the risks of death are much higher than in a younger patient undergoing elective surgery. Elective surgery under the age of 80 years has an overall in-hospital mortality of 8% compared with a 16% mortality in those over the age of 80. An elderly patient over the age of 80 years with malignant large bowel obstruction has a 1 in 3 chance of in-hospital mortality.[8] Similarly, the in-hospital mortality in the presence of an anastomotic leak is much higher than when there has been no leak.[9]

There is thus enormous scope for a skilled surgeon to make a very great difference to in-hospital outcome in patients with rectal cancer. Anastomotic leak rate is a surgeon-related variable. The organisation of a dedicated daytime operating list for the treatment of urgent cases by a senior team has now largely been achieved. From time to time the decision to adopt a local approach, for example local excision, transanal endoscopic microsurgery (TEM) or even local radiotherapy, will be influenced by knowledge of the likely cost benefit of the alternative (local excision of a tumour confined to the rectal wall has an approximately 15% chance of leaving involved lymph nodes behind compared with an approximate 16% mortality for radical surgery in those aged over 80).

Local recurrence

Local recurrence arises for one of the following reasons:

1. The primary tumour was disrupted in some way at the time of the original operation.
2. Local excision was inadequate.
3. Viable exfoliated cells have implanted into the wound/tumour bed/port site/anastomosis.

Tumour disruption

Clearly, cutting into a primary tumour while mobilising it will run a very high risk of spilling viable cancer cells. The occasions when this may happen in rectal cancer surgery include the following:

1. When an adherent loop of intestine is thought to be stuck onto the tumour by 'inflammatory' adhesions. The loop should be resected en bloc with the primary tumour rather than pinched off.[10]
2. Through fragmentation of the envelope of the mesorectum. Heald has done more than anyone else to popularise the importance of maintaining the integrity of the mesorectal envelope.[11] It has been claimed that rough traction, blunt dissection and less-than-total mesorectal excision contribute to disruption of the mesorectal envelope, which on removal will look ragged and shredded. Precise surgery using sharp or diathermy dissection under vision will avoid this problem.
3. Injudicious exploration of the anterior plane in a man with an anterior encroaching tumour.

Anterior encroaching tumour in the male

Rectal cancer rarely penetrates through Denonvillier's fascia to involve the seminal vesicles, prostate or base of bladder. However, all surgeons have experience of cases where this has proved to be the case. The problem does not really arise in women, as the vagina acts as a barrier to involvement of the bladder, and surgeons are used to performing en-bloc hysterectomy when the uterus/back of the vagina is involved.

 Specialised imaging using magnetic resonance (MRI) has transformed the preoperative evaluation of rectal cancer in the UK.

In the best hands,[12,13] exquisite images can be obtained that clearly show the mesorectal envelope and which allow assessment of the circumferential resection margin (**Fig. 5.1**). Whereas endoanal ultrasound permits local evaluation of depth and may help predict cases suited to local excision, MRI examines the margin and helps the clinician choose those most likely to benefit from preoperative chemoirradiation or those males with anterior encroachment sufficient to warrant primary exenteration. In the past, surgeons largely encountered the problem of anterior encroachment unexpectedly during the operation. Given surgeons' natural reluctance to embark unnecessarily on synchronous en-bloc removal of the bladder with construction of an ileal conduit, the fairly modest results of such extensive surgery[14] and the lack of confidence of many surgeons in their own skills in this area, the natural response was to remain in the normal anterior dissection plane, hoping that the tumour and the seminal vesicles could be shaved off the back of the prostate/bladder.

This situation should no longer arise if a standard preoperative work-up (Box 5.1) for all cases of rectal cancer includes first-class MRI. For the now hopefully rare occasion when a surgeon is confronted by such a conundrum, it would be wise to pause and take stock. Would it be better to back out, give a long course of chemoradiotherapy and then return at a later date, when hopefully tumour shrinkage

Box 5.1 • Standard preoperative work-up for rectal cancer

- Full blood count, electrolytes, liver function tests
- Serum carcinoembryonic antigen (optional)
- Group and save serum
- Colonoscopy
- Rectal cancer protocol MRI
- Transrectal ultrasound (if considering local therapy)
- Chest and abdominal computed tomography (CT) scan
- Preoperative discussion at multidisciplinary team meeting

may allow an uninvolved plane to be found? (In these circumstances, a wait of 3 months would be advised; see below.) Is the patient young enough and fit enough to be considered for pelvic exenteration? Such an operation should be preceded in all cases by chemoradiotherapy and performed by a joint colorectal surgical and urological surgical team.

Inadequate local excision

How radical does the pelvic clearance need to be in a standard case of rectal cancer? The issues to be addressed here are total mesorectal excision, extended pelvic lymphadenectomy[15,16] and high vs. low vascular ligation (with or without a pre-aortic strip).[17,18] In addition, the role of local excision needs to be considered.

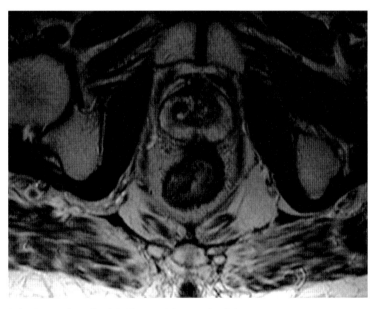

Figure 5.1 • An anterior tumour invading into the prostate can clearly be seen.

Total mesorectal excision

The history of gastric cancer surgery included a vigorous debate on whether total excision of the stomach should always be done or whether it should be undertaken only when it was essential. The debate was summarised as total *gastrectomie de principale* vs. total *gastrectomie de necessitaire*. The debate on total mesorectal excision is identical in its content, the two views being (i) total mesorectal excision should be used but only in certain circumstances and (ii) total mesorectal excision should always be used in all cases of rectal cancer. Few surgeons would now doubt the advisability of performing total mesorectal excision when operating on a case of low or mid-rectal cancer. The debate is focused on upper rectal cancer.

First, there is a lack of clear cancer-related evidence when dealing with upper rectal cancer. Heald et al. have shown that in some cases satellite deposits of cancer, not always in lymph nodes, may be present in the mesorectum distal to the lower palpable margin of the tumour.[19] Does this apply to cases of cancer of the upper rectum? How often? And how far below the lower palpable border of the tumour can some of these deposits be found? The answers to these questions are not very clear from reading the literature. One recent study suggests that extension in the mesorectum may be as much as 3 cm below the distal margin of the tumour,[20] whereas Heald et al. described them extending as far as 4 cm below.[19] Extrapolating from these figures, it would seem reasonable in oncological terms to perform a mesorectal clearance 5 cm below the tumour, which in an upper rectal cancer would not always involve total mesorectal excision.

It might be argued that the good results of total mesorectal excision make these questions redundant but, in practice, function in the absence of a small colonic pouch (see below) or a short rectal remnant is inferior when total mesorectal excision is performed, and complications are high, making a temporary stoma advisable in all cases.

Thus, given this background, there are many surgeons who, when confronted with an upper rectal cancer, would perform a less-than-total mesorectal excision. Nevertheless, they would all perform quite an extensive distal clearance of mesentery, of the order of at least 5 cm, thereby making their anastomosis effectively somewhere in the region of the junction of the mid and lower thirds of the rectum.

Extended pelvic lymphadenectomy

There seems little doubt, at least in the Japanese literature, that lymph nodes are involved in cases of rectal cancer along the internal iliac vessels. These involved lymph nodes lie outside the boundaries of a conventional total mesorectal excision and should, on the face of it, be responsible for local recurrence in cases where they have not been removed.

As an example, one Japanese paper has shown these lymph nodes to be involved in 18% of cases overall and in 36% of Dukes' C cases. In addition, in 6% of cases lateral pelvic side-wall lymph nodes were the only lymph nodes involved. That is to say, if an extended pelvic side-wall lymphadenectomy had not been performed, these cases would have been considered Dukes' A or B.[16] Based on this evidence, the biological rate of local recurrence for total mesorectal excision should be around 18%, not the 3–5% claimed by its protagonists. What are the possible explanations for these discrepancies?

First, the Japanese literature does not make it clear whether the majority of these involved lymph nodes are along the main trunk of the internal iliac vessels (where they would indeed be left behind by total mesorectal excision) or whether they are in fact in the vicinity of the lateral ligaments, where conceivably they would be removed as part of a total mesorectal excision anyway.

Second, post-mortem studies have clearly identified instances of local recurrence in terminal cases not identified in life as they caused no clinical problem. Thus a patient dying with disseminated disease may have undetected recurrence in the pelvic side-wall lymph nodes: the clinical rate of local recurrence will inevitably be quite a lot smaller than the biological rate. Perhaps where the tumour burden is excessive and the patient is doomed anyway, pelvic side-wall lymph nodes may be involved, but their removal in these circumstances will add nothing to the patient's cancer-related outcome.

Third, there is the charge of selection. Perhaps the cases operated upon by those with a low local recurrence rate are not representative of those seen by the rest of us. My own view is to reject this as anything but a most marginal explanation. There is growing evidence that surgeons who have adopted total mesorectal excision have significantly reduced their local recurrence rates, and independent review of Heald's cases does not support selection as a reasonable explanation for his very good results.[11]

Extended pelvic lymphadenectomy is unlikely to become popular in the West, largely because of the poor functional result and because of the perceived success of total mesorectal excision. Half the cases reported in one series had the operation performed unnecessarily, as they did not have any lymph nodes involved at all. Operating times were lengthy, averaging 5.5 hours, and blood loss was excessive (average 1.5 L). All patients had sexual and urinary disturbance, 10% needing a permanent urinary catheter.[16]

Nerve-sparing operations are being developed that combine the potential advantages of an extended lymph node dissection with less collateral nerve damage.[21] Nevertheless, the excellent results of total mesorectal excision make it unlikely that they will ever become popular. Indeed, a recent Swedish study found that only 2 of 33 pelvic recurrences after total mesorectal excision surgery might be attributed to lateral pelvic side-wall lymph node involvement.[22]

High vs. low vascular ligation

The inferior mesenteric artery can be divided either flush on the aorta (high ligation) or at the level of the sacral promontory, in effect preserving the left colic artery (low ligation). There have been quite a number of studies that have compared these two approaches in terms of cancer survival and have found no benefit to high ligation.[17]

About 20% of cases with apical lymph node involvement will be cured. Presumably, had they had a ligation that left the involved apical lymph node behind, they would all have died. A possible explanation for a lack of benefit in studies of high ligation is that the operation was not simultaneously extended in a lateral direction, i.e. lateral pelvic side-wall lymphadenectomy was not also performed at the same time. Presumably, cases with extensive lymph node involvement in one plane will also have extensive lymph node involvement in another, so leaving one set of lymph nodes untreated while solely concentrating on the treatment of the other is unlikely to show benefit.

When performing an anastomosis to the anus it has generally been the view that the descending colon should be used in preference to the sigmoid colon. Not only does the sigmoid colon generate fairly high pressures, which could therefore lead to relatively poor function, but more importantly the marginal artery is absent in the sigmoid colon, which is thus prone to ischaemia if it is used for anastomosis. However, the descending colon will not reach the anus unless the splenic flexure is mobilised in all cases, and there is a flush tie of the inferior mesenteric artery on the aorta. This is because the left colic artery is too short and will not permit the descending colon to reach the anus if a low ligation that preserves the left colic artery is performed. Hence a low anastomosis will always need a high ligation, but for technical rather than cancer-specific reasons. A high anastomosis can be achieved quite easily with either a high or a low ligation.

An international randomised controlled trial comparing colonic pouches with straight coloanal anastomoses employed the sigmoid colon in 42% of cases and these showed no functional or complication disadvantage.[23] It would seem that the earlier favouring of descending colon for anastomosis can now be tempered by issues of practicality: where the splenic flexure is easy to mobilise, then it would still seem appropriate to do so and use descending colon; but with a high and difficult splenic flexure, sigmoid colon might be the best choice, avoiding a difficult mobilisation.

Blood supply at the splenic flexure

There is one other point of importance when preparing the left colon for anastomosis, and that is to do with the precariousness of the marginal artery blood supply in the region of the splenic flexure (Griffiths' point).[24] Between the terminal two branches of the left colic artery the marginal artery can be quite thin (**Fig. 5.2**). It is important when mobilising the blood supply at the splenic flexure to preserve these two branches to act as a support for the marginal artery at this point.

Role of local excision

A tumour confined to the bowel wall has an approximately 15–20% chance of lymph node involvement,[25] whereas a tumour penetrating through the full thickness of the bowel wall has an approximately 40% chance. In addition, a well-differentiated tumour has about a 25% chance of having lymph node involvement, whereas a poorly differentiated tumour has a greater than 50% chance. Thus a well-differentiated tumour, confined to the bowel wall, would have a reasonably low prospect of lymph node involvement.

An analysis of 151 malignant polyps showed that pedunculated polyps had no risk of lymph node

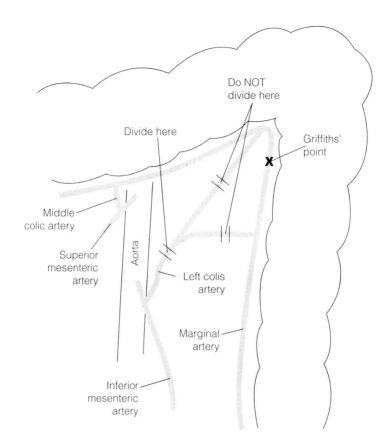

Figure 5.2 • When mobilising the vascular supply to the splenic flexure, it is important not to divide the two terminal branches of the left colic artery, but rather to leave them supporting the marginal artery at the splenic flexure, where it can be deficient, and instead divide the main trunk of the left colic artery as indicated. Frequently, the inferior mesenteric vein also needs to be divided again at the inferior border of the pancreas to gain further length.

involvement when the degree of spread was limited to the head, neck or stalk of the polyp, but was 27% when invasion reached the base of the polyp (however, numbers were small, 3 of 11 having lymph node involvement). Patients with sessile polyps had a 10% chance of lymph node invasion.[21]

A small (say <3 cm in diameter) low rectal cancer, which on biopsy was well differentiated, would be a potential candidate for local excision, whether by TEM or by a conventional transanal approach. As mentioned earlier, the preoperative biopsy may not be truly representative of the histology of the whole tumour once it has been excised, but this has to be accepted.

Assessment of depth of primary tumour penetration with the examining finger is notoriously unreliable. Rectal endosonography is extremely accurate[2] but not all surgeons have ready access to the technique. The alternative is simply to treat the excised specimen as a large biopsy and allow the patholo-

gist to report on the depth of primary tumour penetration and the completeness of excision, as well as commenting finally on the tumour grade. Using this approach, the surgeon can then decide, based on the full histology report, either to continue with a policy of local excision or to advise the patient that further, more radical surgery is advisable.

The updated results of local excision from St Mark's Hospital have been reported. Of 152 patients with tumours confined to the bowel wall, 11% died of cancer.[26] Against this background, it would be hard to advise a young and fit patient to have local excision. However, in the elderly and less fit there does still seem to be a place for this technique. Furthermore, local excision does not require a pelvic dissection, with all its attendant risks to erection, ejaculation and bladder function. Bowel function is also significantly better afterwards than with a straight coloanal anastomosis. For these reasons there will still be some younger patients who, while adequately informed, may nevertheless prefer to avoid conventional surgery and opt for local excision, however performed. This issue has recently been addressed using decision analysis, paying particular attention to comparison between abdominoperineal excision and local excision.[27] As expert colorectal surgeons are more likely than general surgeons to have a choice between sphincter-preserving local excision and sphincter-preserving radical surgery, the conclusion in favour of local excision for early low rectal cancer may not be so applicable to them.

Local excision as practised in the UK has not usually been followed by the application of postoperative radiotherapy, unlike in France[28] and the USA,[29] or sometimes chemoradiotherapy.[30] This is because surgeons have been concerned that any metastases in lymph nodes are unlikely to be eradicated by radiotherapy and because function in an irradiated rectum may become suboptimal, thereby obviating one of the specific advantages of a local approach. Finally, detection of recurrence in an irradiated pelvis may be more difficult than in the absence of postoperative radiotherapy, making the potential for salvage in the presence of recurrence less likely. Nevertheless, although radiotherapy in general will certainly make function worse,[31] it does reduce failure. Its role may apply particularly to the higher risk surgical patient.[32]

Implantation of viable tumour cells

The role of implantation remains controversial. On the one hand, there is clear experimental evidence that colorectal cancer cells are shed into the lumen of the bowel, that they are viable and that they represent clones of cells capable of transplanting.[33] On the other hand, most North American surgeons ignore the risk when operating conventionally, and all surgeons ignore the risk (in fact, they cannot avoid it) when performing any form of transanal local excision, whether conventionally or by TEM.

Not only are viable colorectal cancer cells present in the lumen of the bowel, where presumably they may give rise to anastomotic recurrence if left untreated, but they are also able to cross an otherwise watertight anastomosis, where they potentially might result in the much more common locoregional recurrence.[34] In the test tube, colorectal cancer cells are effectively killed by povidone iodine, mercuric

perchloride and chlorhexidine/cetrimide. Other agents such as water are not effective.[35] However, blood makes povidone iodine and chlorhexidine/cetrimide much less efficient at killing colorectal cancer cells.[36]

Most British surgeons would strongly recommend steps to prevent implantation. The use of tapes both proximally and distally is no longer advised, but a right-angled clamp should be placed across the bowel just distal to the tumour and the bowel then washed out below the clamp. This means that unprotected cross-stapling below a low rectal cancer is considered inadvisable in the UK. Instead, a right-angled clamp should be introduced first and cross-stapling should be done beyond the clamp, after a cytocidal washout.

However, there are circumstances where it is simply not possible to place a right-angled clamp distal to a rectal cancer and then to manage to place a cross-stapling instrument below that. What should the surgeon then do? There are also some circumstances where a tongue of tumour extends down towards the dentate line, when transanal division of the bowel and internal sphincter at this level would permit an otherwise impossible restorative operation to be done (**Fig. 5.3**), but only if a clamp is not used below the tumour.

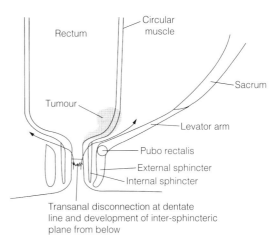

Transanal disconnection at dentate line and development of inter-sphincteric plane from below

Figure 5.3 • A fairly small, well-differentiated tumour close to the anus may have a superficial extension into the upper anal canal. Transanal full-thickness division of the anus and underlying internal sphincter at the level of the dentate line permits entry to the intersphincteric space and may assist completion of an ultra-low attempt at restorative surgery. However, in these circumstances it is impossible both to gain the necessary anal access and to use a right-angled clamp below the tumour with a cytocidal washout below that.

Some surgeons would argue that a restorative operation should not be attempted in these circumstances, and argue in favour of abdominoperineal excision. Others would argue that, in the first example, a right-angled clamp should be applied and the anus washed out below the clamp, before the gut tube is then divided either from above or from below and an endoanal coloanal anastomosis constructed.

However, there are occasions when a restorative operation is technically possible but the application of a distal clamp and washout below this clamp would not be possible. In these circumstances, I (and others[37,38]) think it reasonable to continue with a restorative operation, although cytocidal agents should be instilled after specimen removal and before anastomosis. Thus the use of a distal clamp with washout below it is in my view relative and not absolute. In support of the relative rather than absolute nature of this choice is the very obvious advantage of a restorative operation as against a permanent stoma, the fact that there are many surgeons, particularly in the USA, who think the risk of implantation metastases has been exaggerated, and the fact that British surgeons, who have vehemently argued in favour of protecting the anastomotic line from exposure to viable tumour cells, have still been prepared in certain circumstances to entertain local excision, where all these potential risks apply.

Quality of life

In rectal cancer surgery quality of life issues include preservation of continence, preservation of reasonable bowel frequency and avoidance, as far as possible, of permanent sexual and urinary disturbance.

Preservation of continence

The reasons for abdominoperineal excision include the following:

1. Cancer involves the sphincter or is so near to it that attempts to preserve it are unjustified.
2. The functional result of restorative surgery is likely to be so poor that a colostomy would be an advantage.
3. The potential complications of attempts to restore intestinal continuity are not worth risking, particularly in the frail and elderly.

Distal clearance margin

It is not always clear from an examination of the literature what is meant by the distal margin. A distance of 5 cm at rigid sigmoidoscopy in the living may expand to 8 cm after rectal mobilisation, then shrink to 3 cm after specimen removal, simply because of contraction of the longitudinal muscle. If an attempt is then made to pin out the specimen, a margin of 4.5 cm may be achieved after fixation, but without pinning out the final margin may measure only 2 cm.[39]

Against this background, it is very uncommon for rectal cancer to spread more than 1.5 cm below the distal palpable margin of the tumour, and then only when the tumour is poorly differentiated, when distances as far as 4.5 cm have rarely been reported.[40] Of course, the preoperative biopsy may not accurately represent the final tumour histology, but given this caveat it is usually advised that a 5-cm distal clearance margin should still be considered for a poorly differentiated tumour, whereas a 2-cm margin should suffice otherwise.

In practice, the distal margin is now largely irrelevant for most rectal cancer, as the amount of bowel removed is determined more by a policy of performing total mesorectal excision than it is by considering the distal clearance margin. Nevertheless, the issue does apply when considering cancer in the lower third of the rectum, where it has been argued that, given a tumour that is not poorly differentiated, being able to apply a right-angled clamp below the lower margin of the tumour is clearance enough.[41]

From time to time, the histology report will describe the tumour abutting the distal margin (i.e. being within 1 cm or less of the margin) but not involving it. Studies of resected specimens have shown that so long as the margin itself is uninvolved then the risk of recurrence is not increased,[42] provided that adequate lateral clearance has been achieved. There is a tendency for the inexperienced surgeon to cone in on the distal clearance margin, thereby leaving some of the mesorectum behind on the pelvic side walls. This practice is considered likely to increase the chance of local recurrence and should therefore be avoided.

Tumour height

It has been commonplace to advise measuring the height of the lower border of the tumour from the anal verge. I have always been puzzled by this advice, as the anal verge is often a variable point, for example being much further from the dentate line (in my view the critical point) in patients with a funnel anus.

In fact the dentate line can be felt with the examining finger. The mucosa above is more slippery to the examining finger than is the skin of the pecten (just as the mucosa of the inside of the mouth is more slippery than the skin of the lip). This difference in slipperiness can be appreciated with the examining finger, which allows a much more meaningful relationship of the lower border of the tumour to be assessed.

What actually matters in the critical case is not the measured height of the lower border of the tumour to the dentate line, but rather whether in the case in question there is a sufficient margin either for a clamp to be placed below the tumour and above the dentate line or for the dentate line to be divided transanally (see Fig. 5.3) without going too close to any palpably indurated tongue of tumour projecting downwards towards the dentate line. Added to this is a general assessment of the bulk of the tumour, the accessibility of the pelvis, the quality of the anus and the potential for improving tumour characteristics by the application of preoperative radiotherapy.

Quality of the anus

A woman with a prior history of multiple vaginal deliveries, particularly if there has been a forceps delivery or a complication of episiotomy, has a fairly high chance of an occult sphincter injury, detectable by anal ultrasonography. In practice, one is usually guided to the quality of a good anus by a history of flatus continence and an absence of episodes of faecal incontinence in the past. In more recent times the tumour itself may have contributed to a sense of urgency and thereby may lead to unreasonable pessimism as to the true state of the anus.

Nevertheless, a patient with an undoubtedly poor-quality anus will not be well served by an ultra-low anastomosis and would be very much better off with a colostomy. When the tumour itself is reasonably high in the rectum, then a low Hartmann operation will avoid the complications of a perineal wound, but with a lower tumour an abdominoperineal excision would seem safest.

Abdominoperineal excision of the rectum

Even in the best hands abdominoperineal excision gives worse results than perhaps it should. Surgeons familiar with deep pelvic dissection and total mesorectal excision are now far less familiar with the bottom end of an abdominoperineal excision, particularly in the male. The scope for technical error is high as there is no clear anatomical plane from below, except anteriorly, where it is difficult. When performing total mesorectal excision the rectosacral fascia should be divided in order to dissect the rectum anteriorly, thereby exposing the anal canal, whereas this may compromise the lateral clearance margin when performing abdominoperineal excision. Pathologists report 'coning' or 'waisting' of the specimen at the level of the levators.

To some extent this is to be expected, as any cut voluntary muscle will contract and naturally give some impression of 'coning', but it is probable that surgeons are not excising the pelvic floor widely enough. Unless tumour is in the distal anal canal, when there will be a threat of inguinal lymphatic spread, wide excision of ischiorectal fat is probably unnecessary, although it is important to excise widely at the level of the pelvic floor, particularly as this is the point where any cancer is likely to be situated (if it were not, then total mesorectal excision would likely be feasible). It is possible that the more modern tendency of not routinely excising the coccyx at the time of abdominoperineal excision for cancer lessens the muscle clearance and should be reconsidered.

 Performing the perineal part of the operation in the prone position is increasingly favoured.[43]

The risk of local recurrence can be addressed by applying preoperative radiation therapy in all cases of abdominoperineal excision, regardless of stage, but this approach is associated with very high rates of perineal wound infection and breakdown, so judgement can be difficult.

The colonic pouch

Straight coloanal anastomosis results in fairly poor function, certainly for a number of months and on occasion for a year or two. In a study of 84 cases treated at St Mark's Hospital by proctectomy with endoanal coloanal anastomosis, 8% went on to have a permanent colostomy constructed.[44]

A colonic pouch does not have the same objective as an ileal pouch. The consistency of the stool is different, the harder stool being much more difficult to expel than the semiliquid content of an ileal pouch. Early colonic pouches tended to copy ileal pouches in having a large capacity, but all the early authors had patients who had difficulty evacuating.[45,46] As experience has been gained, so the size of colonic pouches has fallen, now being recommended to be around 5–8 cm in length.[47]

There have been a number of reports that have confirmed that early function with a colonic pouch is superior to a straight coloanal anastomosis.[45–48] This is particularly important in elderly patients, in those with a slightly compromised anus and in those with a relatively short life expectancy.

The more difficult group to evaluate is the young. This is because the results of a straight coloanal anastomosis improve quite markedly with time, and nobody knows to what extent colonic pouches will dilate and decompensate over time. We do not know whether good function in the first few years might be followed by increasing problems with evacuation later as colonic pouches become floppy and dilated.

One argument in favour of the routine use of a colonic pouch is the possible lower anastomotic leak rate from side-to-end rather than end-to-end anastomosis in these circumstances.[23] Should this suggestion be borne out, it will prove a strong argument in favour of the routine use of a small colonic pouch in all cases after total mesorectal excision. The study in question found a clinical anastomotic leak in 15% of patients having a straight coloanal anastomosis and in only 2% with a pouch ($P = 0.03$). However, radiotherapy had been used more frequently (27% vs. 16%) and a covering stoma less frequently (59% vs. 71%). As radiotherapy may be damaging to anastomotic healing, and as a stoma protects against the clinical manifestations of an anastomotic leak, the question of safer anastomoses when a colonic pouch is constructed remains undecided.

An alternative is to use a coloplasty instead of a colon pouch. An 8–10 cm incision is made, which is 4–6 cm proximal to the divided end of the colon, vertically along the antemesenteric border of the colon. The incision is then closed transversely,[49] forming the pouch. End-to-end coloanal anastomosis is then performed.

Sexual and urinary disturbance

The presacral nerves give rise to ejaculation in the male. They lie like a wishbone, joined at the sacral promontory and parting as they run distally on either pelvic side wall. They can be identified at the start of the posterior dissection and preserved in most cases.

Erection in the male is innervated through the nervi erigentes. These nerves lie anterolaterally in the angle between the seminal vesicles and the prostate. Control of bleeding in this area may be followed by erectile failure subsequently, even when only unilateral damage has occurred. With a posteriorly situated tumour early division of Denonvillier's fascia will protect the nerves, but in an anteriorly placed tumour it is important to remove as much Denonvillier's fascia as possible, as it acts as a barrier to tumour penetration, and it is in these circumstances that the nerves are at risk of damage.[50]

Laparoscopic rectal mobilisation has been associated with greater male sexual dysfunction in two studies.[51,52]

 Patients should be warned that urinary and sexual difficulties may follow rectal excision, whether for benign or malignant disease.

Temporary stomas

Anastomotic leakage after ultra-low anastomosis is regrettably quite common, occurring in 10–20% of cases. One can either take the view that an elective stoma would be a burden to the 80–90% of patients unlikely to develop a leak or one can consider that the risks to health and subsequent function from an unprotected anastomotic leak are such that a stoma should be employed in all cases. I favour the latter argument.

The choice then lies between using a loop transverse colostomy or a loop ileostomy. The right upper quadrant is a poor place for siting a stoma, but it is a simple matter to mobilise the hepatic flexure and place a transverse loop colostomy in the right iliac fossa. However, even if this is done, a transverse loop colostomy is a bulky stoma that is prone to prolapse.

In many ways a loop ileostomy after rectal cancer surgery is a better stoma to have. After ileal pouch surgery for inflammatory bowel disease or familial adenomatous polyposis, the small bowel mesentery is pulled taut across the posterior abdominal wall to allow the ileal pouch to reach the anus. Thus it is often difficult to get a loop of small bowel to reach the anterior abdominal wall, making a loop ileostomy in these circumstances at times a pretty poor stoma to experience.

The situation when using a loop ileostomy to defunction a distal colonic anastomosis is entirely different. There is no difficulty in achieving a tension-free spout as the small bowel is freely mobile within the peritoneal cavity. However, a loop ileostomy can be a more difficult stoma to close than a loop transverse colostomy.

In my view, the point that swings the whole debate in favour of a loop ileostomy relates to the blood supply of the distal colon. After coloanal anastomosis, effectively a sine qua non of total mesorectal excision, a high vascular ligation is necessary in order for the descending colon to reach the anus. This means that the blood supply of the distal colon is from the middle colic artery via the marginal artery. The marginal artery is potentially at risk when a loop transverse colostomy is closed, particularly if the colostomy is resected at the time of closure. Any damage would lead to ischaemic necrosis of the distal colon, an avoidable complication if a loop ileostomy is used as a routine.

Role of radiotherapy

This issue is covered in more detail in Chapter 6. Nevertheless, it is important to distinguish between radiotherapy as an adjuvant and radiotherapy as a treatment.

Radiotherapy as an adjuvant is taken to mean radiotherapy applied to a freely mobile tumour that could easily be removed technically without any radiotherapy. When using preoperative radiotherapy in these circumstances, there need be no delay between finishing the course of radiotherapy and embarking on surgery. When confronted by a fixed or tethered tumour, preoperative radiotherapy may allow tumour shrinkage and thus permit the tumour to be excised, but it will of course have no effect on the way the original stage of the tumour predicted the possibility of occult hepatic metastases, and therefore incurability. All it will do is from time to time permit local therapy that might otherwise prove technically impossible.

In these circumstances where radiotherapy is used as a treatment, it is important to leave a sufficient interval between the radiotherapy and the attempted surgery that will maximise any tumour shrinkage. This period is of the order of 2–3 months, when

tumour shrinkage is beginning to be balanced by continuing tumour growth of resistant cells. An interval of only 1 month may deny the potential opportunity of tumour excision in some patients.

The lowest rates of local recurrence reported in the literature have come from surgeons who have not employed any radiotherapy. Indeed, although randomised trials have shown a significant reduction in local recurrence rates, these trials have been conducted against an unacceptably high rate of local recurrence in the control arms.[11]

 The Dutch total mesorectal excision radiotherapy trial has ostensibly addressed the question of whether routinely applied preoperative radiotherapy is an advantage when employing total mesorectal excision.[53] At first glance the case seems well established: at 2 years the radiotherapy group reported a 2.4% rate of local recurrence, statistically significantly better than the 8.2% for surgery alone. However, local recurrence rates have been shown to be constant until 4.5 years from surgery,[10] so the anticipated local recurrence rate at 5 years in the surgery-alone group may be of the order of 15%, far higher than that reported by others for total mesorectal excision alone. If one then takes into account the 108 different hospitals taking part, that only 77% of eligible cases ended up with tumour-free margins without tumour spillage, and that only 65% of cases actually had a low anterior resection (as opposed to abdominoperineal excision or Hartmann's operation), then the assertion that this was a trial of the application of radiotherapy to high-quality total mesorectal excision becomes somewhat suspect. Recently, this trial has reported that 5 years after surgery at least some faecal incontinence was seen in 62% receiving radiation therapy[54] compared with 39% without ($P < 0.001$).

Follow-up

There are three issues that need to be considered during follow-up:

1. Was a synchronous tumour overlooked preoperatively?
2. How should metachronous tumours be looked for?
3. Is there any value at all to follow-up of this cancer?

Synchronous tumours

There is about a 3% chance of a synchronous cancer at the time of the original resection. Of these synchronous cancers, only about 10% are likely to be so small that they would be difficult to feel during a careful laparotomy. Perhaps 1 in 3 of these small and difficult-to-feel tumours might be amenable to removal at colonoscopy using a snare. Preoperative barium enema or colonoscopy is thus seeking to identify these 2 in 1000 cases where the original surgical management might have involved a more extensive or even an additional resection.

The problem is that preoperative investigation is often incomplete and may also be inaccurate. An obstructing tumour in the rectum may make proximal visualisation impossible. Even where it is possible to attempt complete colonic examination, preparation may be poor, thereby masking in particular any smaller synchronous tumours, or colonoscopy may be less than total. Against this background, intraoperative colonoscopy has been attempted. One study showed that even this was inaccurate, missing lesions as large as 2 cm detected at postoperative colonoscopy 3 months later.[55]

For all these reasons, postoperative colonoscopy at about 3 months after resection (and anyway within the first year) will start follow-up with the knowledge that the remaining colon does not already harbour an overlooked polyp or cancer.

Metachronous tumours

The risk of a metachronous tumour is again about 3%, although it will be higher in cases where there is a family history. It would seem sensible to screen the colon at intervals by colonoscopy, perhaps every 3 years in cases where there have been prior polyps and every 5 years otherwise. As any screening examination should 'protect' for about 5 years, a final screen at the age of 75 should protect the patient until at least the age of 80 years, when the risks of routine surveillance colonoscopy will start to outweigh any benefit. Nevertheless, such an approach has never been shown to be worthwhile and many colonoscopies will need to be performed for a very small return.

Surveillance for local and distant recurrence

Surgeons are divided between those who feel follow-up is worthwhile, if only for the emotional health of the patient and to allow an accurate and long-term audit to be kept, and those who are not so convinced.

Before the advent of safe liver resection, the issue of intensive vs. symptomatic follow-up was addressed in a number of studies that failed to show any real benefit for intensive follow-up.[56,57] More recently, a randomised trial of intensive follow-up using monthly carcinoembryonic antigen (CEA) monitoring failed to show any survival benefit to those screened, although it did show a lead time in the diagnosis of recurrence of about 1 year in those screened with CEA. The problem was that this average of 1-year lead time did not translate into lives saved by re-operative surgery (J.M.A. Northover, personal communication). CEA monitoring may yet allow patients with recurrence to be treated earlier with chemotherapy, and this may itself lead to longer survival.

From an examination of first principles, it would seem that few pelvic recurrences after a properly conducted total mesorectal excision would be amenable to re-operative surgery anyway. After all, what is there left to remove that was not removed originally at the time of the first operation? Sacrectomy has a very small role in a few highly selected cases; morbidity is high and longer-term outcome modest. Clearly, anastomotic recurrence might be treated by salvage abdominoperineal excision, but true anastomotic recurrence is rare. Furthermore, anastomotic recurrence, particularly after rectal cancer surgery, is likely to present with symptoms that would make screening for it largely unnecessary.

Sometimes after restorative surgery for a very low rectal cancer there may be recurrence on the lateral pelvic side wall, for example in obturator lymph nodes. Salvage abdominoperineal excision may be technically possible with removal of these lymph nodes, but overall salvage surgery for local recurrence has disappointing results, most patients still ultimately dying from their cancer.

This really leaves the issue of the liver as the only area where follow-up might be beneficial. The problem is that even here it is not known whether regular screening will identify the particular sorts of liver recurrence amenable to curative resection, or whether these more biologically favourable tumours might not present symptomatically, regardless of screening.

The natural history of even solitary hepatic metastases will see a few survivors untreated at 5 years, but probably no more than 16%.[58] The results of liver resection are substantially better, with a low operative mortality and around 40% living for 5 years.[59] Despite this, many surgeons remain unconvinced of the value of regular ultrasound examination of the liver during follow-up. Perhaps, by recognising that

chemotherapy for advanced unresectable disease improves quality of life and is more effective when applied early, more surgeons will undertake regular liver surveillance after colorectal cancer surgery.

Against this background, two recent meta-analyses of all randomised trials of follow-up have shown improved survival for those followed up intensively.[60,61] To address this important question the FACS (Follow-up After Colorectal Surgery) trial has been launched.

Key points

- Most fit patients with rectal cancer should have total mesorectal excision.
- Endorectal ultrasound assesses the advisability of local excision by gauging invasive depth and thus the chance of occult lymph node involvement.
- MRI assesses the circumferential margin and helps decide whether preoperative chemoradiotherapy is worthwhile and whether pelvic exenteration in a young male with an anterior tumour is called for.
- The Dutch trial of total mesorectal excision with and without radiotherapy supports radiotherapy. However, there are still doubts as to whether the surgical standard, although better than in the past, was really good enough.
- After decades of doubt about the value of intensive follow-up, meta-analysis suggests benefit, spawning the FACS trial.

References

1. Finlay IG, Meek DR, Gray HW et al. The incidence and detection of occult hepatic metastases in colorectal carcinoma. Br Med J 1982; 284:803–5.

2. Beynon J, Foy DMA, Roe AM et al. Endoluminal ultrasound in the assessment of local invasion in rectal cancer. Br J Surg 1986; 73:474–7.

3. Blenkinsopp WK, Stewart-Brown S, Blesovsky L et al. Histopathology reporting in large bowel cancer. J Clin Pathol 1981; 34:509–13.

4. Williams NS, Durdey P, Quirke P et al. Preoperative staging of rectal neoplasm and its impact on clinical management. Br J Surg 1985; 72:868–74.

5. Wood DA, Robbins GF, Zippin C et al. Staging cancer of the colon and rectum. Cancer 1979; 43:961–8.

6. Dukes CE. The classification of cancer of the rectum. J Pathol Bacteriol 1932; 35:323–32.

7. Jass JR, Love SB, Northover JMA. A new prognostic classification of rectal cancer. Lancet 1987; i:1303–6.

8. Fielding LP, Phillips RKS, Fry JS et al. Prediction of outcome after curative surgery for large bowel cancer. Lancet 1986; ii:904–6.

9. Fielding LP, Stewart-Brown S, Blesovsky L et al. Anastomotic integrity after operations for large bowel cancer: a multicentre study. Br Med J 1980; 281:411–14.

10. Phillips RKS, Hittinger R, Blesovsky L et al. Local recurrence after 'curative' surgery for large bowel cancer. 1. The overall picture. Br J Surg 1984; 71:12–16.

11. McFarlane JK, Ryall RD, Heald RJ. Mesorectal excision for rectal cancer. Lancet 1993; i:457–60.

12. Brown G, Richards CJ, Newcombe RG et al. Rectal carcinoma: thin-section MR imaging for staging in 28 patients. Radiology 1999; 211:215–22.

13. Beets-Tan RG, Beets GL, Vliegen RF et al. Accuracy of magnetic resonance imaging in prediction of tumour-free resection margin in rectal cancer surgery. Lancet 2001; 357:497–504.

14. Shirouzu K, Isomoto H, Kakegawa T. Total pelvic exenteration for locally advanced colorectal carcinoma. Br J Surg 1996; 83:32–5.

15. Enker WE, Philipshen SJ, Heilwell ML et al. En bloc pelvic lymphadenectomy and sphincter preservation in the surgical management of rectal cancer. Ann Surg 1986; 293:426–33.

16. Moriya Y, Hojo K, Sawada T et al. Significance of lateral node dissection for advanced rectal carcinoma at or below the peritoneal reflection. Dis Colon Rectum 1989; 32:307–15.

17. Surtees P, Ritchie J, Phillips RKS. High versus low ligation of the inferior mesenteric artery in rectal cancer. Br J Surg 1990; 77:618–21.

18. Corder AP, Karanjia ND, Williams JD et al. Flush aortic tie versus selective preservation of the ascending left colic artery in low anterior resection for rectal carcinoma. Br J Surg 1992; 79:680–2.

19. Heald RJ, Husband EM, Ryall D. The mesorectum in rectal cancer surgery: the clue to recurrence? Br J Surg 1982; 69:613–16.

20. Scott N, Jackson P, Al-Jaberi T et al. Total mesorectal excision and local recurrence: a study of tumour spread in the mesorectum distal to rectal cancer. Br J Surg 1995; 82:1031–3.

21. Nivatvongs S, Rojanasakul A, Reiman H et al. The risk of lymph node metastasis in colorectal polyps with invasive adenocarcinoma. Dis Colon Rectum 1991; 34:323–8.

22. Syk E, Torkzad MR, Blomqvist L et al. Radiological findings do not support lateral residual tumour as a major cause of local recurrence of rectal cancer. Br J Surg 2006; 93:113–19.

23. Hallbook O, Paholman L, Krog M et al. Randomized comparison of straight and colonic J pouch anastomosis after low rectal excision. Ann Surg 1996; 224:58–65.

24. Griffiths JD. Surgical anatomy of the blood supply of the distal colon. Ann R Coll Surg Engl 1956; 19:241–56.

25. Huddy SP, Husband EM, Cook MG et al. Lymph node metastases in early rectal cancer. Br J Surg 1993; 80:1457–8.

26. Lock MR, Ritchie JK, Hawley PR. Reappraisal of radical local excision for carcinoma of the rectum. Br J Surg 1993; 80:928–9.

27. Temple LFF, Naimark D, McLeod RS. Decision analysis as an aid to determining the management of early low rectal cancer for the individual patients. J Clin Oncol 1999; 17:312–18.

28. Rouanet P, Saint Aubert B, Fabre JM et al. Conservative treatment for low rectal carcinoma by local excision with or without radiotherapy. Br J Surg 1993; 80:1452–6.

29. Chakravarti A, Compton CC, Shellito PC et al. Long term follow-up of patients with rectal cancer managed by local excision with and without adjuvant irradiation. Ann Surg 1999; 230:49–54.

30. Wagman R, Minsky BD, Cohen AM et al. Conservative management of rectal cancer with local excision and postoperative adjuvant therapy. Int J Radiat Oncol Biol Phys 1999; 44:841–6.

31. Dahlberg M, Glimelius B, Graf W et al. Preoperative irradiation affects functional results after surgery for rectal cancer. Results from a randomised study. Dis Colon Rectum 1998; 41:543–51.

32. Hershman MJ, Sun Myint A, Makin CA. Multimodality approach in curative local treatment of early rectal carcinomas. Colorectal Dis 2003; 5:445–50.

33. Umpleby HC, Fermor B, Symes MO et al. Viability of exfoliated colorectal carcinoma cells. Br J Surg 1984; 71:659–63.

34. Leather AJM, Yiu CY, Baker LA et al. Passage of shed intraluminal colorectal cancer cells across a sealed anastomosis. Br J Surg 1991; 78:756.

35. Umpleby HC, Williamson RCN. The efficacy of agents employed to prevent anastomotic recurrence in colorectal carcinoma. Ann R Coll Surg Engl 1984; 66:192–4.

36. Docherty JG, McGregor JR, Purdie CA et al. Efficacy of tumouricidal agents in vitro and in vivo. Br J Surg 1995; 82:1050–2.

37. Tiret E, Poupardin B, McNamara D et al. Ultralow anterior resection with intersphincteric dissection: what is the limit of safe sphincter preservation? Colorectal Dis 2003; 5:454–7.

38. Portier G, Ghouti L, Kirzin S et al. Oncological outcome of ultra-low coloanal anastomosis with and without intersphincteric resection for low rectal carcinoma. Br J Surg 2007; 94:341–5.

39. Phillips RKS. Adequate distal margin of resection for adenocarcinoma of the rectum. World J Surg 1992; 16:463–6.

40. Williams NS, Dixon M, Johnston D. Reappraisal of the 5cm rule of distal excision for carcinoma of the rectum: a study of distal intramural spread and of patients' survival. Br J Surg 1983; 70:150–4.

41. Karanjia ND, Schache DJ, North WRS et al. 'Close shave' in anterior resection. Br J Surg 1990; 77:510–12.

42. Phillips RKS, Hittinger R, Blesovsky L et al. Local recurrence after 'curative' surgery for large bowel cancer. 2. The rectum and rectosigmoid. Br J Surg 1984; 71:17–20.

43. Holm T, Ljung A, Haggmark T et al. Extended abdominoperineal resection with gluteus maximus flap reconstruction of the pelvic floor for rectal cancer. Br J Surg 2007; 94:232–8.

44. Sweeney JL, Ritchie JK, Hawley PR. Resection and sutured peranal anastomosis for carcinoma of the rectum. Dis Colon Rectum 1989; 32:103–6.

45. Lazorthes F, Fages P, Chiotasso P et al. Resection of the rectum with construction of a colonic reservoir and colo-anal anastomosis for carcinoma of the rectum. Br J Surg 1986; 73:136–8.

46. Nicholls RJ, Lubowski DZ, Donaldson DR. Comparison of colonic reservoir and straight coloanal reconstruction after rectal excision. Br J Surg 1988; 75:318–20.

47. Seow-Choen F, Goh HS. Prospective randomised trial comparing J colonic pouch–anal anastomosis and straight coloanal reconstruction. Br J Surg 1995; 82:608–10.

48. Mortensen NJM, Ramirez JM, Takeuchi N et al. Colonic J pouch–anal anastomosis after rectal excision for carcinoma: functional outcome. Br J Surg 1995; 82:611–13.

49. Fazio VW, Mantyh CR, Hull TL. Colonic 'coloplasty'. Novel technique to enhance low colorectal or coloanal anastomosis. Dis Colon Rectum 2000; 43:1448–50.

50. Heald RJ, Moran BJ, Brown G et al. Optimal total mesorectal excision for rectal cancer is by dissection in front of Denonvilliers' fascia. Br J Surg 2004; 91:121–3.

51. Quah HM, Jayne DG, Eu KW et al. Bladder and sexual dysfunction following laparoscopically assisted and conventional open mesorectal resection for cancer. Br J Surg 2002; 89:1551–56.

52. Jayne DG, Brown JM, Thorpe H et al. Bladder and sexual function following resection for rectal cancer in a randomized clinical trial of laparoscopic versus open technique. Br J Surg 2005; 92:1124–32.

53. Kapiteijn E, Marijnen CAM, Nagtegaal ID et al. Preoperative radiotherapy combined with total mesorectal excision for respectable rectal cancerf. N Engl J Med 2001; 345:368–46.

54. Lange MM, Der Dulk M, Bossema ER et al. Risk factors for faecal incontinence after rectal cancer treatment. Br J Surg 2007; 94:1278–84.

55. Finan PJ, Donaldson DR, Allen-Mersh T et al. Experience with perioperative colonoscopy in patients with primary colorectal cancer. Gut 1988; 29:A730.

56. Cochrane JPS, Williams JT, Faber RG et al. Value of outpatient follow-up after curative surgery for carcinoma of the large bowel. Br Med J 1980; 280:593–5.

57. Tornquist A, Ekelund G, Leandder L. The value of intensive follow-up after curative resection for colorectal carcinoma. Br J Surg 1982; 69:725–8.

58. Greenway B. Hepatic metastases from colorectal cancer: resection or not. Br J Surg 1988; 75:513–19.

59. Sugihara K, Hojo K, Moriya Y et al. Patterns of recurrence after hepatic resection for colorectal metastases. Br J Surg 1993; 80:1032–5.

60. Renehan AG, Egger M, Saunders MP et al. Impact on survival of intensive follow-up after curative resection for colorectal cancer: systematic review and meta-analysis of randomised trials. Br Med J 2002; 324:813.

This meta-analysis has readdressed the value of intensive follow-up and finds significant benefit. The FACS trial should help decide this issue.

61. Jeffrey GM, Hickey BE, Hider P. Follow-up strategies for patients treated for non-metastatic colorectal cancer. Cochrane Library, IssueRef611. Oxford: Update Software, 2002.

6

Adjuvant therapy for colorectal cancer

Paul Hatfield
David Sebag-Montefiore

Introduction

Only chemotherapy and radiotherapy have an established role as adjuvant treatment for colorectal cancer. They are given either before or after definitive surgical treatment to specific groups of patients (usually those at highest risk of relapse) in an attempt to improve the outcome of the group as a whole. As with other adjuvant treatments in cancer, the majority of patients receiving treatment (with all the associated side-effects and inconvenience) will not actually benefit, either because surgery alone would be curative or because the disease will ultimately relapse despite the additional treatment. However, the policy is justified because in a common cancer, with a significant rate of relapse, altering the outcome in even a small proportion of individuals translates into many hundreds or thousands of lives saved. When counselling individual patients it is therefore important to outline some of these uncertainties, and carefully to evaluate any comorbid factors that may increase the risks of treatment.

Chemotherapy

Chemotherapy based on 5-fluorouracil (5-FU) is widely used as an adjuvant treatment in stage III colon cancer, where it confers a 5–10% improvement in absolute survival.[1] This is based on a considerable body of published evidence from the last 15–20 years. More recently 5-FU has increasingly been combined with oxaliplatin, especially in fitter patients at higher than average risk of relapse.

The largest evidence base supporting the use of chemotherapy exists in patients with colon cancer and its applicability to patients with rectal cancer remains controversial. Nevertheless, in the UK it is common to use the same criteria to select patients, irrespective of the primary site within the large bowel.

Many uncertainties remain, such as the optimum regimen, the benefit of adding further chemotherapeutic or biological agents, the best route of administration and the role of chemotherapy in stage II disease.

Why 5-FU?

Various trials were performed before 1990 attempting to show a benefit with adjuvant chemotherapy in colon cancer. Many included 5-FU, which had a long history in metastatic colorectal cancer dating back to the 1950s.[2] However, a meta-analysis of 25 such studies in 1988 failed to show any significant survival benefit,[3] although the overall quality of studies was poor.

In 1989 and 1990 two important studies were published which changed the situation.[4,5] These large randomised trials clearly showed a survival benefit for 12 months of 5-FU plus levamisole over observation alone. The results from INT-0035 were updated in 1995[6] with similar results. The USA National Institutes of Health therefore recommended this combination strategy in stage III colon cancer patients.[7]

In the years that followed, there was increasing interest in combining 5-FU with folinic acid (FA), which potentiates its effect on the target enzyme thymidylate synthase. Indeed, a meta-analysis in 1992 had shown this combination to have an increased effect in metastatic disease.[8] There was also scepticism about the role of levamisole (an antihelminthic with immunostimulatory properties that had been proposed to enhance the effect of 5-FU). Studies were also performed addressing the optimum duration of therapy. In summary, these trials concluded that 6 months of chemotherapy with 5-FU/FA was equivalent to 12 months of 5-FU/levamisole, and superior to 6 months of 5-FU/levamisole. Furthermore, combining 5-FU/FA with levamisole gave no extra benefit.

Particularly influential in the UK was the Quick and Simple and Reliable (QUASAR) study,[9] which compared high- and low-dose FA with or without levamisole. Nearly 5000 patients were recruited and no significant difference was shown between groups, which suggested that levamisole is not necessary and that low-dose FA provides adequate modulation of 5-FU. In this study, patients were given either weekly bolus chemotherapy or five consecutive days every 4 weeks (the so-called 'Mayo regimen'). Although not randomly allocated, the weekly schedule appeared much less toxic, with equivalent efficacy. This very large trial encouraged widespread adoption of the weekly regimen in the UK.

Recent developments

In the last few years a variety of trials have combined 5-FU/FA with other chemotherapy agents (with proven efficacy in metastatic disease) in an attempt to increase the impact of adjuvant chemotherapy. Interestingly, three large studies (one published and two presented in abstract form) have shown no benefit to the combination of 5-FU and irinotecan.[10–12]

More importantly, however, two large randomised trials (MOSAIC and NSABP-C07) have now shown a benefit to combining oxaliplatin with different 5-FU/FA regimes in the adjuvant setting.[13,14] Both have shown improved disease-free survival rates for the combination, at the expense of increased toxicity (see below). Furthermore, subgroup analysis of MOSAIC has also shown a small but statistically significant 4.6% (72.9% vs 68.3%) improvement in overall survival for stage III (but not stage II) patients, after a median follow-up of 6 years.[15]

There has also been interest in using oral fluoropyrimidines (the group of drugs to which 5-FU belongs) to avoid the inconvenience and risks of intravenous 5-FU administration. Capecitabine is one such drug, which has been compared to the Mayo regimen of 5-FU/FA in stage III patients, with equivalent outcome and a favourable toxicity profile.[16] It has now been approved as an alternative adjuvant treatment to 5-FU/FA in the UK. Currently, however, capecitabine has not been compared to less toxic weekly 5-FU regimens, and its use in combination regimes for adjuvant therapy remains unproven (although relevant trial data are awaited).

Toxicity

5-FU can cause several side-effects such as fatigue, nausea, vomiting, diarrhoea, stomatitis, plantar–palmar erythema, epistaxis and sore eyes. Alopecia and significant myelosuppression are uncommon. The severity and site-specific side-effects are dependent on the regimen used. Capecitabine tends to mimic infusional 5-FU, with plantar–palmar erythema and diarrhoea being particularly common. A rare complication is angina, which may be related to coronary artery spasm and is commoner in those receiving continuous infusions of 5-FU or capecitabine. This does not necessarily occur in patients with known coronary artery disease, although there is some evidence that this slightly increases the risk.[17]

A small proportion of people are deficient for the enzyme dihydropyrimidine dehydrogenase (DPD), which is important in metabolising 5-FU.

Such individuals will be otherwise healthy but have extremely severe and early toxicity with standard doses of 5-FU. When such toxicity is observed, it is normally within the first 2–3 weeks of treatment and patients usually experience severe manifestations of all the listed side-effects. Such cases require emergency admission to the oncology centre. Whilst most of these toxicities can be controlled symptomatically, or by reducing the dose by around 50% after recovery from toxicity, each patient clearly needs to be evaluated carefully before embarking on further treatment.

Oxaliplatin in combination with 5-FU/FA increases toxicity. In the MOSAIC trial, significant neutropenia was much commoner in the combined arm (41.1% vs. 4.7%), but was complicated by infection/fever in only 1.8%. However, perhaps the biggest problem in the clinic is the increased incidence of sensory neuropathy with oxaliplatin, which can be somewhat unpredictable in onset. This was sufficiently severe to interfere with function in 12.4% of patients receiving combined treatment in MOSAIC, although for the majority this resolved in the subsequent months (down to 0.7% after 4 years median follow-up[18]).

Patient selection

Decisions concerning adjuvant therapy are often complex. Clinicians vary in their interpretation of the published evidence and patients have different attitudes to the level of inconvenience or toxicity they are willing to accept for given levels of potential benefit. Patients also vary in their medical fitness for different sorts of treatment and their life expectancy from other comorbid conditions. These factors all impact on the ultimate choice that is made.

Most oncologists would now give high-risk (e.g. heavily node-positive) stage III patients the choice of combination oxaliplatin/5-FU/FA if they are sufficiently fit and aware of the toxicities. For others, however, 6 months of 5-FU/FA or capecitabine remains the mainstay of treatment.

Controversy persists in some areas. For instance, elderly patients are generally under-represented in clinical trials and yet form the majority of patients in clinic. There is some evidence to suggest that the magnitude of benefit in the elderly is the same as in younger patients,[19–21] but subgroup analyses from influential randomised trials have often shown little benefit in older patients (>65–70).[14,22] Frequently,

there can also be concerns over comorbid conditions or the toxicity of treatment. Ultimately this leads to a lower proportion of such patients being treated, although clearly this is a decision that needs to be individualised.

Another area of considerable debate is the role of chemotherapy in stage II colorectal cancer. Such patients already have a reasonable prognosis and very large studies are required to detect any benefit from chemotherapy.

 Perhaps the most significant individual trial to address this issue is the QUASAR study, which randomised 3239 patients with colon or rectal cancer, where the indication for chemotherapy was uncertain, between 5-FU-based chemotherapy or observation.[22] The majority of patients were stage II (91%). Overall, the relative risk of death reduced by a similar amount to higher risk patients (18%), but due to the better overall prognosis this translates into only a small absolute survival benefit at 5 years (3.6% assuming a recurrence rate of 20% without chemotherapy).

Although not directly addressed by this study, it is known that some stage II tumours have a worse prognosis, such as those presenting with perforation, obstruction, extramural vascular invasion, peritoneal involvement or poorly differentiated histology.[23–28] Many clinicians would target this group of patients for adjuvant chemotherapy, on the basis that their absolute risk of relapse is higher and therefore the likely benefit is greater. Nevertheless, careful discussion of the pros and cons is required in each case. Molecular features such as microsatellite stability and loss of heterozygosity at chromosome 18q are also associated with a worse outcome and current trials are investigating the targeted use of chemotherapy after the resection of such tumours.

Many patients are referred for chemotherapy with a defunctioning stoma after resection of their primary. Despite their obvious desire to have a reversal as soon as possible, this is commonly deferred until after chemotherapy. This is to allow chemotherapy to commence as soon as possible after surgery, as most of the clinical trials have required chemotherapy to commence within 6–8 weeks. There is little evidence for giving chemotherapy at later time points or for interrupting chemotherapy to allow reversal.

Can current treatments be improved?

Adjuvant chemotherapy could be improved if:

- it was better tolerated;
- it was more effective;
- it was targeted more closely to the patients who would benefit/respond.

Increasing tolerability

The increasing use of capecitabine in adjuvant therapy is one approach to improving the acceptability of chemotherapy for patients (by avoiding the need for intravenous access or in-dwelling line complications) but it is not without its own problems. Indeed, for some patients diarrhoea and plantar–palmar erythema can be particular problems with this approach. Furthermore, agents such as oxaliplatin continue to require intravenous access, meaning that some of the convenience is lost when contemplating combination approaches.

Much of the toxicity with conventional 6-month regimens could be reduced by treating for a shorter period. An interesting approach would be to determine if less chemotherapy had equivalent efficacy. This forms the basis of a large, multicentre trial (SCOT), due to open in the UK in 2008, comparing 3 or 6 months of oxaliplain/5-FU-based chemotherapy.

Increasing effectiveness

In advanced colorectal cancer, a range of targeted biological agents have been shown to enhance the response to conventional chemotherapy. Of particular interest are antibodies specific to the epidermal growth factor receptor (EGFR) and vascular endothelial growth factor (VEGF). The cellular pathways triggered by EGFR are important in cellular growth, proliferation and programmed cell death, whilst VEGF is a key mediator of angiogenesis (the process by which growing tumours develop their own blood supply to facilitate further growth). Cetuximab and panitumumab are licensed products (in metastatic disease) targeting EGFR, whilst bevacizumab targets VEGF. Despite only relatively modest improvements in outcome in metastatic disease, a range of ongoing trials are evaluating the benefit of adding these agents to conventional adjuvant chemotherapy.[29] Theoretically, these agents may be particularly effective in the adjuvant setting, interfering with the processes that allow residual tumour

cells to proliferate, so it will be interesting to see if this is borne out in practice.

Better targeting

Various molecular markers have been examined as potential predictive factors for response to adjuvant treatment. Examples include thymidylate synthase (the target enzyme of 5-FU), the *DCC* (deleted in colorectal cancer) gene, microsatellite instability, as well as markers of angiogenesis or cellular proliferation. Others have performed sensitive assays for the detection of micrometastases to try and identify high-risk individuals.[30] However, none of these strategies is sufficiently accurate to use in clinical practice at the present time.

Radiotherapy

Radiotherapy is the use of ionising radiation to eliminate cancer cells. In modern practice it is usually delivered with linear accelarators that can target tumours with great accuracy (**Fig. 6.1**). Due to the dose-limiting effects of the small bowel in the abdominal cavity, and the problems that can arise treating more mobile targets outside the pelvis, radiotherapy is used almost exclusively for the

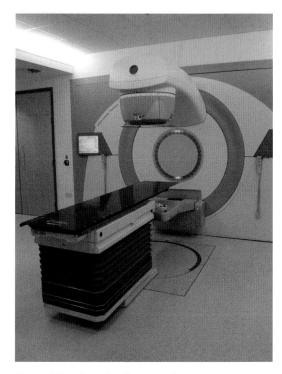

Figure 6.1 • A modern linear accelerator.

treatment of rectal cancer, rather than colon cancer. Local pelvic recurrence is also a particularly unpleasant feature of rectal cancer which is ideally prevented if possible.

Over the last three decades there has been a considerable effort to define the role of radiotherapy. Until the mid-1990s randomised controlled trials included a standard arm of surgery alone.

However, two overviews of these early trials, published in 2000 and 2001, demonstrated unequivocal evidence that adjuvant radiation reduced the risk of local recurrence in resectable rectal cancer.[31,32]

As well as a dose effect, analysis of these data also demonstrated that preoperative treatment seemed more effective than postoperative radiotherapy. Only one of these overviews[32] demonstrated an improvement in overall survival, although both reported improvements in cancer-specific mortality.

With the widespread adoption of total mesorectal excision (TME) for rectal cancer, the outcome of surgery alone has improved significantly in recent years. The evidence comes directly from individual surgical series,[33] population-based studies[34,35] and indirectly from a recently published randomised controlled trial.[36] This development alone is sufficient to make a distinction between the randomised trial evidence discussed above, where the local recurrence rates following surgery alone were commonly greater than 20%, and the current situation, where surgeons often report local recurrence rates of 10% or less. Furthermore, the strong evidence supporting the hypothesis that local recurrence of rectal cancer is predicted by the presence of microscopic cancer cells within 1 mm of the circumferential resection margin (CRM)[35,37–39] has also been very influential.

Therefore, the question in this new era is how to define a routine policy for adjuvant therapy when several choices exist (e.g. routine short-course preoperative radiotherapy (SCPRT), selective SCPRT, neoadjuvant chemoradiotherapy (CRT) or selective postoperative (chemo)radiotherapy). A distinction also needs to be drawn between tumours that are initially felt to be resectable and those where the planned resection margins are threatened by tumour.

Indications

There are three main indications for adjuvant radiation in rectal cancer:

- reducing the risk of local recurrence in patients with resectable rectal cancer;
- shrinking locally advanced rectal cancer to facilitate successful resection (although this is confused by a lack of agreement about how to define the local extent of disease);
- using radiation to shrink or 'downsize' resectable disease to achieve sphincter-preserving surgery.

Reducing local recurrence in resectable disease

In this context radiotherapy can either be administered before or after surgery. The advantage of preoperative radiotherapy is that the pelvic anatomy is undisturbed. As a result, there is usually less small bowel in the radiation field, which results in reduced gastrointestinal toxicity and higher compliance. The tissues are also likely to be well oxygenated and tumour radiosensitivity may consequently be increased. Disadvantages include over-treatment when a routine policy of preoperative radiotherapy is used, exposing some patients to the risks of late radiation damage without benefit.

In contrast, postoperative strategies allow a targeted approach in patients with high-risk pathological features, albeit with poorer compliance, increased toxicity and a need for higher doses.

Development of the '25 Gy in five fractions' preoperative schedule

The potential use of preoperative radiation was approached cautiously. One key requirement was the development of a short, accelerated schedule that minimised any delay in definitive (surgical) treatment. This led to a number of trials that used 5 Gy per fraction, including two in the UK and three in Sweden.[40–44] Overall, this approach was well tolerated, although it became clear during the follow-up of the earliest trials that careful planning, using a three- or four-field arrangement and a superior border no higher than the L4/5 junction, was required to reduce toxicity (**Fig. 6.2**). Modern radiotherapy techniques allow target volumes and organs at risk to be outlined with great accuracy in three dimensions (**Fig. 6.3**).

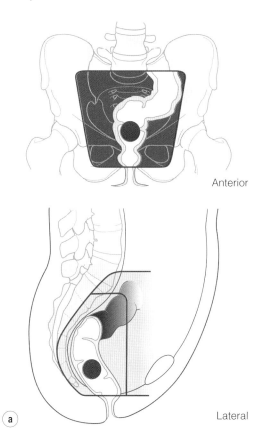

Anterior

Lateral

a

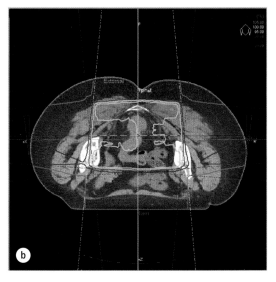

b

Figure 6.2 • Planning radiotherapy for rectal cancer. **(a)** Diagram showing radiation portals used to irradiate the posterior pelvis (purple: mid-rectal tumour; shaded blue area: treated volume). **(b)** Representative slice through the treated volume showing 'isodoses' (i.e. lines joining points receiving equivalent proportions (%) of the prescribed dose, where the target must receive at least 95% – pale blue line) and the four intersecting radiation beams (diverging lines from top, bottom and both sides) used for treatment.

 The Swedish Rectal Cancer Trial was the largest of these studies and was particularly influential, since it showed improved survival with SCPRT, compared to surgery alone, as well as reduced local recurrence rates.[44]

It could be hypothesised that radiotherapy in these early studies was simply compensating for inadequate surgery, before the introduction of routine TME. Therefore, to establish the role of SCPRT in the TME era, the Dutch Colorectal Cancer Study Group trial and the Medical Research Council (MRC) CR07 trial were both designed to compare SCPRT with selective postoperative approaches, based on CRM status (radiotherapy alone in the Dutch study, chemoradiotherapy in CR07).

 Results from the Dutch trial[36,45] and early data from the CR07 study[46] (presented in abstract form) both showed a reduction in local recurrence with routine SCPRT, which was associated with minimal complications. CR07 also demonstrated a 5% improvement in 3-year disease-free survival. Absolute benefit was greatest in those patients at highest risk of relapse. Overall, the proportional reduction in local recurrence appeared very similar to the pre-TME era, but the absolute reduction was that much smaller due to the better surgical outcomes.

SCPRT does have some well-established, long-term complications, including permanent sterility for men and premenopausal women. There is

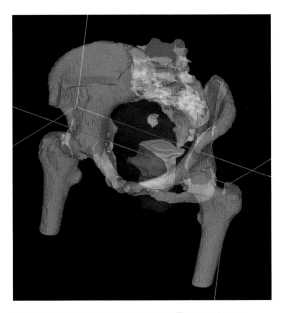

Figure 6.3 • Modern radiotherapy. Target volumes (e.g. macroscopic tumour, in primary and mesorectal nodes – orange; planning target volume, including surrounding areas at risk – red) and organs at risk (e.g. bladder – blue) can be outlined on a series of computed tomography (CT) scan slices to build up composite three-dimensional volumes. This facilitates more accurate treatment planning.

also an increased incidence of erectile dysfunction and impaired bowel function,[47–49] although rates of pelvic fractures and bowel obstruction do not appear to be increased.[47] It is therefore important to weigh up the pros and cons of SCPRT in different groups of patients. Many clinicians would not treat patients with stage I disease but opinions vary on where the threshold should be set for more advanced tumours.

'Long-course' preoperative radiation schedules

An alternative approach to SCPRT is to use a longer course of radiation with a lower (more conventional) dose per fraction. This is an approach favoured in much of mainland Europe. Most current long-course schedules use 45–50.4 Gy over 5–5.5 weeks using 1.8–2.0 Gy per fraction. As with SCPRT, there is evidence for improved local control using this strategy but no trial evidence for improved survival. There has been an increasing interest in long-course CRT regimes, an approach that maximises response rates when used in locally advanced disease.

Recent randomised trials have shown that concurrent chemotherapy given with radiotherapy (CRT) is more effective than radiotherapy alone, when used preoperatively in resectable disease. The EORTC 22921[50] and FFCD 9203 trials[51] both showed that local recurrences were reduced using CRT, with no difference in disease-free survival.

As yet it is not clear what the advantage of preoperative CRT may be over SCPRT, although the former is clearly more expensive and resource intensive. Only one trial, from Poland, has been performed to compare these strategies[52] and this was powered to detect differences in sphincter preservation rather than local recurrence or survival. Unsurprisingly, CRT followed by a 4- to 6-week wait led to greater tumour downstaging, pathological complete response rates and CRM-negative resections, but was also associated with higher rates of acute toxicity. Nevertheless, there was no significant difference seen in the rate of sphincter-preserving surgery and, interestingly, no statistical difference in local recurrence or late toxicity.

Postoperative radiation alone for resectable disease

Eight evaluable randomised trials were identified in the overview[31] that assessed postoperative radiation and included surgery alone as a control arm. The MRC3 trial[53] was the only trial that demonstrated a statistically significant reduction in local recurrence, with no impact in overall survival. Taken together, however, there was a significant reduction in local recurrence and cancer-specific mortality, although the proportional reduction of these events was smaller than that found for preoperative radiation. Most of the postoperative trials were underpowered to detect small improvements.

Development of postoperative chemoradiation

The relatively disappointing results of the trials of postoperative radiation alone, and the hope of improving overall survival, led to trials that integrated chemotherapy. Interpretation is difficult, however, mainly due to heterogeneous trial design.

Most of these studies were from North America and the results of three[54–56] led to a consensus statement from the National Institutes of Health in 1990, making postoperative chemoradiation (adjuvant chemotherapy + concurrent CRT) for patients with pT3/4 or N-positive disease (TNM stage II and III) the standard of care.[7] This policy was more selective than routine preoperative radiotherapy but only spared patients with stage I disease the morbidity of treatment. Furthermore, the acute toxicities were more severe, making its applicability to the general population less certain. There was particular concern about older patients.[57] However, until recently this was the standard approach in North America.

Preoperative versus postoperative radiation in resectable disease

Both the CR07 and Dutch trials have compared routine SCPRT with selective postoperative treatments (as described above), and both have shown less local recurrence with the preoperative approach. Nevertheless, many oncologists around the world remain wary of SCPRT because of a perception that it increases long-term toxicity.[58]

 Of particular significance, however, are the results of the recent German CAO/ARO/AI0 94 trial,[59] comparing pre- and postoperative CRT. This influential study, using standardised TME surgery and postoperative chemotherapy in all patients, showed that the preoperative approach resulted in lower local recurrence rates (6% vs. 12%) and reduced complications (both acute and late). Overall survival was unaffected.

This study (combined with the preoperative superiority of CRT over long-course radiotherapy alone, described above) appears to have decisively changed the treatment paradigm in rectal cancer to a preoperative approach and is already influencing practice in North America.[58,60] Nevertheless, whether preoperative CRT in resectable disease is superior to SCPRT, or justifies the extra costs, remains to be proven. Furthermore, with TME surgery producing very low local recurrence rates, it is likely that for many patients the extra toxicities of treatment are hard to justify. Therefore, if we accept that we have shown when to treat these patients, then the next challenge is to further define who should be treated, as well as how.

Radiotherapy for locally advanced rectal cancer

Definitions of 'locally advanced' disease have varied over time. However, the development of preoperative imaging has allowed attempts to predict T and N stage, with transrectal ultrasound generally accepted as the reference investigation for assessing the transmural extent of tumour.

Recognition of the importance of the CRM in predicting local recurrence has also led to increased interest in cross-sectional imaging, particularly magnetic resonance imaging (MRI), to demonstrate the relationship of the tumour to the mesorectal fascia (the intended 'CRM' for a mesorectal excision).

Development of pelvic MRI

A number of early studies[61–66] reported the value of high-resolution pelvic MRI using phased-array surface coils in the preoperative staging of rectal cancer. By identifying patients whose disease extends beyond the mesorectal fascia (commonly described as T4 disease) or is threatening the mesorectal fascia (**Fig. 6.4**) it was hoped that MRI could be used to select patients for more intensive preoperative CRT regimens (to downsize the tumour and facilitate complete excision at subsequent surgery).

 The MERCURY trial[67,68] has now confirmed the validity of this approach, showing a strong correlation between the MRI-predicted CRM status and pathological findings. MRI staging is now considered routine before surgery, allowing informed decisions to be made concerning preoperative treatment.

Randomised controlled trials assessing radiotherapy in locally advanced disease

Given the difficulty of surgery alone in this group of patients, there is limited randomised evidence to support the use of radiotherapy. Two trials from the UK have evaluated the addition of preoperative radiation to surgery alone.[41,69] Both demonstrated a significant reduction in local recurrence but no difference in overall survival.

A small trial from Uppsala[70] randomised 70 patients with fixed, unresectable disease between 46 Gy radiation alone and a complex CRT schedule using 40 Gy and methotrexate, leucovorin and 5-FU over 8 weeks. There was a statistically significant reduction in local recurrence with CRT but no difference in overall survival.

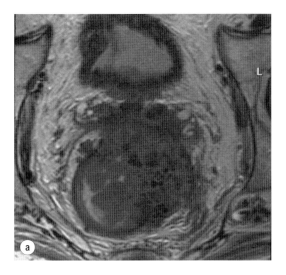
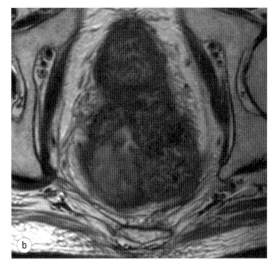

Figure 6.4 • MRI staging of rectal cancer. MRI is now a standard preoperative technique to identify tumours (outlined in red) that either **(a)** extend beyond the expected CRM (green dashed line) or **(b)** threaten it. Such patients can then be selected for more aggressive preoperative treatment to try and downsize the tumour and facilitate complete resection.

Phase II studies

In recent years neoadjuvant concurrent chemo-radiotherapy has become a standard treatment for locally advanced rectal cancer, because of increased response rates seen in the very large number of phase II studies that have been performed (**Fig. 6.5**). Many have used either infusional 5-FU[71] or bolus 5-FU with leucovorin,[72–74] but no direct comparison has been performed and there remains considerable uncertainty as to how to derive the optimum regimen[75] or the most useful end-point.[76]

Currently there is considerable interest in the use of other drugs such as capecitabine, oxaliplatin, irinotecan and the targeted biologicals in chemoradiation schedules. Many studies utilising these agents are under way but no phase III data have yet been reported comparing them to standard 5-FU-based regimens.

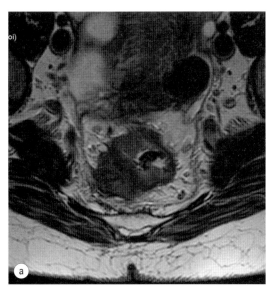
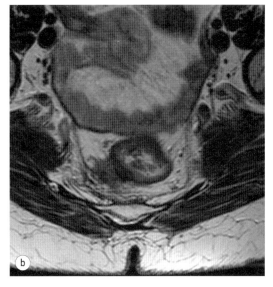

Figure 6.5 • Response to neoadjuvant chemoradiotherapy. **(a)** A bulky tumour (red outline) threatens the expected CRM (green dashed line). **(b)** Following neoadjuvant CRT a small tumour residuum remains, although this no longer involves the CRM. The mesorectal envelope has also contracted as the tumour has reduced in size.

There is considerable uncertainty as to the benefit of adjuvant chemotherapy following prior neo-adjuvant CRT. If it is to be used, should it be given to those who have responded well to CRT[77] (and therefore have chemosensitive disease) or should combination treatment be given to those that have not responded to CRT containing a single agent?[60] Ongoing trials are addressing this issue.

Improving sphincter preservation

It remains controversial whether preoperative treatment (usually with CRT) can increase rates of sphincter-preserving surgery in low rectal cancer (i.e. converting a planned abdomino-perineal resection into a low anterior resection). Indeed, a systematic review[78] has found no evidence of increased sphincter preservation following preoperative treatment. The authors argue that surgeons are reluctant to change their initial plan, even after a good response, because of understandable concern over residual microscopic disease at the original site of the tumour. There is also concern about the functional outcome following very low anterior resections. Nevertheless, some series have shown it to be possible, without excessive local recurrence, and the debate continues.[79]

The future

Radiotherapy has a well-established role in the adjuvant treatment of rectal cancer. The next few years are likely to see increased refinement of our current techniques. For instance, we may be able to achieve better patient selection through the use of imaging or even molecular markers. More effective regimens of chemoradiotherapy are likely to be developed (incorporating new agents) and trials designed to show when they should be used. There is even interest in avoiding surgery for subgroups of patients with complete clinical responses after CRT.[80] More targeted use of short-course preoperative radiotherapy in the TME era may also be possible, with maturing evidence from the Dutch trial and the results of CR07.

Key points

- Six months of adjuvant chemotherapy with 5-FU/leucovorin or capecitabine is currently standard treatment for patients with stage III colorectal cancer.
- Fit, high-risk patients are now routinely offered the combination of oxaliplatin/5-FU/leucovorin.
- The use of chemotherapy in stage II disease produces only a small improvement in overall survival. Therefore, chemotherapy is not routinely offerred, although many clinicians would treat selected 'high-risk' patients.
- The role of additional agents (particularly antibodies) in adjuvant chemotherapy remains to be clarified.
- Adjuvant radiotherapy is widely used in rectal cancer to reduce the risk of local recurrence. The benefit persists even with TME surgery.
- Worldwide, preoperative rather than postoperative radiotherapy is increasingly considered a standard treatment for resectable rectal cancer, although whether SCPRT or long-course CRT is used varies.
- With improvements in rectal surgery, low-risk patients can probably be spared the toxicity of radiotherapy, although there is no universal definition of this group.
- Neoadjuvant chemoradiotherapy is frequently used in fit patients with unresectable rectal cancer to try and downstage the disease before surgery and allow complete resection. It remains controversial whether this really enables sphincter-preserving surgery in low rectal cancer.

References

1. Haydon A. Adjuvant chemotherapy in colon cancer: what is the evidence? Intern Med J 2003; 33(3):119–24.

2. Moertel CG. Chemotherapy for colorectal cancer. N Engl J Med 1994; 330(16):1136–42.

3. Buyse M, Zeleniuch-Jacquotte A, Chalmers TC. Adjuvant therapy of colorectal cancer. Why we still don't know. JAMA 1988; 259(24):3571–8.

4. Laurie JA, Moertel CG, Fleming TR et al. Surgical adjuvant therapy of large-bowel carcinoma: an evaluation of levamisole and the combination of levamisole and fluorouracil. The North Central Cancer Treatment Group and the Mayo Clinic. J Clin Oncol 1989; 7(10):1447–56.

   Large randomised trial that was important in proving the principle of adjuvant chemotherapy.

5. Moertel CG, Fleming TR, Macdonald JS et al. Levamisole and fluorouracil for adjuvant therapy of resected colon carcinoma. N Engl J Med 1990; 322(6):352–8.

   Along with Ref. 4, led to the NIH Consensus Statement recommending adjuvant chemotherapy for stage C colon cancer.

6. Moertel CG, Fleming TR, Macdonald JS et al. Fluorouracil plus levamisole as effective adjuvant therapy after resection of stage III colon carcinoma: a final report. Ann Intern Med 1995; 122(5):321–6.

   An update of the trial patients in Ref. 5 that continued to show ongoing benefit to adjuvant treatment.

7. NIH Consensus Conference. Adjuvant therapy for patients with colon and rectal cancer. JAMA 1990; 264(11):1444–50.

   A very influential guide to practice in North America, that was widely followed until recently.

8. Advanced Colorectal Cancer Meta-Analysis Project. Modulation of fluorouracil by leucovorin in patients with advanced colorectal cancer: evidence in terms of response rate. J Clin Oncol 1992; 10(6):896–903.

9. QUASAR Collaborative Group. Comparison of flourouracil with additional levamisole, higher-dose folinic acid, or both, as adjuvant chemotherapy for colorectal cancer: a randomised trial. Lancet 2000; 355(9215):1588–96.

   An influential UK study which showed that low-dose FA was equivalent to high-dose FA, and also demonstrated no benefit for levamisole. Led to weekly bolus 5-FU/FA becoming widely used in the UK.

10. Saltz LB, Niedzwiecki D, Hollis D et al. Irinotecan fluorouracil plus leucovorin is not superior to fluorouracil plus leucovorin alone as adjuvant treatment for stage III colon cancer: results of CALGB 89803. J Clin Oncol 2007; 25(23):3456–61.

11. Ychou MR, Raoul JL, Douillard JY. A phase III randomized trial of LV5FU2 + CPT-11 vs. LV5FU2 alone in adjuvant high risk colon cancer (FNCLCC Accord02/FFCD9802). J Clin Oncol 2005; 23 (Suppl):16s, Abstract 3502.

12. Van Cutsem E, Labianca R, Hossfeld G. Randomized phase III trial comparing infused irinotecan/5-fluorouracil (5-FU)/folinic acid (IF) versus 5-FU/FA (F) in stage III colon cancer patients (PETACC 3). J Clin Oncol 2005; 23(Suppl):3s, Abstract 8.

13. Wolmark N, Wieand HS, Keubler JP. A phase III trial comparing FULV to FULV + oxaliplatin in stage II or III carcinoma of the colon: results of the NSABP protocol C-07. 2005; 23(Suppl):16s, Abstract 3500.

   One of two large randomised trials addressing the addition of oxaliplatin to adjuvant 5-FU/FA (in this case as a weekly bolus regime 6 weeks out of every 8). The combination gave improved disease-free survival.

14. Andre T, Boni C, Mounedji-Boudiaf L et al. Oxaliplatin, fluorouracil, and leucovorin as adjuvant treatment for colon cancer. N Engl J Med 2004; 350(23):2343–51.

   The other large randomised trial combining oxaliplatin with 5-FU/FA, in this case using a 48-hour infusional regime of 5-FU every 2 weeks. In this paper the improvement in disease-free survival is reported.

15. de Gramont A, Boni C, Navarro M et al. Oxaliplatin/5FU/LV in adjuvant colon cancer: updated efficacy results of the MOSAIC trial, including survival, with a median follow-up of six years. J Clin Oncol 2007; 25(Suppl):18S, Abstract 4007.

   Updated results from the MOSAIC trial which described an overall survival benefit, for the oxaliplatin-containing combination arm, in a subgroup analysis of stage III patients.

16. Twelves C, Wong A, Nowacki MP et al. Capecitabine as adjuvant treatment for stage III colon cancer. N Engl J Med 2005; 352(26):2696–704.

17. Labianca R, Beretta G, Clerici M et al. Cardiac toxicity of 5-fluorouracil: a study on 1083 patients. Tumori 1982; 68(6):505–10.

18. de Gramont A, Boni C, Navarro M et al. Oxaliplatin/5FU/LV in the adjuvant treatment of stage II and stage III colon cancer: efficacy results with a median follow-up of 4 years. J Clin Oncol 2005; 23:16S, Abstract 3501.

19. Sargent DJ, Goldberg RM, Jacobson SD et al. A pooled analysis of adjuvant chemotherapy for resected colon cancer in elderly patients. N Engl J Med 2001; 345(15):1091–7.

20. Iwashyna TJ, Lamont EB. Effectiveness of adjuvant fluorouracil in clinical practice: a population-based cohort study of elderly patients with stage III colon cancer. J Clin Oncol 2002; 20(19):3992–8.

21. Jessup JM, Stewart A, Greene FL et al. Adjuvant chemotherapy for stage III colon cancer: implications of race/ethnicity, age, and differentiation. JAMA 2005; 294(21):2703–11.

22. QUASAR Collaborative Group, Gray R, Barnwell J, McConkey C et al. Adjuvant chemotherapy versus observation in patients with colorectal cancer: a randomised study. Lancet 2007; 370 (9604):2020–9.

This large randomised trial addressed the benefit of adjuvant chemotherapy in patients where the benefit was uncertain (predominantly stage II patients). It showed a small but statistically significant improvement in overall survival.

23. Wolmark N, Wieand HS, Rockette HE et al. The prognostic significance of tumor location and bowel obstruction in Dukes B and C colorectal cancer. Findings from the NSABP clinical trials. Ann Surg 1983; 198(6):743–52.

24. Steinberg SM, Barkin JS, Kaplan RS et al. Prognostic indicators of colon tumors. The Gastrointestinal Tumor Study Group experience. Cancer 1986; 57(9):1866–70.

25. Steinberg SM, Barwick KW, Stablein DM. Importance of tumor pathology and morphology in patients with surgically resected colon cancer. Findings from the Gastrointestinal Tumor Study Group. Cancer 1986; 58(6):1340–5.

26. Shepherd NA, Baxter KJ, Love SB. Influence of local peritoneal involvement on pelvic recurrence and prognosis in rectal cancer. J Clin Pathol 1995; 48(9):849–55.

27. Talbot IC, Ritchie S, Leighton M et al. Invasion of veins by carcinoma of rectum: method of detection, histological features and significance. Histopathology 1981; 5(2):141–63.

28. Talbot IC, Ritchie S, Leighton MH et al. Spread of rectal cancer within veins. Histologic features and clinical significance. Am J Surg 1981; 141(1):15–17.

29. de Gramont A, Tournigand C, Andre T et al. Targeted agents for adjuvant therapy of colon cancer. Semin Oncol 2006; 33(6, Suppl 11):S42–5.

30. Bilchik AJ, Hoon DS, Saha S et al. Prognostic impact of micrometastases in colon cancer: interim results of a prospective multicenter trial. Ann Surg 2007; 246(4):568–75; discussion 575–7.

31. Adjuvant radiotherapy for rectal cancer: a systematic overview of 8,507 patients from 22 randomised trials. Lancet 2001; 358(9290):1291–304.

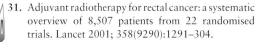

A very important overview of the many early trials of adjuvant radiotherapy in rectal cancer that clearly demonstrated a reduction in local recurrence and also suggested a reduction in cancer-related mortality. Used individual patient data for analysis.

32. Camma C, Giunta M, Fiorica F et al. Preoperative radiotherapy for resectable rectal cancer: a meta-analysis. JAMA 2000; 284(8):1008–15.

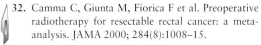

Another important meta-analysis of adjuvant radiotherapy trials with similar results to Ref. 31.

33. Heald RJ, Moran BJ, Ryall RD et al. Rectal cancer: the Basingstoke experience of total mesorectal excision, 1978–1997. Arch Surg 1998; 133(8):894–9.

34. Martling AL, Holm T, Rutqvist LE et al. Effect of a surgical training programme on outcome of rectal cancer in the County of Stockholm. Stockholm Colorectal Cancer Study Group, Basingstoke Bowel Cancer Research Project. Lancet 2000; 356(9224):93–6.

35. Wibe A, Rendedal PR, Svensson E et al. Prognostic significance of the circumferential resection margin following total mesorectal excision for rectal cancer. Br J Surg 2002; 89(3):327–34.

36. Kapiteijn E, Marijnen CA, Nagtegaal ID et al. Preoperative radiotherapy combined with total mesorectal excision for resectable rectal cancer. N Engl J Med 2001; 345(9):638–46.

Initial report of the Dutch trial of SCPRT combined with TME surgery (versus a policy of TME followed by selective post-op radiotherapy). Showed that routine SCPRT continued to have an effect on local recurrence despite the excellent results with TME alone.

37. Adam IJ, Mohamdee MO, Martin IG et al. Role of circumferential margin involvement in the local recurrence of rectal cancer. Lancet 1994; 344(8924):707–11.

38. Birbeck KF, Macklin CP, Tiffin NJ et al. Rates of circumferential resection margin involvement vary between surgeons and predict outcomes in rectal cancer surgery. Ann Surg 2002; 235(4):449–57.

39. Nagtegaal ID, Quirke P. What is the role for the circumferential margin in the modern treatment of rectal cancer? J Clin Oncol 2008; 26(2):303–12.

40. Goldberg PA, Nicholls RJ, Porter NH et al. Long-term results of a randomised trial of short-course low-dose adjuvant pre-operative radiotherapy for rectal cancer: reduction in local treatment failure. Eur J Cancer 1994; 30A(11):1602–6.

41. Marsh PJ, James RD, Schofield PF. Adjuvant preoperative radiotherapy for locally advanced rectal carcinoma. Results of a prospective, randomized trial. Dis Colon Rectum 1994; 37(12):1205–14.

42. Stockholm Colorectal Cancer Study Group. Randomized study on preoperative radiotherapy in rectal carcinoma. Ann Surg Oncol 1996; 3(5):423–30.

43. Cedermark B, Johansson H, Rutqvist LE et al. The Stockholm I trial of preoperative short term radiotherapy in operable rectal carcinoma. A prospective randomized trial. Stockholm Colorectal Cancer Study Group. Cancer 1995; 75(9):2269–75.

44. Swedish Rectal Cancer Trial. Improved survival with preoperative radiotherapy in resectable rectal cancer. N Engl J Med 1997; 336(14):980–7.

A large randomised trial of 1168 patients that demonstrated both a reduction in local recurrence and an improvement in overall survival for routine SCPRT in resectable rectal cancer.

45. Peeters KC, Marijnen CA, Nagtegaal ID et al. The TME trial after a median follow-up of 6 years: increased local control but no survival benefit in irradiated patients with resectable rectal carcinoma. Ann Surg 2007; 246(5):693–701.

    Longer-term follow-up of patients in Dutch TME/SCPRT trial. Confirmed sustained improvement in local control but found no effect on overall survival.

46. Sebag-Montefiore D, Steele R, Quirke P. Routine short course pre-operative radiotherapy or selective post-op chemoradiotherapy for resectable rectal cancer? Preliminary results of the MRC CR07 trial. ASCO Annual Meeting 2006(24):Abstract 3511.

    Large, international, multicentre randomised trial, coordinated in the UK, comparing routine SCPRT with a selective policy of post-op chemoradiotherapy. Reinforced the results of the Dutch trial, with improved local control after routine SCPRT. Also showed a small but statistically significant improvement in disease-free survival at 3 years.

47. Peeters KC, van de Velde CJ, Leer JW et al. Late side effects of short-course preoperative radiotherapy combined with total mesorectal excision for rectal cancer: increased bowel dysfunction in irradiated patients – a Dutch colorectal cancer group study. J Clin Oncol 2005; 23(25):6199–206.

48. Marijnen CA, van de Velde CJ, Putter H et al. Impact of short-term preoperative radiotherapy on health-related quality of life and sexual functioning in primary rectal cancer: report of a multicenter randomized trial. J Clin Oncol 2005; 23(9):1847–58.

49. Pollack J, Holm T, Cedermark B et al. Late adverse effects of short-course preoperative radiotherapy in rectal cancer. Br J Surg 2006; 93(12):1519–25.

50. Bosset JF, Collette L, Calais G et al. Chemotherapy with preoperative radiotherapy in rectal cancer. N Engl J Med 2006; 355(11):1114–23.

    Large European trial showing that the addition of chemotherapy to conventionally fractionated preoperative radiotherapy improves local control rates. Interestingly, postoperative chemotherapy conferred no survival benefit after long-course preoperative treatments.

51. Gerard JP, Conroy T, Bonnetain F et al. Preoperative radiotherapy with or without concurrent fluorouracil and leucovorin in T3–4 rectal cancers: results of FFCD 9203. J Clin Oncol 2006; 24(28):4620–5.

    A further large trial which also showed improved local control with the addition of chemotherapy to preoperative long-course radiotherapy. It did not address the role of adjuvant chemotherapy.

52. Bujko K, Nowacki MP, Nasierowska-Guttmejer A et al. Long-term results of a randomized trial comparing preoperative short-course radiotherapy with preoperative conventionally fractionated chemoradiation for rectal cancer. Br J Surg 2006; 93(10):1215–23.

53. Medical Research Council Rectal Cancer Working Party. Randomised trial of surgery alone versus surgery followed by radiotherapy for mobile cancer of the rectum. Lancet 1996; 348(9042):1610–4.

54. Gastrointestinal Tumor Study Group. Prolongation of the disease-free interval in surgically treated rectal carcinoma. N Engl J Med 1985; 312(23):1465–72.

55. Krook JE, Moertel CG, Gunderson LL et al. Effective surgical adjuvant therapy for high-risk rectal carcinoma. N Engl J Med 1991; 324(11):709–15.

56. Fisher B, Wolmark N, Rockette H et al. Postoperative adjuvant chemotherapy or radiation therapy for rectal cancer: results from NSABP protocol R-01. J Natl Cancer Inst 1988; 80(1):21–9.

57. Neugut AI, Fleischauer AT, Sundararajan V et al. Use of adjuvant chemotherapy and radiation therapy for rectal cancer among the elderly: a population-based study. J Clin Oncol 2002; 20(11):2643–50.

58. Kachnic LA. Should preoperative or postoperative therapy be administered in the management of rectal cancer? Semin Oncol 2006; 33(6, Suppl 11):S64–9.

59. Sauer R, Becker H, Hohenberger W et al. Preoperative versus postoperative chemoradiotherapy for rectal cancer. N Engl J Med 2004; 351(17):1731–40.

    A very influential study which has led to the widespread adoption of preoperative rather than postoperative CRT, after showing improved local control and reduced toxicity.

60. Minsky BD. Adjuvant management of rectal cancer: the more we learn, the less we know. J Clin Oncol 2007; 25(28):4339–40.

61. Botterill ID, Blunt DM, Quirke P et al. Evaluation of the role of pre-operative magnetic resonance imaging in the management of rectal cancer. Colorectal Dis 2001; 3(5):295–303.

62. Blomqvist L, Machado M, Rubio C et al. Rectal tumour staging: MR imaging using pelvic phased-array and endorectal coils vs endoscopic ultrasonography. Eur Radiol 2000; 10(4):653–60.

63. Brown G, Richards CJ, Newcombe RG et al. Rectal carcinoma: thin-section MR imaging for staging in 28 patients. Radiology 1999; 211(1):215–22.

64. Bissett IP, Fernando CC, Hough DM et al. Identification of the fascia propria by magnetic resonance imaging and its relevance to preoperative assessment of rectal cancer. Dis Colon Rectum 2001; 44(2):259–65.

65. Beets-Tan RG, Beets GL, Vliegen RF et al. Accuracy of magnetic resonance imaging in prediction of tumour-free resection margin in rectal cancer surgery. Lancet 2001; 357(9255):497–504.

66. Brown G, Radcliffe AG, Newcombe RG et al. Preoperative assessment of prognostic factors in rectal cancer using high-resolution magnetic resonance imaging. Br J Surg 2003; 90(3):355–64.

67. Diagnostic accuracy of preoperative magnetic resonance imaging in predicting curative resection of rectal cancer: prospective observational study. BMJ 2006; 333(7572):779.

Powerful data supporting the accuracy of preoperative MRI scanning when predicting circumferential resection margin status. Has led to the widespread adoption of pelvic MRI as a standard staging procedure for rectal cancer.

68. Extramural depth of tumor invasion at thin-section MR in patients with rectal cancer: results of the MERCURY study. Radiology 2007; 243(1):132–9.

Further data from the MERCURY study showing the accuracy of MRI when predicting the depth of extramural spread around rectal cancers.

69. Medical Research Council Rectal Cancer Working Party. Randomised trial of surgery alone versus radiotherapy followed by surgery for potentially operable locally advanced rectal cancer. Lancet 1996; 348(9042):1605–10.

70. Frykholm GJ, Pahlman L, Glimelius B. Combined chemo- and radiotherapy vs. radiotherapy alone in the treatment of primary, nonresectable adenocarcinoma of the rectum. Int J Radiat Oncol Biol Phys 2001; 50(2):427–34.

71. Rich TA, Skibber JM, Ajani JA et al. Preoperative infusional chemoradiation therapy for stage T3 rectal cancer. Int J Radiat Oncol Biol Phys 1995; 32(4):1025–9.

72. Minsky B, Cohen A, Enker W et al. Preoperative 5-fluorouracil, low-dose leucovorin, and concurrent radiation therapy for rectal cancer. Cancer 1994;73(2): 273–80.

73. Minsky BD, Kemeny N, Cohen AM et al. Preoperative high-dose leucovorin/5-fluorouracil and radiation therapy for unresectable rectal cancer. Cancer 1991; 67(11):2859–66.

74. Bosset JF, Pavy JJ, Hamers HP et al. Determination of the optimal dose of 5-fluorouracil when combined with low dose D,L-leucovorin and irradiation in rectal cancer: results of three consecutive phase II studies. EORTC Radiotherapy Group. Eur J Cancer 1993; 29A(10):1406–10.

75. Glynne-Jones R, Sebag-Montefiore D. Chemoradiation schedules – what radiotherapy? Eur J Cancer 2002; 38(2):258–69.

76. Glynne-Jones R, Mawdsley S, Pearce T et al. Alternative clinical end points in rectal cancer – are we getting closer? Ann Oncol 2006; 17(8):1239–48.

77. Collette L, Bosset JF, den Dulk M et al. Patients with curative resection of cT3–4 rectal cancer after preoperative radiotherapy or radiochemotherapy: does anybody benefit from adjuvant fluorouracil-based chemotherapy? A trial of the European Organisation for Research and Treatment of Cancer Radiation Oncology Group. J Clin Oncol 2007; 25(28):4379–86.

78. Bujko K, Kepka L, Michalski W et al. Does rectal cancer shrinkage induced by preoperative radio(chemo)therapy increase the likelihood of anterior resection? A systematic review of randomised trials. Radiother Oncol 2006; 80(1):4–12.

79. Rullier E, Sebag-Montefiore D. Sphincter saving is the primary objective for local treatment of cancer of the lower rectum. Lancet Oncol 2006; 7(9):775–7.

80. O'Neill BD, Brown G, Heald RJ et al. Non-operative treatment after neoadjuvant chemoradiotherapy for rectal cancer. Lancet Oncol 2007; 8(7):625–33.

7

Anal cancer

John H. Scholefield

Introduction

Anal cancer is rare, accounting for approximately 4% of large bowel malignancies; however, there is some evidence that its incidence is increasing. Most anal cancers arise from the squamous epithelium of the anal margin or anal canal, although a few arise from anal glands and ducts.

Traditionally, the anal region is divided into the anal canal and the anal margin or verge. The natural history, demography and surgical management of anal cancer differ between these areas. There is controversy regarding the exact definition of the anal canal. Anatomists see it as lying between the dentate line and the anal verge, whereas surgically it is defined as lying between the anorectal ring and the anal verge. For pathologists, the canal has been defined as corresponding to the longitudinal extent of the internal anal sphincter. The canal above the dentate line is lined by rectal mucosa, except for a small zone immediately above the line called the transitional or junctional zone. Inferiorly, the canal is covered by stratified squamous epithelium. Further confusion relates to the definition of the anal canal and anal margin as sites for cancer. The anal margin is variously described as the visible area external to the anal verge, or as the area below the dentate line. This argument has become less important as surgery plays a lesser role in treatment, but reports of surgical results from past decades are confused by this variation in definition.

Over 80% of anal cancers are of squamous origin, arising from the squamous epithelium of the anal canal and perianal area; 10% are adenocarcinomas arising from the glandular mucosa of the upper anal canal, the anal glands and ducts. A very rare and particularly malignant tumour is anal melanoma. Lymphomas and sarcomas of the anus are even less common but have increased in incidence in recent years, particularly among patients with human immunodeficiency virus (HIV) infection. There has also been a rise in the incidence of other anal epidermoid tumours among patients with HIV.

Epidermoid tumours

Aetiology and pathogenesis

Anal squamous cell carcinomas are relatively uncommon tumours; there are between 250 and 300 new cases per year in England and Wales. Based on these figures each consultant general surgeon might expect to see one anal carcinoma every 3–4 years. However, anal cancers are probably underreported, since some anal canal tumours are misclassified as rectal tumours and some perianal tumours as squamous carcinomas of skin.

The SEER data (2005) quote an incidence of 1.5 per 100 000 population in the USA; similar incidence rates apply for the UK. The average age at presentation was 57 years for both sexes.

There is wide geographical variation in the incidence of anal cancers around the world, but figures must be interpreted with caution for the reasons given above. Nevertheless, a low incidence (0.2 per 100 000 of population) is reported by Rizal in the Philippines, while the highest incidence (3.6 per 100 000 of population) is in Geneva, Switzerland. Areas with a high incidence of anal cancer usually also have a high incidence of cervical, vulval and penile tumours (reflecting the common aetiological agent – papillomaviruses).

The increasing incidence of HIV infection in the USA has resulted in a rise in the incidence of anal cancer, areas such as San Francisco, with a large gay population, reportedly seeing a dramatic increase. A recent study from Denmark has reported a doubling in the incidence of anal cancer over the last 10 years, particularly in women.[1] No other countries have reported similar increases to date, but the Cancer Registry data in Denmark are renowned for their remarkable accuracy and completeness.

The occurrence of a disproportionately high incidence of anal cancer among male homosexual communities was reported from San Francisco and Los Angeles. Daling et al.[2] identified risk factors for the development of squamous cell carcinoma of the anus, a history of receptive anal intercourse in males increasing the relative risk of developing anal cancer by 33 times compared with controls with colon cancer. A history of genital warts also increased the relative risk of developing anal cancer (27-fold in men and 22-fold in women). These studies suggest that a sexually transmissible agent may be an aetiological factor in anal squamous cell carcinoma.

Similarly, epidemiological and molecular biological data have shown an association between a sexually transmissible agent and female genital cancer. Using nucleic acid hybridisation techniques, human papillomavirus (HPV) type 16 DNA, and less commonly types 18, 31 and 33 DNA, were consistently found to be integrated into the genome in genital squamous cell carcinomas. The same HPV DNA types have also been identified in a similar proportion of anal squamous cell carcinomas.[3] HPVs, which are DNA viruses, comprise more than 60 types capable of causing a wide variety of lesions on squamous epithelium. Common warts can be found on the hands and feet of children and young adults, and are caused by the relatively infectious HPV types 1 and 2. Anogenital papillomaviruses are less infective than types 1 and 2 and are exclusively sexually transmitted. The epidemiology of genital papillomavirus infection is poorly understood, largely due to the social and moral taboos surrounding sexually transmissible infections. Anogenital papillomavirus-associated lesions range from condylomas through intraepithelial neoplasias to invasive carcinomas. The most common HPV types causing genital warts are types 6 and 11, which may also be isolated from low-grade intraepithelial neoplasia. HPV types 16, 18, 31 and 33 are much less commonly associated with genital condylomas but are more commonly found in high-grade intraepithelial neoplasias and invasive carcinomas. Once one area of the anogenital epithelium is infected, spread of papillomavirus infection throughout the rest of the anogenital area probably follows, but remains occult in the majority of individuals. Therefore the commonly held belief that anal cancer occurs only in individuals who practise anal intercourse is probably unfounded.

Premalignant lesions

Anal and genital papillomavirus-associated lesions may be identified clinically either by naked eye inspection or more usually with an operating microscope (colposcope) and the application of acetic acid to the epithelium, resulting in an 'aceto-white' lesion. Colposcopic examination may suggest the degree of dysplasia and permits targeted biopsy of a lesion, but histological examination remains the diagnostic standard. Although the natural history of cervical papillomavirus infection and intraepithelial neoplasia is reasonably well understood, the same is not true for anal lesions, probably because they have been diagnosed only over the last 5–10 years. Consequently, the natural history and malignant potential of anal intraepithelial neoplasia are both uncertain.

Anogenital intraepithelial neoplasia of the cervix (CIN), vulva (VIN), vagina (VAIN) and anus (AIN) is graded from I to III, according to the number of thirds of epithelial depth that appear dysplastic on histological section. Thus in grade III the cells of the whole thickness of the epithelium appear dysplastic, being synonymous with carcinoma in situ.

High-grade anal intraepithelial lesions may be characterised by hyperkeratosis or changes in the pigmentation of the epithelium. Thus carcinoma in situ may appear white, red or brown, the pigmentation commonly being irregular. The lesions may be flat or raised, but ulceration is suggestive of invasive disease. It is important that any suspicious area is biopsied and examined histologically. The terms 'Bowen's disease of the anus' and 'leucoplakia' are best avoided as they are confusing and convey no specific information, the malignant potential of both being uncertain.

At present, multifocal genital intraepithelial neoplasia represents a difficult clinical problem, which may be further complicated by the occurrence of synchronous or metachronous AIN.[4] The management of these patients is uncertain as the natural history of these lesions remains poorly understood.

Co-carcinogens

Carcinogenesis is a multistep process, papillomaviruses probably being only one of a number of factors in the pathogenesis of these tumours. Other potential co-carcinogens are being investigated, including other sexually transmissible infective agents such as herpes simplex type II and chlamydia.

There are few published data on the prevalence of HPV infection among HIV-infected patients, but it appears that anogenital HPV infection is particularly common in this group. The dramatic increase in the incidence of anal cancer in areas where HIV infection is prevalent suggests that suppression of cell-mediated responses to HPV infection may be important in the pathogenesis of anal cancer; this is also supported by the increased incidence of squamous carcinomas in patients receiving systemic immunosuppression following organ transplantation.

Histological types

Included within the category of epidermoid tumours are squamous cell, basaloid (or cloacogenic) carcinomas and muco-epidermoid cancers. The different morphological types of anal cancer do not appear to have different prognoses. Tumours arising at

the anal margin tend to be well differentiated and keratinising, whereas those arising in the canal are more commonly poorly differentiated. Basaloid tumours arise in the transitional zone around the dentate line and form 30–50% of all anal canal tumours.

Patterns of spread

Anal canal cancer spreads locally, mainly in a cephalad direction, so that the tumour may appear to have arisen in the rectum. The tumour also spreads outwards into the anal sphincters and into the rectovaginal septum, perineal body, scrotum or vagina in more advanced cases (**Fig. 7.1**). Lymph node metastases occur frequently, especially in tumours of the anal canal. Spread occurs initially to the perirectal group of nodes and thereafter to inguinal, haemorrhoidal and lateral pelvic lymph nodes. The frequency of nodal involvement is related to the size of the primary tumour together with its depth of penetration. Approximately 14% of patients will present with inguinal lymph node involvement, but this rises to approximately 30% when the primary tumour is greater than 5 cm in diameter. Only 50% of patients with enlarged nodes at presentation will subsequently be shown to contain tumour. Synchronously involved nodes carry a particularly poor prognosis, whereas when metachronous spread develops the salvage rate is much higher.

Haematogenous spread tends to occur late and is usually associated with advanced local disease. The principal sites of metastases are the liver, lung and bones. However, metastases have been described in the kidneys, adrenals and brain.

Clinical presentation

The predominant symptoms of epidermoid anal cancer are pain and bleeding, which are present in about 50% of cases. The presence of a mass is noted by a minority of patients, around 25%. Pruritus and discharge occur in a similar proportion. Advanced tumours may involve the sphincter mechanism,

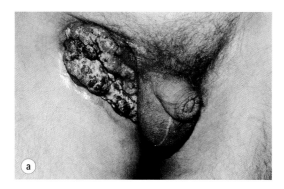

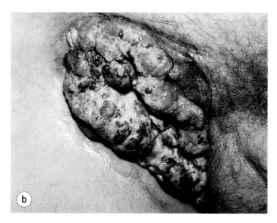

Figure 7.1 • Locally advanced anal cancer involving the anal canal, perianal skin, perineal skin and base of scrotum. Treatment with chemo-irradiation failed to control the disease and the patient underwent a salvage abdominoperineal excision.

causing faecal incontinence. Invasion of the posterior vaginal wall may cause a fistula.

Cancer of the anal margin usually has the appearance of a malignant ulcer, with a raised, everted, indurated edge. Lesions within the canal may not be visible, though extensive lesions spread to the anal verge, or can extend via the ischiorectal fossa to the skin of the buttock. Digital examination of the anal canal is usually painful, and may reveal the distortion produced by the tumour. Since anal cancer tends to spread upwards, there may be involvement of the distal rectum, perhaps giving the impression that the lesion has arisen there. Involvement of the perirectal lymph nodes may be palpable on digital examination, rather more than may be apparent in disseminating rectal cancer. If the tumour has extended into the sphincter muscles, the characteristic induration of a spreading malignancy may be felt around the anal canal.

 Although up to one-third of patients will have inguinal lymph nodes that are enlarged, biopsy will confirm metastatic spread in only 50% of these; the rest are due to secondary infection. Biopsy or fine-needle aspiration is recommended by many to confirm involvement of the groin nodes if radical block dissection is contemplated. Distant spread is unusual in anal cancer, so hepatomegaly, though it must be looked for, is very uncommon. Frequently, other benign perianal conditions will exist in association with anal cancer, such as fistulas, condylomas or leucoplakia.

Investigation

 The most important investigation in the management of anal cancer is examination under anaesthetic. Examination under anaesthesia permits optimum assessment of the tumour in terms of size, involvement of adjacent structures and nodal involvement, and also provides the best opportunity to obtain a biopsy for histological confirmation. Sigmoidoscopic examination is probably best performed at this examination.

Clinical staging

No one system of staging for anal tumours has been adopted universally. However, that of the UICC is the most widely used. For anal canal lesions this system has been criticised as it has required assessment of involvement of the external sphincter. To overcome this a system has been suggested by Papillon et al.[5] as follows:

T1	<2 cm;
T2	2–4 cm;
T3	>4 cm, mobile;
T4a	invading vaginal mucosa;
T4b	extension into structures other than skin, rectal or vaginal mucosa.

In recent years magnetic resonance imaging (MRI) has taken over from endoanal ultrasound in staging these lesions. MRI is better than endoanal ultrasound, providing information on spread beyond the anal canal.

Serum tumour markers are unhelpful as they do not provide reliable information.

Treatment

Historical

Traditionally, anal cancer has been seen as a 'surgical' disease. Anal canal tumours were treated by radical abdominoperineal excision and colostomy, whereas anal margin lesions were treated by local excision. Over the past decade, non-surgical radical treatments, i.e. radiotherapy with or without chemotherapy, have taken over as primary treatments of choice in most cases.

Overall, the results of surgery for anal cancer are disappointing for what is essentially a locoregional disease. For decades radical abdominoperineal excision of the rectum and anus was the preferred method of treatment at most centres around the world. Abdominoperineal excision for anal canal cancer differs little from the procedure used for rectal cancer, but particular care is taken to clear the space below the pelvic floor. Around 20% of cases are incurable surgically at presentation. Results published since the mid-1980s reporting series collected over the previous several decades have varied widely in their survival outcome, but on average the 5-year survival has been around 55–60%. Most postsurgical relapses occur locoregionally.

Around 75% of cancers at the anal margin have been treated in the past by local excision. The rationale for this was based on the perception that margin lesions rarely metastasise, though this has not always been confirmed by prolonged follow-up. It may be postulated that disappointing 5-year survival rates (around 50–70%) might have been better if radical surgery had been applied more frequently.

Current

Radiotherapists have been treating anal tumours for many years, achieving equivalent survival rates but with the advantage of stoma avoidance in the majority of cases which might otherwise have required radical surgery. Ironically it was a surgeon, Norman Nigro, reporting the use of combined chemotherapy and radiotherapy to try to turn inoperable cases into candidates for surgical salvage, who began to turn surgeons away from operation as first-choice therapy.[6]

Radiation-alone therapy

The initial treatment for anal cancer was radiotherapy because the mortality and morbidity of surgical treatment of anal carcinoma were unacceptable. By the 1930s, however, it was recognised that the low-voltage radiotherapy used frequently produced severe radionecrosis. As surgery became safer, abdominoperineal excision for invading lesions, and local excision for small growths, became the standard treatment for the next four decades.

The development in the 1950s of equipment that could deliver high-energy irradiation by the cobalt source generator or, more recently, by linear accelerators enabled radiotherapists to deliver higher penetrating doses to deeper placed structures with less superficial expenditure of energy. Radiation damage to surrounding tissues was consequently reduced while simultaneously delivering an enhanced tumoricidal effect. Interstitial irradiation alone may produce local tumour control rates of 47%. Improved results have been described using a technique of external beam irradiation, combined with interstitial therapy: two-thirds survived for 5 years, the majority maintaining adequate sphincter function. In the UK high-dose external beam radiotherapy is most commonly used, for which 5-year survival rates of 75% at 3 years have been described.

Chemo-irradiation therapy (combined modality therapy)

Combined modality therapy for anal cancer was championed by Norman Nigro. Nigro chose to use 5-fluorouracil (5-FU) and mitomycin C empirically as a preoperative regimen aimed at improving the results of radical surgery.[6] The radiotherapy then consisted of 30 Gy of external beam irradiation over a period of 3 weeks. A bolus of mitomycin C was given on the first day of treatment, and 5-FU was delivered in a synchronous continuous 4-day infusion during the first week of radiotherapy. After completion of radiotherapy, a further infusion of 5-FU was administered and patients later proceeded to abdominoperineal excision. It was evident to Nigro that the majority had quite dramatic tumour shrinkage: in his 1974 publication the tumour was reported to have disappeared completely in all three patients. No tumour was found in the surgical specimen in both of the patients who underwent abdominoperineal excision; the third refused surgery. Nigro's experience over the ensuing 10 years bore out his early enthusiasm. As he became more confident, he no longer routinely pressed his patients to undergo radical surgery, initially confining himself to excising the site of the primary tumour after combined modality therapy. Later, he dropped even this relatively minor surgical step if the primary site looked and felt normal after treatment.[7]

A variety of similar techniques have subsequently been described. With wider experience, it became clear that higher doses of radiotherapy (45–60 Gy) could be applied, usually split into two courses to minimise morbidity. Chemotherapy comprised intravenous infusion of 5-FU at the beginning and end of the first radiotherapy course, and a single bolus of mitomycin C given on the first day of treatment.[8] Modifications of chemotherapy dosage and prophylactic antibiotic therapy were necessary in elderly or frail patients, and those with extensive ulcerated tumours.

All the reported series describe excellent results, but there was a debate about whether chemotherapy added any advantage over radiotherapy alone.

The most recent data on combined modality therapy from the UK Coordinating Committee on Cancer Research compared chemo-irradiation with radiotherapy alone in a randomised multicentre study.[9] This study randomised 585 patients, making it the largest single trial in anal cancer. The trial showed that combined modality therapy gave superior local control of disease compared with radiotherapy alone. Only 36% of patients receiving combined therapy had 'local failure' compared with 59% of those receiving radiotherapy alone. Although there was no significant overall survival advantage for either treatment regimen, the risk of death from anal cancer was significantly less in the group receiving combined modality therapy (**Fig. 7.2**). As a result of this trial it seems that the standard treatment for anal squamous carcinoma should be a combination of radiotherapy and intravenous 5-FU with mitomycin, which remains the gold standard.

Mitomycin causes much of the toxicity of chemoradiation (a problem particularly in elderly patients) and thus trials of the use of cisplatin as an alternative to mitomycin have been performed (RTOG, 2006). This trial randomised 652 patients but showed that cisplatin had no advantage over mitomycin and may be inferior. The search for the optimal regimen goes on.

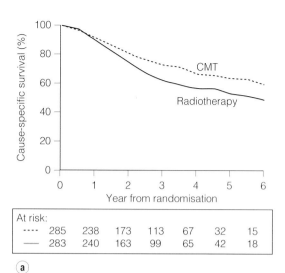

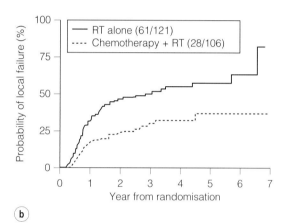

Figure 7.2 • **(a)** Deaths from anal cancer. Number of events: radiotherapy 105, combined modality therapy (CMT) 77 (RR = 0.71, 95% CI 0.53–0.95, *P* = 0.02). Number at risk = number alive. **(b)** UKCCCR Anal Cancer trial: risk of local failure (T1–2 and N0). Part **(a)**: UKCCCR Anal Cancer Trial Working Party. Lancet 1996; 348:1055, Figure 5. With permission from Elsevier. Part **(b)**: Northover J, Meadows A, Ryan C et al., on behalf of UKCCCR Anal Cancer Trial Working Party. Lancet 1996; 349:206. With permission from Elsevier.

Complications of chemoradiation for anal carcinoma include diarrhoea, mucositis, myelosuppression, skin erythema and desquamation. Late complications include anal stenosis and fistula formation.

HIV patients with anal epidermoid cancers are probably best treated with chemoradiation, but have increased toxicity.[10]

Role of surgery today

Although surgeons no longer play the central thera-peutic role, they nevertheless have important contri-butions to make.

Initial diagnosis

Most patients present to surgeons, who are best suited to perform examination under anaesthesia to confirm diagnosis and assess local extent.

Lesions at the anal margin

Small lesions at the anal margin may still best be treated by local excision alone, obviating the need for protracted courses of non-surgical therapy. There is some evidence that the risk of regional lymph node metastasis is not related to primary tumour size, which may explain the disappointing results sometimes reported after local excision; this conflicts with the view that tumour size is related to stage, which explains the excellent results of local excision in small tumours.

Treatment complications and disease relapse

Surgeons retain an important role in the treatment of anal cancer after failure of primary non-surgi-cal therapy, either early or late. Four situations may require surgery after primary non-surgical treat-ment: residual tumour, complications of treatment, incontinence or fistula after tumour resolution, and subsequent tumour recurrence.

1. The appearance of the primary site is often misleading after radiotherapy. In most patients complete remission is indicated by the tumour disappearing completely. In some, however, an ulcer may remain, occasionally looking like an unchanged primary tumour. Only generous biopsy will reveal whether the residual ulcer contains tumour or consists merely of inflammatory tissue. Histological proof of residual disease is essential before radical surgery is recommended to the patient. For patients with proven residual disease, a salvage abdominoperineal resection may be the only option. In fit patients with extensive pelvic disease extending around the vagina or bladder, pelvic exenteration may need to be considered. This type of surgery carries a high morbidity with impaired wound healing due to the radiotherapy. A primary reconstruction of the perineal area using a myocutaneous flap is strongly recommneded in these cases.

2. Complications of non-surgical treatment for anal cancer do occur in a proportion of patients, including radionecrosis, fistula and incontinence. Severe anal pain due to radionecrosis of the anal lining may necessitate either a colostomy, in the hope that the lesion may heal after faecal diversion, or radical anorectal excision with a flap used to reconstruct the perineum.

3. Occasionally, a tumour is so locally extensive that the patient will be rendered incontinent as a consequence of primary tumour shrinkage. Although rectovaginal fistula may be amenable to repair, sphincter damage is unlikely to improve with local surgery, necessitating abdominoperineal excision of the anorectum. Abdominoperineal excision of the rectum under these circumstances is usually best undertaken in conjunction with a rectus abdominis myocutaneous flap to aid perineal wound healing.

4. When there is recurrent disease developing after initial resolution, biopsy is mandatory before surgical intervention. These biopsies need to be of reasonable size, number and depth as the histological appearances following radiotherapy can make histopathological interpretation difficult. If high-dose radiotherapy was used for primary treatment, further non-surgical therapy for recurrence is usually contraindicated, making radical surgical removal necessary.

Inguinal metastases

Inguinal lymph nodes are enlarged in 10–25% of patients with anal cancers. Although inguinal lymph node involvement may be treated by radiotherapy, some argue in favour of surgery; however, histological confirmation is advisable before radical groin dissection as up to 50% of cases of inguinal lymphadenopathy may be due to inflammation alone. Enlargement of groin nodes some time after primary therapy is most likely to be due to recurrent tumour; radical groin dissection is indicated in this situation, with up to 50% 5-year survival.

Treatment of intraepithelial neoplasia

HPV infection of the anogenital area is very common; it is reported that over 70% of sexually active adults have at some time had occult or overt genital HPV infection. In most individuals the infection remains occult, but in a minority the infection manifests itself as either condylomas or intraepithelial neoplasia. As with other viral infections, it is impossible to eradicate HPV infection by surgical excision; for this reason, surgical excision of condylomas is effectively performed more for relief of symptoms and cosmesis.

Similarly, the natural history of low-grade AIN (I and II) is relatively benign and therefore a policy of observation alone is adequate. This is likely to be particularly advisable when large areas of the anogenital epithelium are affected. However, for high-grade AIN (III) the advice is more circumspect as we do not know the natural history of this condition. If the area of AIN III is small, it is probably prudent to excise it locally and then to observe the patient at regular intervals for a number of years. If the area of AIN III is too large for local excision without risk of anal stenosis, then a careful observational policy with 6-monthly review may be an option.

Aggressive surgical excision of the whole perianal skin and anal canal and resurfacing with split skin with a defunctioning colostomy has been used to treat wide areas of AIN III. This sort of surgery necessitates multiple procedures and carries significant morbidity, which for a condition of uncertain malignant potential may make the treatment worse than the disease.

The use of immunomodulators in AIN has been investigated as a potential therapeutic option. While some authors report encouraging results, these are all small studies of short duration. Photodynamic therapy using topical photosensitisers may be useful, but experience is currently very limited. All these treatments are painful and this often limits their use.

Rarer tumours

Adenocarcinoma

Adenocarcinoma in the anal canal is usually a very low rectal cancer that has spread downwards to involve the canal; however, true adenocarcinoma of the anal canal does occur, probably arising from the anal glands which arise around the dentate line and pass radially outwards into the sphincter muscles. This is a very rare tumour, quite radiosensitive, and is increasingly being treated by chemoradiation.

Malignant melanoma

Another very rare tumour, this accounts for just 1% of anal canal malignant tumours. The lesion may mimic a thrombosed external pile due to its colour, although amelanotic tumours also occur. Anal melanomas have a dismal prognosis; the literature suggests a median survival of around 18 months after diagnosis and only 10–20% 5-year survival. All treatment options appear to be equally unsuccessful. Liver and lung metastases are common. As the chances of cure are minimal, radical surgery as primary treatment should be abandoned, but local excision may provide useful palliation.[11]

Key points

- HPV is an aetiological factor in anal squamous cell carcinomas. Women with previous gynaecological lesions on the cervix and vulva and the immunosuppressed (transplant recipients and HIV patients) are at risk for AIN. These premalignant lesions may be rapidly progressive in immunocompromised patients.
- The management of anal squamous carcinoma has changed dramatically in the last few years. Chemo-irradiation is the treatment of first choice for most lesions.
- Surgery may be the primary treatment modality for small perianal lesions that can be locally excised.
- Melanoma of the anus is very rare and has a dismal prognosis. Radical surgery, chemotherapy and radiotherapy are of little benefit. Local excision may provide useful palliation.

References

1. Frische M, Melbye M. Trends in the incidence of anal carcinoma in Denmark. Br Med J 1993; 306:419–22.

2. Daling J, Weiss N, Hislop T et al. Sexual practices, sexually transmitted diseases and the incidence of anal cancer. N Engl J Med 1987; 317:973–7.

   Excellent epidemiological paper on anal squamous cell carcinoma.

3. Palmer JG, Scholefield JH, Shepherd N et al. Anal cancer and human papillomaviruses. Dis Colon Rectum 1989; 32:1016–22.

4. Scholefield J, Hickson W, Smith J et al. Anal intraepithelial neoplasia: part of a multifocal disease process. Lancet 1992; 340:1271–3.

5. Papillon J, Mayer M, Mountberon J et al. A new approach to the management of epidermoid carcinoma of the anal canal. Cancer 1987; 51:1830–7.

6. Nigro N, Vaitkevicius V, Considine B Jr et al. Combined therapy for cancer of the anal canal. A preliminary report. Dis Colon Rectum 1974; 27:354–6.

   A classic paper – the first experience of using chemoradiation in anal cancer.

7. Nigro N. An evaluation of combined therapy for squamous cell cancer in the anal canal. Dis Colon Rectum 1984; 27:763–6.

8. Cummings B, Keane T, O'Sullivan B et al. Mitomycin in anal canal carcinoma. Oncology 1993; 50(Suppl 1):63–9.

9. UKCCCR Anal Cancer Trial Working Party. Epidermoid anal cancer: results from the UKCCCR randomised trial of radiotherapy alone versus radiotherapy, 5-fluorouracil, and mitomycin. Lancet 1996; 348:1049–54.

   A large well-run randomised trial that changed the management of this cancer in the UK.

10. Uronis HE, Bendell JC. Anal cancer – an overview. Oncologist 2007; 12:524–34.

11. Ross M, Pezzi C, Pezzi T et al. Patterns of failure in anorectal melanoma. A guide to surgical therapy. Arch Surg 1990; 125:313–16.

8

Diverticular disease

Zygmunt H. Krukowski

Introduction

Diverticular disease has a lowly status in the surgical and public psyche. Perceived as self-inflicted, it is often a diagnosis of dismissal following exclusion of more 'major' pathology, yet there is such diversity of opinion in both elective and emergency surgery that its management has never been more challenging.

Right-sided colonic diverticula are common in the Orient,[1] but in Western society the problem is predominantly left-sided and sigmoid. The incidence increases with age with a prevalence based on flexible sigmoidoscopy exceeding 75% of those over 70 years.[2] Symptomatic complications occur in 10–30% of patients,[3–5] although the reliability of these historical data, based as they were on symptoms and not imaging, is debatable. Knowledge is hampered by the lack of consistent documentation.[6] A recent prospective Swedish study[7] of acute diverticulitis demonstrated an annual admission rate of 47 and operation rate of 12 per 100 000 population. There are issues relating to patient management after an episode of sepsis requiring hospitalisation,[8] as well as in those with symptomatic but uncomplicated diverticular disease.[9]

Sickness and even death in diverticulitis are caused by sepsis in often frail and elderly patients. Mortality may be minimised, yet not eliminated, by optimal operative and supportive treatment. Whilst it is increasingly accepted that most people do not need emergency surgery, identifying who does and when and how to perform it is essential. Unnecessary, inappropriate or poorly performed emergency intervention may mean that morbidity from bad surgery exceeds that of conservatively managed disease. Often, when managing emergencies, a conservative initial approach should be favoured, although excessive reluctance subsequently to operate electively in some patients may disadvantage them.[10,11] Resection rates between the UK, Europe and the USA reflect different systems and their political and financial pressures, yet the clinical issues are the same – who, when and how.

Evidence base in surgery for diverticular disease

Despite much literature, the quality is poor.[8,12]

 There are only two published randomised controlled trials in the management of complicated diverticulitis[13,14] and two consensus documents from the American Society of Colon and Rectal Surgeons[15] and the European Association of Endoscopic Surgeons,[16] the latter relying on the expert synthesis. Papers proliferate, yet a systematic review of acute diverticultitis[8] found only 21 of 1360 potentially relevant papers met the inclusion criteria. Likewise a review of 49 articles on diagnostic accuracy found only three with a level of evidence of IIb or better.[17] A recent critical review[18] challenges even the advice in the consensus documents and the conclusion of the systematic review[17] of diagnostic imaging is hard to justify.

Pathology

Aetiology

A recent comprehensive review[19] supports acquired sigmoid diverticular disease being a consequence of deficient dietary vegetable fibre.[20] Hyperelastosis[21] and altered collagen structure[22] in the colon wall related to ageing and disordered motility contribute. An active lifestyle and the reduced intraluminal pressure associated with a high-fibre diet together reduce the incidence of diverticular disease.[23] Segmentation of the narrow sigmoid colon predisposes to high intraluminal pressure (Laplace's law) with characteristic protrusion of the mucosa at weak points where the terminal arterial branches penetrate the circular muscle adjacent to the taenia (**Fig. 8.1**). The rectum, with its complete layer of longitudinal muscle and larger diameter, rarely develops diverticula.

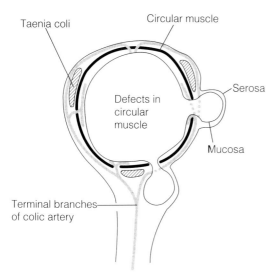

Figure 8.1 • Diagrammatic cross-section of colon showing sites of diverticulum formation.

Complications

Increased wall tension and colonic luminal pressure aggravated by visceral hypersensitivity account for the pain experienced by patients with uncomplicated diverticular disease.[19] The major complications of sigmoid diverticular disease follow bacterial infection with local or generalised sepsis. Subsequent fibrosis and mural thickening compounded by inflammatory oedema may cause stricture formation and obstruction. Fistula formation between the sigmoid colon and any contiguous structure is possible. Infrequently profuse bleeding may arise from a diverticulum. Both smoking[24] and ingestion of non-steroidal anti-inflammatory agents (NSAIDs)[25] have been implicated as aggravating factors in the development of complications. Sometimes other pathologies may coexist or mimic the symptoms of diverticular disease. Gangrenous sigmoiditis, sometimes blamed on prolonged muscular spasm, is probably a vascular occlusive problem and, whilst inflammatory bowel disease can coexist with diverticular disease, longitudinal fistulous tracks with granulomas suggest Crohn's disease.

Obstruction of a diverticular ostium promotes bacterial proliferation in a sealed space with the risk of abscess formation. Minor episodes with surrounding cellulitis may be self-limiting, but progression occurs in a variable and unknown proportion. Infection may involve a length of colon and spread into surrounding tissue to produce an inflammatory phlegmon. The rate of septic progression and the initial site dictate the degree of containment – a diverticulum within the mesocolon being more confined than one on the antimesenteric border. Slow development of infection allows adherence of inflamed adjacent structures, production of fibrinous exudate and localisation of peritoneal infection. At its worst a complex suppurative mass incorporating colon, small bowel, bladder, uterus, ovaries, tubes and occasionally ureter may develop. The extent of peritonitis associated with diverticular masses varies and, although there may be extensive fibrinous exudate and inflammatory peritoneal fluid, this may contain few bacteria.

When an uninflamed diverticulum ruptures, a punched-out defect communicating directly with the colonic lumen may result (**Fig. 8.2**) – but such free perforation resulting in faecal peritonitis is uncommon. Purulent peritonitis is more often the result of rupture of a previously contained abscess.

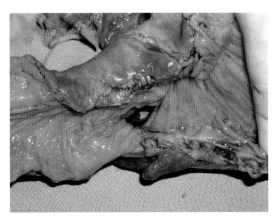

Figure 8.2 • Punched-out defect characteristic of uninflamed divertiuculum rupture.

Large communicating perforations occasionally release faecal boluses directly into the peritoneal cavity, but this sort of faecal peritonitis is probably due to stercoral ulceration secondary to pressure necrosis. Whether such a perforation is inappropriately attributed to the diverticular disease which often coexists is a moot point. Equally, when a single perforation due to a scyballous mass in the colon is encountered, this may or may not be included, influencing subsequent analysis.

The highly variable inflammatory response and extent of peritoneal contamination which is a feature of diverticulitis may result in inaccurate classification. A considerable inflammatory exudate may be present, which on Gram staining shows scant bacterial contamination. Whilst appearing dramatic, such reactive peritonitis has a different prognosis from a purulent generalised peritonitis resulting from the rupture of a previously localised abscess – for here the peritoneal fluid will be highly contaminated with millions of bacteria per millilitre of fluid. Similarly, although faecal peritonitis is notoriously associated with the highest mortality, early intervention may allow removal of solid faecal masses before peritoneal inflammatory changes become established. This will mean that residual contamination after peritoneal toilet is minor. However, when treatment is delayed faecal contamination of the general peritoneal cavity is lethal.

Occasionally, a diagnosis of Crohn's disease is made in conjunction with that of sigmoid diverticular disease. This may be suggested by a preoperative barium enema which shows sigmoid diverticula and one or more fistulous tracks, which often run along the length of the bowel, or by the presence of granulomatous changes on histological examination of sigmoid colon resected for diverticula. Whilst this may indeed be the coincidence of two relatively common diseases, there is some evidence that a granulomatous reaction, histologically similar to Crohn's disease, can occur in association with diverticular disease that is limited to the sigmoid colon and is not associated with any other current or subsequent manifestations of Crohn's disease[26,27] (granulomatous sigmoiditis).

Severe diverticular disease can cause liver abscesses and prompt subsequent resection of the sigmoid colon.

Classification of diverticular disease

Comparison between both elective and emergency series is difficult because of inconsistency in diagnosis, description of gross and radiological pathology and peritoneal contamination encountered. Most elective series subdivide patients into uncomplicated (i.e. diverticulosis) and complicated cases with previous episodes of acute diverticulitis, abscess, stricture and fistulas. The situation is more complex in the emergency situation, and whilst Killingback's classification of the pathology[28,29] permits accurate description, the coexistence of some of these features requires a simpler classification. Hinchey's classification[30] is the most widely used but is based on operative findings and only applies to perforated diverticulitis. Preoperative imaging categorises[31,32] the extent of sepsis without surgery. The relationship between the various systems is shown in Table 8.1. The importance of defining the nature and extent of the inflammatory process is well illustrated by Haglund et al.[33] Of 392 patients admitted with acute diverticulitis, 97 (25%) underwent emergency operation. Within the operated group, 31 had phlegmonous inflammation with no evidence of suppuration or perforation; mortality was 3%. By contrast, 66 patients had evidence of perforation; mortality was 33%. The relevance is that, if the threshold for operation is inappropriately low, more patients with mild disease and an intrinsically good prognosis are subjected to surgery and a spuriously low mortality for surgery is reported. The overall number of emergency admissions, the number undergoing surgery

Table 8.1 • Relationship between pathological, operative and classifications of diverticulitis

Pathology[28]		Hinchey et al.[30]	Hansen and Stock[32]	Ambrosetti et al.[31]
Diverticulosis – no inflammation			0	
Acute diverticulitis	Non-perforated		I	
Phlegmonous/peridiverticulitis			IIa	Mild
Mesenteric/pericolic abscess		I	IIb	
Pelvic abscess	Perforated – non-communicating	II		Severe
Purulent peritonitis		III	IIc	
Faecal peritonitis	Perforated – communicating	IV		
Chronic/recurrent diverticulitis – stricture/fistula			III	

and an accurate classification of the extent of sepsis must be recorded in any systematic analysis of the outcome of management of acute diverticular disease. Furthermore, the declining rate of autopsy in the UK must mean that some elderly patients dying with 'peritonitis' in whom surgery was considered inappropriate will have perforated diverticulitis.

Presentation

The spectrum of pathology encountered in sigmoid diverticular disease results in a wide variety of clinical presentations.

Elective

Many patients who present with symptoms of lower abdominal pain, distension and altered bowel habit prove to have diverticular disease during the course of exclusion of neoplastic disease by endoscopy and contrast radiology. In the majority, advice to increase dietary soluble fibre coupled with reassurance will suffice. Failure of medical management with continuing symptoms over a number of years may justify surgery in the absence of specific complications of diverticular disease. In a study of 261 patients with a radiological diagnosis of diverticular disease, only 6.5% subsequently required antibiotics for presumed diverticulitis, although 36% experienced recurrent episodes of pain.[34] Unfortunately, elective resection of the colon does not relieve the pain in all these patients,[35] and by inference this is because of a persisting underlying functional bowel problem.

Emergency

Acute diverticulitis

The typical presentation of acute diverticulitis is with a few days' history of increasing lower abdominal pain that localises in the left iliac fossa,[36] variably accompanied by nausea, altered bowel habit and irritation of pelvic viscera. Pain and tenderness can be maximal to the right of the midline, depending on the disposition of the sigmoid colon, which is a trap for the unwary.

In the majority, left iliac fossa signs suggest a working diagnosis of acute diverticulitis, but there is a differential diagnosis which includes processes affecting the large or small bowel, the genitourinary system, major arteries (e.g. ruptured iliac aneurysms) and abdominal wall (e.g. rectus sheath haematoma). Initial clinical assessment of the extent of peritoneal inflammation may be misleading and overestimate it. Once patient anxiety is relieved following resuscitation and analgesia, an apparently diffuse process often becomes more localised. In a minority of patients there are clinical and radiological signs of generalised peritonitis and systemic sepsis, but even then the indications for operation are not absolute.[37] In all patients a vigorous trial of conservative therapy is initially appropriate with surgical intervention reserved for those who fail to improve.

Fistula

The potential exists for fistulation between an inflamed diverticulum and any adjacent viscus. Although fistulas have been described between

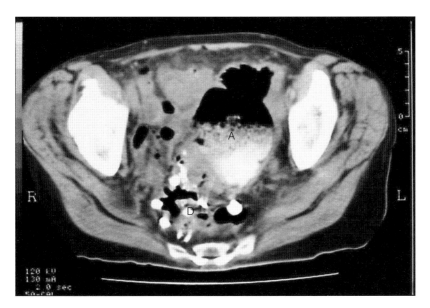

Figure 8.3 • CT scan showing large abscess (A) secondary to sigmoid diverticular disease (D).

colon and appendix, ovarian tube, uterus, ureter, skin and both large and small bowel, the most common are colovesical and colovaginal.[38] The latter may be more common after hysterectomy.[39] When a pericolic abscess, usually at the apex of the sigmoid colon, adheres to and subsequently ruptures into the vault of the bladder, a vesicocolic fistula results, with the typical symptoms of urinary tract infection and pneumaturia. Whilst sigmoid diverticular disease is the most likely cause, Crohn's disease and colon and bladder cancer must be excluded.

Abscess

Patients with pericolic, pelvic or mesocolic abscesses secondary to diverticular disease usually present with signs of localised lower abdominal sepsis and systemic upset. Although a classical pelvic abscess palpable through the anterior rectal wall may be clinically obvious, most diverticular abscesses are detected on computed tomography (CT) scanning (**Fig. 8.3**) or contrast enema (**Fig. 8.4**). In some patients the development of an abscess is more insidious and identified only in retrospect by outpatient barium enema.

Haemorrhage

Bleeding from colonic diverticular disease is characteristically painless and profuse, with the colour depending on the level of bleeding in the colon. Bleeding from the left side of the colon presents as

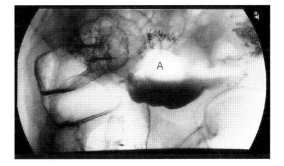

Figure 8.4 • Contrast enema showing a large abscess (A) with a gas–fluid level secondary to diverticular disease.

bright red blood with clots, whereas that arising on the right side is often darker and plum-coloured. Colonic bleeding is rarely exsanguinating, although it may be repeated or persistent requiring transfusion and ultimately operation.[40]

Obstruction

Patients with left-sided colonic obstruction due to fibrous stricturing in the sigmoid colon present in a manner identical to that due to the progressive obstruction developing in a carcinoma. If obstruction is complete, investigation and management are essentially identical and depend on the demonstration of typical features on plain abdominal radiographs with confirmation of the site of the obstruction on an urgent contrast study. The differentiation between a malignant and a benign stricture may be suspected on the radiological features but is normally confirmed only after resection, examination of the opened bowel and subsequent histology.

Intestinal obstruction also results from adhesion of loops of small bowel to an inflammatory mass in the pelvis and occasionally the features of small bowel obstruction are more striking than those of the initiating colonic pathology.[41]

Investigation

Acute diverticulitis/abscess

Clinical features in patients with mild disease may permit management with only minimal investigation.[42,43] Plain abdomen and chest radiography often provide indirect evidence of major inflammation, the most obvious being a pneumoperitoneum. However, the demonstration of a small amount of subdiaphragmatic gas, a traditional sign of generalised peritonitis, is not an absolute indication for operation[37] and management should be based on the clinical assessment of the patient, not the radiology. Occasionally soft tissue changes, including evidence of obstruction, thickening of bowel wall and extraluminal masses, suggest acute diverticulitis.

Digital rectal examination but not sigmoidoscopy is essential before an emergency contrast study. However, sigmoidoscopy is mandatory before laparotomy and patient discomfort is minimised if this is performed under general anaesthesia before opening the abdomen. Sigmoidoscopy is necessary to exclude anorectal conditions that might influence the proposed operation, the most important of which is a coincidental rectal neoplasm.

When the clinical features do not require immediate laparotomy, it is necessary actively to confirm the provisional diagnosis of acute diverticulitis and exclude alternative diagnoses to avoid prolonging inappropriate therapy. There has been a major shift towards spiral CT with bowel contrast when investigating possible acute diverticulitis (Figs 8.3 and **8.5**).

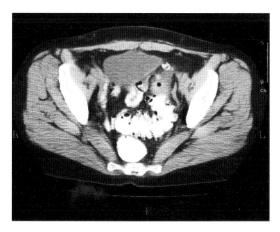

Figure 8.5 • CT scan of pelvis showing contrast in the colonic lumen and sigmoid diverticula.

Concerns about exposure to ionising radiation, particularly if usage is 'early and frequent',[44] must be set against the quality of images and impact on management.

If access to spiral CT is limited, a water-soluble contrast enema remains a practical alternative. A contrast enema may show thickening, mucosal oedema, irregularity and extravasation of contrast (Fig. 8.4). Extravasation, if present, is usually localised, but free perforation into the peritoneal cavity may be seen. The examination should be limited to confirming the diagnosis, and possible synchronous pathology must subsequently be excluded by formal colonoscopy or barium enema in the convalescent period. It is important to remember that the information derived from an urgent enema, although valuable in determining management, cannot be considered definitive. The possibility of carcinoma coexistent with the inflammatory mass or elsewhere in the colon must be excluded after resolution of the acute episode (**Fig. 8.6**). Indeed, when the left colon is excised as an emergency for presumed diverticular disease, a colon cancer may be found within the mass in 20–25% of cases.[29]

The threshold for requesting CT varies between clinicians, so suspected acute diverticulitis was confirmed in only 43% (64 of 150 patients) in one series,[44] compared with 66–77% in others.[45,46]

 Despite the poor evidence base,[17] the arguments in favour of CT over ultrasound or single-contrast enema are persuasive.[31]

 Specificity is high, greater than 97%,[44] and alternative pathology can be shown, explaining why CT is now the first-line investigation.

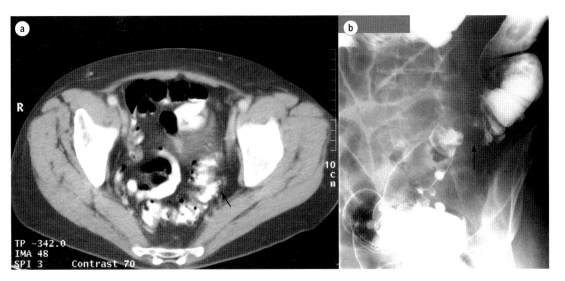

Figure 8.6 • **(a)** CT scan showing diverticulitis and colonic wall abnormality. **(b)** Subsequent barium enema showing carcinoma within diverticular disease.

Radiologists are undecided about the relative merits of rectal or oral contrast. The former can be performed rapidly and will confirm extravasation, whereas the latter requires 48 hours delay but yields extra information as it opacifies the small bowel.

CT aids diagnosis, but its impact on management is less striking. Extravasation of contrast on either enema[47] or CT[48] increases the chance of early surgery, but of itself is not an absolute indication for operation. Between 1990 and 1999 the routine first investigation in our unit was a water-soluble contrast enema, with CT reserved for patients for whom management was not adequately clarified: the overall operation rate was 15% (**Fig. 8.7**), being somewhat less than the 24% reported when CT is used as routine or the national average of 23% for England and Wales.[49] CT does detect more abscesses than would otherwise be diagnosed, but only a minority of these require intervention.[48]

Ultrasound scanning has been employed effectively in some centres, but the variability of interpretation and dependence on operator skill reduces its general applicability as the first investigation. When the surgical staff themselves deliver ultrasound, then it significantly enhances diagnostic accuracy.[50]

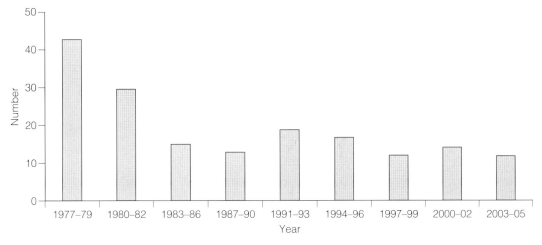

Figure 8.7 • Percentage of patients admitted with acute diverticulitis undergoing surgery during their emergency admission.

Sonography has a role in monitoring the progression of known abscesses or masses.

Contrast enema, CT and ultrasound scanning are looking for different things in acute diverticulitis. A contrast enema will show intraluminal changes and leakage of contrast, but may underestimate extramural disease; even so, sensitivity is high (approximately 90%).[51] CT and ultrasound are better at demonstrating bowel wall thickening, non-communicating abscesses and extraluminal disease than a contrast enema. Nevertheless, the overall impact on patient management should be similar, so the selection of imaging modality can justifiably reflect local expertise and facilities. All imaging investigations must be interpreted within the patient's clinical context to minimise unnecessary intervention.

Obstruction

If left-sided colonic obstruction is suspected on plain abdominal radiography, a single-contrast enema will help determine the level of obstruction and exclude pseudo-obstruction.

Fistula

Barium enema is often sufficient to diagnose the underlying pathology in patients with a colovesical fistula, although to exclude carcinoma may require biopsy, necessitating flexible endoscopy and cystoscopy. But increasingly a CT scan is used as the first investigation and may reveal some of the rarer fistulas. Colovaginal fistula is much more common if a patient has had a prior hysterectomy and rigid sigmoidoscopy of the vagina or a vaginal fistulogram may be more sensitive.[39]

Haemorrhage

Continuing or repeated episodes of bleeding require urgent mesenteric angiography, which should include visualisation of both the superior and inferior mesenteric circulation. Demonstration of a bleeding point (**Fig. 8.8**) permits targeted resection[40] limited to one-half of the colon, rather than blind subtotal colectomy. When angiography fails to identify the source of bleeding or has not been possible to arrange before surgery, on-table colonic irrigation with colonoscopy may identify the source and avoid subtotal colectomy. Passage of the colonoscope per

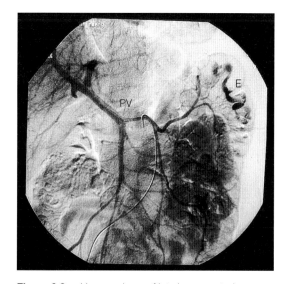

Figure 8.8 • Venous phase of interior mesenteric angiography with the portal vein (PV) labelled and extravasation of contrast into the colonic lumen (E) secondary to bleeding from a diverticulum at the splenic flexure.

anum and advancement to the caecum is straightforward when the abdomen is open and the instrument can be directed by the operating surgeon. Furthermore, transillumination of the colon may show the characteristic features of angiodysplasia. In a debilitated patient unfit for resection there may be a role for endoscopic haemostasis in some cases, but only if the bleeding diverticulum can be identified.[52] Embolisation of bleeding colonic lesions risks infarction of the colonic wall.

Management

Different places and healthcare systems manage diverticular disease differently. Yesterday's heresy evolves into current convention, with increasing conservatism in some institutions contrasting with high rates of surgery in others. Whereas individual and institutional interest, and possibly wealth, can positively influence the rate of treatment, lack of resource may be a subtle brake. Optimal patient selection and timing of surgery remains contentious, so the proportion of cases operated on as emergencies or electively varies widely. Unlike colonic cancer, where surgery almost automatically follows diagnosis, relatively few patients with sigmoid diverticular disease need surgery, and the boundary between those who need an operation and those who do not is imprecise. This means that decision-making is difficult, requiring experience and judgement. Although diverticular disease is often perceived to be a common problem, a recent prospective audit from 30 UK hospitals indicated that on average only 10 patients with complicated diverticular disease were admitted to each unit over a 4-year period.[6] An individual consultant general surgeon, therefore, is unlikely to admit more than two or three patients with the more severe forms of acute diverticulitis in a year. Accumulating and maintaining experience is difficult for both trainee and consultant.

Elective

In the absence of complications, elective surgery is reserved for so-called failed medical treatment with persistent pain. However, careful follow-up after elective resection for uncomplicated sigmoid diverticular disease reveals continuing symptoms in a quarter of patients,[35] which probably reflects an underlying problem in gut motility, sigmoid diverticula simply being the most easily demonstrated abnormality. The possibility of postoperative symptoms should be explained to patients before surgery is considered.

 Recent evidence[8,18] questions whether elective resection is indeed necessary after one or more episodes of acute inflammation requiring hospital admission.

There are accumulating data that major complications are likeliest during the first acute episode, that only a minority of patients continue to have symptoms or further acute episodes, and that the risk of emergency Hartmann's after an acute episode is 1 in 2000 patient-years.[18] Surgery should not automatically follow one or more acute episodes in the absence of ongoing symptoms secondary to repeated sepsis or obstruction due to stricture formation. The increased morbidity and mortality observed in immunosuppressed[53] patients may be a reason for accepting a lower threshold for elective surgery in this group. Whilst sigmoid colectomy for 'uncomplicated' diverticular disease is straightforward at either laparotomy or laparoscopy, a fibrotic mass fused to the pelvic wall often incorporating the ureter can be a different proposition.

Fit patients with a colovesical fistula should undergo surgery, but in the old and infirm an initial trial of conservative management may be worthwhile. Formal resection of the affected colon is essential and pedicled greater omentum should be interposed between the colorectal anastomosis and the bladder defect. The fistulous opening in the bladder wall is usually too small to require suture and catheter drainage is all that is required. Fistula recurrence is rare unless the sigmoid colon is not resected but simply detached with repair of the fistulous opening, in which case there is an unacceptably high recurrence rate of the order of 30–50%.

The extent of resection depends on the extent of the diverticular disease but should never be less than a formal sigmoid colectomy with anastomosis of the colon to the upper rectum. The distal resection must include all the affected colon, for without this the incidence of recurrent disease is unacceptably high. Resection of the entire left colon is required when this is extensively involved, but the occasional diverticulum placed more proximally can be ignored. When there is pancolonic involvement by diverticular disease the aetiology is different to acquired sigmoid diverticular disease and the reasons for operation need to be clear. Subtotal colectomy with ileorectal anastomosis for diverticular disease is rarely indicated.

Emergency

Surgery should be used to control peritoneal sepsis that is overwhelming or has failed to respond to best medical management (Box 8.1). Emergency management may be summarised by answering three questions: when to operate, when to resect and when to anastomose?

When to operate

This is the most difficult of the three questions. When abdominal signs are localised to the left lower

Box 8.1 • Surgical options in perforated diverticulitis

Conservative

Laparoscopic lavage plus drainage
Laparotomy with or without suture, with or without drainage, with or without proximal stoma
Exteriorisation of sigmoid loop

Radical

Resection without anastomosis (Hartmann's procedure)
Resection plus anastomosis
Resection plus anastomosis plus proximal stoma

quadrant and systemic upset is limited, few would advocate urgent surgery. At the other extreme, when there is widespread evidence of peritonitis and free gas, urgent operation for generalised peritonitis of unknown origin would generally be advocated. For the remainder a policy of vigorous resuscitation and antibiotic therapy is appropriate. It is remarkable how rapidly patients with extensive signs of peritoneal contamination can improve on such a regimen. We have successfully managed patients with pneumoperitoneum without an operation,[37] either because clinical improvement was rapid or the risk of surgery unacceptable.

Optimal management demands serial assessment, ideally by the same observer. A trial of conservative management requires a readiness to review the decision not to operate in the light of the evolving clinical response. A trial of conservative management is allowed for up to 3 days before deciding on surgery. Although imaging plays an important role, in contrast to North American practice abscesses are rarely drained percutaneously. The majority of those less than 5 cm in diameter resolve on conservative measures.[48] Although extravasation of contrast on imaging increases the likelihood of surgery during the emergency admission, it is not of itself an absolute indication for urgent operation.[47,48] We initiated a conservative policy in the early 1980s with a sustained reduction (Fig. 8.7) in the frequency of urgent operation for sigmoid diverticular disease over the last 25 years, and a continuing low overall and postoperative mortality.[54]

Diagnostic laparoscopy in the acute setting is unnecessary if the diagnosis is confident. Therapeutic laparoscopy, on the other hand, seems an exciting innovation.

 Initial scepticism of small series[55] of highly selected patients[56] treated by laparoscopic peritoneal lavage describing favourable outcomes has been tempered by the publication of two recent studies[57,58] of patients with generalised and faecal peritonitis. Both these papers suggest that laparotomy can be avoided in the majority of patients with a lower overall morbidity and mortality than is currently reported.[59]

When to resect

With good indications for surgery, resection of the sigmoid has been popular.

 The original review of surgery – i.e. laparotomy, for generalised and faecal peritonitis (Hinchey stages III and IV) – confirmed increased survival if the perforated colon was resected rather than left in situ, relying on drainage and/or proximal colostomy[29] (**Fig. 8.9**).

Whilst this review is now somewhat dated, critical analysis of all subsequent publications including the two randomised studies confirms that when contamination is worst resection improves survival.[13,14] This is why the clear recommendation is to resect the sigmoid colon if laparotomy is necessary. The recent publication by Myers et al.[58] does appear to indicate that preliminary laparoscopy to identify only those with a communicating, free colonic

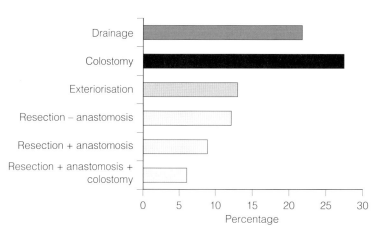

Figure 8.9 • Mortality following conservative and radical surgery for generalised and faecal peritonitis (Hinchey stages III and IV).

perforation who will need laparotomy will reduce the need for laparotomy further.

More problematic is when surgery has been performed prematurely, or where the diagnosis is unexpected, the latter usually resulting from misdiagnosis as gynaecological or appendicular sepsis. Increasingly, however, with the wider use of laparoscopy in assessing the acute abdomen, an inflamed left colon may be found with a variable degree of peritoneal inflammatory response. In these circumstances it is reasonable to avoid resection and rely on postoperative antibiotics, which usually leads to rapid resolution. The alternative choices of stoma formation, drainage or resection are unwarranted. Obsolete surgical dogma might dictate resection to eliminate the source of peritoneal contamination, but this exposes an elderly or compromised patient to a prolonged procedure with a major bowel resection and often a stoma, which itself may prove permanent. Although presented as life-saving by some, the mortality, morbidity, inconvenience and potential for a second major laparotomy for re-anastomosis makes non-resection the much more attractive option in this situation.

With a policy of conservative management with urgent investigation whenever possible, the problem of operating on an inflamed but non-perforated colon rarely arises. Every surgeon with an emergency commitment should be aware that such a conservative option is not only available but preferable.

When to anastomose

Given the above decisions on when to operate and when to resect, when to anastomose requires experience and judgement. In the last quarter of the 20th century considerations of safety led to advocacy of Hartmann's procedure as the safest option in managing left-sided colonic emergencies. Immediate resection without anastomosis eradicates the source of sepsis but without the risk of anastomotic leakage. However, it brings its own peculiar set of problems. Anastomotic avoidance means that a stoma will be required along with closure or exteriorisation of the rectal stump. These manoeuvres demand similar levels of technical skill to anastomosis in unfavourable circumstances. A left iliac fossa colostomy brought out under tension can result in complications as problematic as a

poor anastomosis. Breakdown of the suture line on the rectal stump can lead to significant peritonitis, particularly if the intraperitoneal portion is long and packed with stool.

Widespread experience with immediate anastomosis after resection for the obstructed colon has led to its increasing use in patients after resection for perforated diverticulitis. In our hands the majority of patients now have a primary anastomosis.[37] However, anastomoses should only be made in a fully resuscitated patient, with competent anaesthesia and a surgeon proficient in colorectal anastomoses. The increasing use of primary anastomosis probably reflects improvements in perioperative care and supervision which anticipate and treat cardiovascular instability and hypoxaemia promptly, promoting anastomotic healing in the critical first 48 hours after surgery.

 The recent systematic review comparing outcomes following primary resection and anastomosis (PRA) and Hartmann's procedure in non-elective surgery for acute diverticulitis[59] confirms the earlier observation[29] that mortality after PRA is less. Following emergency surgery mortality after PRA was 7.4% and Hartmann's 15.6%. Interestingly these results have not improved over the intervening 25 years.

It is not plausible that PRA enhances recovery, so these differences reflect selection of patients unlikely to leak. There is little attraction in making a proximal 'covering' stoma following the type of high colorectal anastomosis fashioned in these circumstances. When conditions are suboptimal, considerations of safety should still override surgical enthusiasm and anastomosis should be deferred.

Haemorrhage

Strenuous efforts should be made preoperatively to localise the site either by colonoscopy, angiography if actively bleeding, or by labelled red cell scan if less acute. When this fails, perioperative colonoscopy should be attempted. If a bleeding point still cannot be found and thus targeted resection is not possible then 'blind' subtotal colectomy must be performed. When this is necessary the patient's condition is usually parlous and it is unwise to perform an ileorectal anastomosis.[40] Completion of the operation by ileostomy and closure of the rectal stump is the prudent option. The possibility of subsequent restoration of bowel continuity can be considered later.

Recommendations

 Rapid resolution of apparently extensive peritoneal contamination follows vigorous conservative management with fluid resuscitation, appropriate monitoring and systemic antibiotics, and represents routine practice for most patients.

Conservative management

Although single antibiotic agents may be as effective as combination therapy, none has been shown to be superior and most are more expensive. A tailored response reflecting the degree of contamination has proved successful over the years. A combination of oral metronidazole and trimethoprim is effective against both aerobic and anaerobic organisms and is used for less severe episodes. For major sepsis, combination therapy is favoured: gentamicin (7 mg/kg i.v. once daily) for rapid bactericidal activity against Gram-negative coliform organisms, and metronidazole (500 mg i.v. t.i.d.) for anaerobic organisms. The requirements for activity against enterococci and the use of a penicillin derivative remain unconvincing and are not essential in first-line therapy. Suitable alternative combinations include metronidazole and cefuroxime/cefotaxime or single agents like coamoxiclav, imipenem or cefoxitin.[36]

Although antibiotics are the mainstay of conservative therapy, they must always be instituted before operation: the dramatic impact of systemic antibiotics on reducing the viable bacterial population in peritonitis is well documented.[60]

Operative strategy

Preparation of the patient undergoing laparotomy for advanced intraperitoneal sepsis requires thorough clinical assessment, fluid resuscitation and antibiotics supplemented by appropriate monitoring, which must continue through the postoperative period. We have been impressed by the reported results of laparoscopic lavage in Hinchey stage III patients and provided suitable expertise is available would now recommend preliminary laparoscopy, with a view to avoiding laparotomy and resection, including laparoscopic resection, altogether. There will remain an increasingly small cohort of patients with generalised peritonitis or those who have failed

to respond to more conservative measures in whom laparotomy is unavoidable.

Incision

A midline incision for its simplicity, reliability of mass closure and low wound infection rate is used.[61] The skin incision is to the right of the umbilicus so as not to interfere with a left-sided stoma. Mechanical precautions that minimise contamination of the abdominal parietes from infected intraperitoneal material include wound towels, plastic ring wound protector and institution of a 'red danger towel' technique. Contamination of the abdominal parietes should be minimised by elevating the abdominal wall and aspirating pus and contaminated peritoneal fluid through a small incision in the peritoneum before it percolates over and inoculates the wound.

There are only disadvantages to a short incision in this situation, not least of which is failure to appreciate and document accurately the extent of peritoneal and colonic disease. Restricted exposure and access lead to inadequate surgery with incomplete peritoneal toilet and lavage and limited colonic mobilisation. Thorough access to all quadrants of the abdomen permits accurate assessment and classification of contamination. Inexperience, a desire to justify the decision to operate and anticipation of an unfavourable outcome are common reasons for over-reporting the severity of peritoneal sepsis.

Although the operation is for presumed benign disease, there is little place for wedge excision of a few centimetres of sigmoid colon. Mobilisation of the left colon should be equivalent to a radical cancer operation with routine (although not invariable) mobilisation of the splenic flexure for tension-free formation of a stoma or anastomosis. Preservation of the inferior mesenteric artery to the rectal stump is logical when cancer has been excluded. The limit of proximal resection of the colon is dictated by the extent of inflammation and presence of arterial pulsation at the point of division. The distal resection is always to the upper rectum.

If there is gross faecal loading of the colon, this should be evacuated, even when Hartmann's procedure is chosen, to avoid stercoral perforation and obstruction proximal to a stoma. Access to the rectum is required in emergency left-sided colonic procedures. The rectum should be routinely washed out per anum as a prophylactic measure to reduce the risk of leakage from a closed rectal stump and in case a cancer has been unknowingly resected.

Hartmann's procedure

If conditions preclude safe anastomosis, the divided left colon is brought out through a trephined wound in the left lower quadrant, selecting a flat area of the abdomen and preferably emerging through the rectus abdominis. Parastomal herniation may thereby be reduced. Whenever possible the best site should be marked preoperatively. Avoiding closure of the lateral space simplifies both the operation and subsequent reconstitution of bowel continuity. Closure of the rectal stump can be accomplished by cross-stapling or suturing, although my experience (including closure of the rectal stump after total colectomy for inflammatory bowel disease) suggests fewer leaks in sutured cases. A single layer of continuous 2/0 or 3/0 serosubmucosal monofilament absorbable suture is supplemented with two long non-absorbable sutures at the lateral ends to aid future identification of the rectal stump.

Immediate anastomosis

There is debate about the need for mechanical preparation of the colon, but on-table colonic irrigation achieves near perfect cleansing and has aesthetic appeal. The appendix, or if absent the terminal ileum, is intubated with a Foley catheter. In the absence of a custom collection device, a short section of sterilised corrugated anaesthetic tubing is inserted into the colon proximal to the diseased area and tied in place with nylon tape. This is conveniently connected to a laparoscopic camera sheath to conduct and contain the effluent.

The advantages of radical resection are that unexpected malignancy has been appropriately treated and healthy bowel is obtained for potential anastomosis. After irrigation and division of the rectum between the sacral promontory and peritoneal reflection, and after division of the proximal colon, an open single-layer serosubmucosal end-to-end colorectal anastomosis is made with interrupted 3/0 sutures. I see no place for proximal 'defunctioning' stomata in anastomoses at this level.

Antibiotic policy

For many years it was the practice to lavage the peritoneal cavity and abdominal parietes with tetracycline solution because of the low wound and intraperitoneal infection rates.[61] Difficulty obtaining a suitable parenteral preparation of tetracycline has forced a change to cefotaxime as the lavage agent (1 mg/mL 0.9% saline). This has been used for many years in local paediatric practice with comparable results and continuing audit has confirmed equivalence in adults. The midline incision is closed with a continuous mass suture with 1-polydioxanone and further lavage of the subcutaneous space precedes primary skin closure. This strategy, even in such 'dirty' surgery, is associated with a low wound infection rate and delayed primary closure is not required at a first laparotomy. Postoperative antibiotics are continued for only 3 days, provided peritoneal contamination has been eliminated. Gentamicin levels are checked once daily and if systemic sepsis persists beyond 3 days bacteriology and sensitivities from cultures taken at operation will be available to direct a change of antibiotics.

Controversies

Timing of emergency surgery

If all patients with sigmoid diverticular disease were destined to come to operation, a case could be made for early scheduled intervention with, preferably, a single-stage procedure during the acute admission if it could be accomplished with low mortality and morbidity. However, urgent operation is required increasingly infrequently and the majority of patients do not experience significant recurrent complications over the next 10 years[54,62] to justify resection (**Fig. 8.10**). An excessively interventional approach, whether born

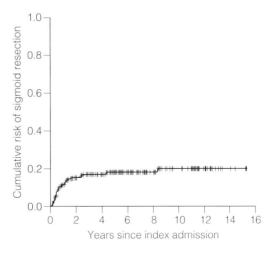

Figure 8.10 • Risk of sigmoid resection following emergency admission with acute diverticulitis in 232 patients.

of enthusiasm or inexperience, can result in the accumulation of a large series of patients treated surgically with low mortality and morbidity and a high rate of single-stage procedures. Perhaps selecting patients with mild disease has fuelled the novelty of a laparoscopic approach. It is likely that substantial numbers of patients with moderate diverticular inflammation are subjected to surgery in the belief, albeit misplaced, that this is life-saving. Consequently data may be produced that support conservative surgery in the management of complicated diverticulitis, yet not performing an operation at all may have been just as effective. Proper interpretation of such accounts requires knowledge of the number of patients managed non-operatively during the study period.

Radical versus conservative procedures

It is noteworthy that, although indirect evidence supports the concept that elimination of the source of sepsis (by resection) in the most severe forms of peritonitis is historically associated with lower mortality,[29] the two randomised comparative trials comparing primary resection with proximal stoma formation and drainage showed a lower mortality in the conservative group,[13,14] with the proviso that the few patients with Hinchey stage IV disease did better with resection.

Primary anastomosis

The role of primary resection and anastomosis during an emergency admission is increasingly being promoted,[59] even in the presence of diffuse or faecal peritonitis.[63] It remains controversial and should be used selectively when circumstances are favourable and not a misguided marker of surgical virtuosity.

 Opinion is divided on the need for surgery following conservative management of an acute episode of diverticulitis. Ambrosetti refined the argument by demonstrating a relation between the severity of the episode as judged on CT scan with the risk of delayed complications. Patients categorised as 'mild' have a risk of recurrent episodes of 14% while 'severe' forms have a risk of 39%.[48] The corollary of this useful observation, however, is that the majority of patients do not suffer a further attack. It is our experience that the long-term risk of requiring

sigmoid resection is low if surgery is not required during or shortly after the index admission (Fig. 8.10). The variability of the acute disease and the wide spectrum of patients affected precludes categorical statements and exercise of clinical judgement remains appropriate. For the majority simple observation and reassurance that a life-threatening recurrence is unlikely is appropriate.[8,18]

Subsequent elective surgery

There is a view that the risk of subsequent episodes in younger patients (variably defined as less than 40 or 50 years of age) is of the order of 25%, but this is then interpreted as either confirming the need for elective surgery[10] or indicating that the majority of patients will not require operation and all should be managed conservatively.[64] Ambrosetti reported a recurrence rate of 60% for young patients with an initial severe episode of sepsis, with even the mild form carrying a 23% risk of further complications.[48] Although such a high risk of recurrence is not universal and the severity of the presenting episode may be more important than the age,[65] it is not unreasonable to discuss elective resection with a patient under the age of 50 years following a severe episode of diverticulitis with continuing symptoms and serious structural changes in the colon.

Any patient admitted twice with acute sepsis should be considered for operation, having taken account of coincidental risk factors. There is some evidence that long-term administration of a poorly absorbed antibiotic and mesalazine may reduce the frequency and severity of episodes of diverticular inflammation,[66] which might be an option to consider in a poor-risk patient. Similarly, increased admission rates in patients on NSAIDs implies critical reassessment of their need in the elderly.

Role of laparoscopic surgery

Laparoscopy is increasingly advocated for both elective and emergency surgery for diverticular disease.[67] There is now ample evidence that the sigmoid colon can be resected laparoscopically in the elective setting. However, the need for the operation in uncomplicated cases, which comprise the vast majority of published series – indeed, 1353 (88%) of 1545 laparoscopic resections in the largest German series[68] – must be questionable. Perhaps predictably the risk of conversion to open surgery is much higher in complicated (61%) than in uncomplicated (14%) cases.[69] Some papers have addressed the comparative costs of laparoscopic surgery for diverticular disease but there has been no sophisticated health economic analysis to support or refute a wholesale change to this approach. Nevertheless, when successful a laparoscopic resection for sigmoid diverticular disease appears to be associated with the usual short-term benefits of shorter hospitalisation and convalescence that follow laparoscopic surgery.[70] There are no randomised trials comparing quality of life in patients with either complicated or uncomplicated diverticular disease treated surgically or medically to inform decision-making.

However, what is new and exciting is the impact of early therapeutic laparoscopy in patients with Hinchey stage III and IV disease. The prospect of a reduced requirement not only for emergency laparotomy with its consequent mortality and morbidity but also the low rate of subsequent resection is enticing, but needs validation.

Conclusion

The threshold for elective surgery for diverticular disease lacks definition and the suspicion exists that surgical preference is the major determinant. The management of complicated acute diverticulitis demands even more thoughtful clinical appraisal, appropriate imaging and a surgical strategy that combines conservatism before operation with a radical approach once committed to laparotomy if low mortality and morbidity are to be achieved.

Key points

- Sigmoid diverticular disease is common.
- Emergency admission is uncommon.
- Contrast CT scan is the best emergency investigation.
- Urgent operation is required in less than 20% of emergency admissions.
- Abscesses less than 5 cm in diameter usually resolve with antibiotics alone.
- In generalised peritonitis laparoscopic lavage should be considered.
- If laparotomy is required resection is the best option.
- Primary anastomosis is safe in selected cases.
- Elective resection should be offered to symptomatic patients.

References

1. Chia JG, Wilde CC, Ngoi SS et al. Trends of diverticular disease of the large bowel in a newly developed country. Dis Colon Rectum 1991; 34: 498–501.

2 Loffeld RJLF, van der Putten ABMM. Diverticular disease of the colon and concomitant abnormalities in patients undergoing endoscopic evaluation of the large bowel. Colorectal Disease 2002; 4:189–192.

3. Pohlman T. Diverticulitis. Gastrointest Clin North Am 1988; 17:357–85.

4. Almy TP, Howell DA. Diverticular disease of the colon. N Engl J Med 1980; 302:325–31.

5. Parks TG. Natural history of diverticular disease of the colon. Clin Gastroenterol 1975; 4:53–69.

6. Tudor RG, Farmakis N, Keighley MRB. National audit of complicated diverticular disease: analysis of index cases. Br J Surg 1994; 81:730–2.

7. Laurell H, Hansson L-E, Gunnarson U. Acute diverticulitis – clinical presentation and differential diagnostics. Colorectal Dis 2007; 9:496–502.

8. Peppas G, Bliziotis IA, Oikonomaki D et al. Outcomes after medical and surgical treatment of diverticulitis: a systematic review of the available evidence. JK Gastroenterol Hepatol 2007; 22:1360–8.

9. Simpson J, Scholefield JH, Spiller RC. Origin of symptoms in diverticular disease. Br J Surg 2003; 90:899–908.

10. Farmakis N, Tudor RG, Keighley MRB. The 5-year natural history of complicated diverticular disease. Br J Surg 1994; 81:733–5.

11. Schoetz DJ. Uncomplicated diverticulitis: indications for surgery and surgical management. Surg Clin North Am 1993; 73:965–74.

12 O'Kelly TJ, Krukowski ZH. Acute diverticulitis. Non-operative management. In: Schein M, Wise L (eds) Crucial controversies in surgery. Lippincott, Williams & Wilkins, 1999; Vol. 3, pp. 109–16.

13. Kronborg O. Treatment of perforated sigmoid diverticulitis: a prospective randomised trial. Br J Surg 1993; 80:505–7.

14. Zeitoun G, Laurent A, Rouffet F et al. Multicentre, randomized clinical trial of primary versus secondary sigmoid resection in generalized peritonitis complicating sigmoid diverticulitis. Br J Surg 2000; 87:1366–74.

15. Wong WD, Wexner SD, Lowry A et al. Practice parameters for the treatment of sigmoid diverticulitis – supporting documentation. Dis Colon Rectum 2000; 43:290–7.

16. Kohler L, Sauerland S, Neugebauer E. Diagnosis and treatment of diverticular disease: results of a consensus development conference. Surg Endosc 1999; 13:430–6.

17. Liljegren G, Chabok A, Wickbom M et al. Acute colonic diverticulitis: a systematic review of diagnostic accuracy. Colorectal Dis 2007; 9:480–8.

18. Janes S, Meagher A, Frizelle FA. Elective surgery after acute diverticulitis. Br J Surg 2005; 92: 133–42.

19. Simpson J, Scholefield JH, Spiller RC. Pathogenesis of colonic diverticula. Br J Surg 2002; 89:546–54.

20. Painter NS, Burkitt DP. Diverticular disease of the colon, a 20th century problem. Clin Gastroenterol 1975; 4:3–22.

21. Whiteway J, Morson BC. Elastosis in diverticular disease of the sigmoid colon. Gut 1985; 26: 258–66.

22. Wess L, Eastwood MA, Wess TJ et al. Cross linkage of collagen is increased in colonic diverticulosis. Gut 1995; 37:91–4.

23. Aldoori WH, Giovannucci EL, Rimm EB et al. Prospective study of physical activity and the risk of symptomatic diverticular disease in men. Gut 1995; 36:276–82.

24. Papagrigoriadis S, Macey L, Bourantas N et al. Smoking may be associated with complications of diverticular disease. Br J Surg 1999; 86:923–6.

25. Campbell K, Steele RJ. Non-steroidal anti-inflammatory drugs and complicated diverticular disease: a case control study. Br J Surg 1991; 78: 190–1.

26. Burroughs SH, Bowrey DJ, Morris-Stiff GJ et al. Granulomatous inflammation in sigmoid diverticulitis: two diseases or one? Histopathology 1998; 33:349–53.

27. Gledhill A, Dixon MF. Crohn's-like reaction in diverticular disease. Gut 1998; 42:392–5.

28. Killingback M. Management of perforated diverticulitis. Surg Clin North Am 1983; 63: 97–115.

29. Krukowski ZH, Matheson NA. Emergency surgery for diverticular disease complicated by generalized and faecal peritonitis: a review. Br J Surg 1984; 71: 921–7.

30. Hinchey EJ, Schaal PG, Richards GK. Treatment of perforated diverticular disease of the colon. Adv Surg 1978; 12:85–109.

31. Ambrosetti P, Becker P, Terrier F. Colonic diverticulitis: impact of imaging on surgical management – a prospective study of 542 patients. Eur Radiol 2002; 12:1145–9.

32. Hansen O, Stock W. Prophylaktische Operation bei der Divertikelkrankheit des Kolons – Stufenkonzept durch exakte Stadienteiloung. Langenbeck's Arch Chir Suppl 199; II:1257.

33. Haglund U, Hellberg R, Johnsen C et al. Complicated diverticular disease of the sigmoid colon: an analysis of short and long term outcome in 392 patients. Ann Chir Gynaecol 1979; 68:41–6.

34. Simpson J, Neal KR, Scholefield JH et al. Patterns of pain in diverticular disease and the influence of acute diverticulitis. Eur J Gastroenterol Hepatol 2003; 15:1005–10.

35. Munson KD, Hensien MA, Jacob LN et al. Diverticulitis: a comprehensive follow-up. Dis Colon Rectum 1996; 39:318–22.

36. Kellum JM, Sugerman HJ, Coppa JF et al. Randomized prospective comparison of cefoxitin and gentamicin/clindamycin in the treatment of acute colonic diverticulitis. Clin Ther 1992; 14:376–84.

37. Shaikh S, Krukowski ZH, O'Kelly TJ. Conservative management of pneumoperitoneum secondary to complicated sigmoid diverticulitis: a prospective observational study. Colorectal Dis 2006; 8(Suppl 4):115–16.

38. Vasilevsky CA, Belliveau P, Trudel JL et al. Fistulas complicating diverticulitis. Int J Colorectal Dis 1998; 13:57–60.

39. Tancer ML, Veridiano NP. Genital fistulas caused by diverticular disease of the sigmoid colon. Am J Obst Gynecol 1996; 174:1547–50.

40. McGuire HH. Bleeding colonic diverticula. A reappraisal of natural history and management. Ann Surg 1994; 220:653–6.

41. Kim AY, Bennett GL, Bashist B et al. Small bowel obstruction associated with sigmoid diverticulitis. Am J Roentgenol 1998; 170:1311–13.

42. Rege RV, Nahrwold DL. Diverticular disease. Curr Probl Surg 1989; 26:128–32.

43. Thompson DA, Bailey HR. Management of acute diverticulitis with abscess. Semin Colon Rectal Surg 1990; 1:74–80.

44. Rao PM. CT of diverticulitis and alternative conditions. Semin Ultrasound CT MR 1999; 20: 86–93.

45. Eggesbo HB, Jacobsen T, Kolmannskog F et al. Diagnosis of acute left sided colonic diverticulitis by three radiological modalities. Acta Radiol 1998; 39:315–21.

46. Brengman ML, Otchy DP. Timing of computed tomography in acute diverticulitis. Dis Colon Rectum 1998; 41:1023–8.

47. Kourtesis GL, Williams RA, Wilson SE. Acute diverticulitis. Safety and value of contrast studies

in predicting need for operation. Aust NZ J Surg 1988; 58:801–4.

48 Ambrosetti P. Diverticulitis of the left colon. In: Taylor I, Johnson CD (eds) Recent advances in surgery. 1997; Vol. 20, pp. 145–60.

49. Kang JY, Hoare J, Tinto A et al. Diverticular disease of the colon – on the rise: a study of hospital admissions in England between 1989/1990 and 1999/2000. Aliment Pharmacol Ther 2003; 17:1189–95.

50. Schwerk WB, Schwarz S, Rothmund M. Sonography in acute colonic diverticulitis: a prospective study. Dis Colon Rectum 1992; 35:1077–84.

51. Smith TR, Cho KC, Morehouse HT et al. Comparison of computed tomography and contrast enema evaluation of diverticulitis. Dis Colon Rectum 1990; 33:1–6.

52. Prakash C, Chokshi H, Walden DT et al. Endoscopic hemostasis in acute diverticular bleeding. Endoscopy 1999; 31:460–3.

53. Tyau ES, Prystowsky JB, Joehl RJ et al. Acute diverticulitis: a complicated problem in the immunocompromised patient. Arch Surg 1991; 126:855–9.

54. Shaikh S, Krukowski ZH. Outcome of a conservative policy for managing acute sigmoid diverticulitis. Br J Surg 2007; 94:876–9.

55. O'Sullivan GC, Murphy D, O'Brien MG et al. Laparoscopic management of generalized peritonitis due to perforated colonic diverticula. Am J Surg 1996; 171:432–4.

56. Mutter D, Bouras G, Forgione M et al. Two stage totally minimally invasive approach for acute complicated diverticulitis. Colorectal Dis 2006; 8:501–6.

57. Taylor CJ, Layani L, Ghusn A et al. Perforated diverticulitis managed by laparoscopic lavage. Aust NZ J Surg 2006; 76:962–5.

58. Myers E, Hurley M, O'Sullivan GC et al. Laparoscopic peritoneal lavage for generalized peritonitis due to perforated diverticulitis. Br J Surg 2008; 95:97–101.

59. Constantinides VA, Tekkis PP, Athanasiou T et al. Primary resection with anastomosis vs. Hartmann's procedure in non-elective surgery for acute colonic

diverticulitis: a systematic review. Dis Colon Rectum 2006; 49:966–81.

60. Krukowski ZH, Al Sayer HM, Reid TMS et al. Effect of topical and systemic antibiotics on bacterial growth kinesis in generalized peritonitis in man. Br J Surg 1987; 74:303–6.

61. Krukowski ZH, Matheson NA. A ten-year computerised audit of infection after abdominal surgery. Br J Surg 1988; 75:857–61.

62. Chautems RC, Ambrosetti P, Ludwig A et al. Long term follow-up after first acute episode of sigmoid diverticulitis: is surgery mandatory? A prospective study of 118 patients. Dis Colon Rectum 2002; 45:962–6.

63. Schilling MK, Maurer CA, Kollmar O et al. Primary vs. secondary anastomosis after sigmoid colon resection for perforated diverticulitis (Hinchey Stage III and IV): a prospective outcome and cost analysis. Dis Colon Rectum 2001; 44:699–703.

64. Vignati V, Welch JP, Cohen JL. Long-term management of diverticulitis in young patients. Dis Colon Rectum 1995; 38:627–9.

65. Biondo S, Pares D, Marti Rague J et al. Acute colonic diverticulitis in patients under 50 years of age. Br J Surg 2002; 89:1137–41.

66. Tursi A, Brandimarte G, Daffina R. Long-term treatment with mesalazine and rifaximin versus rifaximin alone for patients with recurrent attacks of acute diverticulitis of colon. Dig Liver Dis 2002; 34:510–15.

67. Franklin ME, Dorman JP, Jacobs M et al. Is laparoscopic surgery applicable to complicated colonic diverticular disease? Surg Endosc 1997; 11:1021–5.

68. Scheidbach H, Schneider C, Rose J et al. Laparoscopic approach to treatment of sigmoid diverticulitis: changes in the spectrum of indications and results of a prospective multicenter study on 1545 patients. Dis Colon Rectum 2004; 47:1883–8.

69. Vargas HD, Ramirez RT, Hoffman GC et al. Defining the role of laparoscopic-assisted sigmoid colectomy for diverticulitis. Dis Colon Rectum 2000; 43:1726–31.

70. Alves A, Panis Y, Slim K et al. French multicentre prospective observational study of laparoscopic versus open colectomy for sigmoid diverticular disease. Br J Surg 2005; 92:1520–5.

9

Ulcerative colitis

R. John Nicholls
Paris P. Tekkis

Introduction

Ulcerative colitis is a disease of unknown aetiology confined to the large-intestinal mucosa. Medical treatment can control the disease in most cases but about 30% of patients will come to surgery. Criteria for the management of acute and chronic disease are now well established.

Aetiology

The disease chiefly affects the young, has an equal sex distribution and is rare in the tropics. The annual incidence per 100 000 population is similar for males and females up to the fourth decade of life. As a rule of thumb, it is useful to remember incidences of 10 and 5 per 100 000 for ulcerative colitis and Crohn's disease respectively. The incidence of ulcerative colitis has changed little over the last 30 years, whereas that for Crohn's disease has increased about fivefold, although this may now be stabilising and is possibly in decline.

The prevalence of ulcerative colitis is about 160 per 100 000 population (compared with about 50 per 100 000 for Crohn's disease). This means that there are around 100 000 people affected in the UK.

Genetic

Between 10% and 20% of affected individuals have a first-degree relative with inflammatory bowel disease

(IBD). There is a concordance within Jewish families, a low incidence in spouses and absence of IBD in families of adopted probands. In one twin study the association of ulcerative colitis of the twin of a proband with ulcerative colitis was 1 of 20 dizygotic and 1 of 26 monozygotic pairs, less than that for Crohn's disease (1 of 26 and 8 of 18 twin pairs).[1] In another questionnaire study of 150 twin pairs, concordance was reported in 5 of 25 monozygotic and 3 of 46 dizygotic twin pairs for Crohn's disease and in 6 of 38 monozygotic and 1 of 34 dizygotic twin pairs for ulcerative colitis.[2]

Both Crohn's disease and ulcerative colitis can occur in the same family, and the overlap of features of the two diseases (indeterminate colitis) of 10–15% and the change of diagnosis from one to the other in a further 10% may be a feature of genetic heterogeneity. While it has been suggested that both diseases share some similar gene loci with other genes defining each condition, it is noteworthy that there are no reports of mixed Crohn's disease and ulcerative colitis among monozygotic twins.

Extra-alimentary manifestations, including ankylosing spondylitis and primary sclerosing cholangitis, are more common in first-degree relatives of affected propositi; both have HLA associations, including HLA-B27 and HLA-B8 respectively. Ulcerative colitis is more common in whites than in blacks or Arabs. Whether this is genetic or environmental is unknown. IBD has a low incidence in underdeveloped countries.

Environmental factors

The incidence of ulcerative colitis rises about 10 years ahead of Crohn's disease, suggesting environmental influences.

There is evidence that non-steroidal inflammatory drugs can be associated with IBD in humans. It has long been recognised that some patients with ulcerative colitis have a history of infective proctocolitis. Smoking is protective in ulcerative colitis but not in Crohn's disease. This also appears to be true for pouchitis. Data are conflicting on the influence of oral contraceptives and most of the information relates to Crohn's disease. No causative dietary factor has been identified in humans. However, lactose intolerance can accompany ulcerative colitis, although this is rare.

Pathology

Inflammation is confined to the large intestine, which includes the colon, rectum and upper anal canal. The mucosal columnar glandular epithelium extends into the anal canal to the anal transitional zone, which varies in longitudinal length from a few millimetres to over a centimetre.[3] The anatomical extent of ulcerative colitis varies from involvement of the upper anal canal and rectum alone (proctitis) to the colon more proximally (proctocolitis). The rectum is always involved for all practical purposes, although relative rectal sparing can occur in patients receiving local anti-inflammatory treatment. A spared rectum not associated with local treatment should raise the suspicion of Crohn's disease. Backwash ileitis occurs only in cases with colonic extension to the ileocaecal junction. Anal disease occurs in about 10% of cases coming to proctocolectomy. The lesion is usually minor, e.g. a low fistula or fissure. Rectovaginal fistula can occasionally occur in ulcerative colitis.

The inflammation in the colon and rectum is diffuse without intervening normal mucosa. Ulceration causes bleeding and in patients with severe disease the inflammatory exudate results in loss of water, electrolyte and protein, which may be as great as 200 g per 24 hours.

Clinical presentation

At presentation, approximately 50% of cases have disease confined to the rectum (proctitis). In 30%

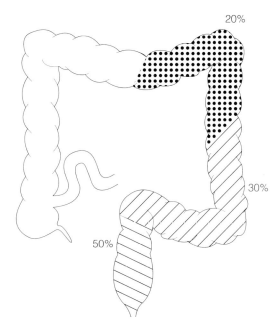

Figure 9.1 • Extent of disease at presentation.

this extends to the left colon (proctosigmoiditis) and in a further 20% disease extends beyond the splenic flexure (extensive colitis) (**Fig. 9.1**). Symptoms are local and general. The severity of the former and the presence of the latter depend largely on the anatomical extent of the disease. Ulcerative colitis is characterised by exacerbations and remissions. Bloody diarrhoea with urgency is the hallmark of colitis.

Proctitis

Symptoms include bleeding and mucus secretion. Sometimes constipation occurs but more often there is increased frequency of defecation. Rectal irritability may result in urgency of defecation. Systemic symptoms are very uncommon. Patients do not suffer from disturbances of growth, and only rarely from extra-alimentary manifestations or subsequent cancer. There is a tendency for proctitis to extend proximally with time.

Proctosigmoiditis and extensive colitis

Proximal extension to the left colon and more proximally leads to worsening local symptoms and systemic disturbances in some cases. Urgency is the most incapacitating local symptom. When severe, patients may have warning of impending defecation of a few seconds only. In such cases, urge incontinence can occur. Severe symptoms often dominate the patient's life and seriously affect work and family life. The protein-losing enteropathy may lead to malnutrition with loss of lean body mass and anaemia. Retardation of growth in children may be a feature of extensive colitis. In acutely ill patients, water and electrolyte loss may cause hypovolaemia, and breakdown of the mucosal barrier may lead to toxicity.

Exacerbations may be precipitated by anxiety or stress but usually there is no recognisable causative factor. The disease may be of the acute relapsing type, with acute episodes interspersed by periods of complete resolution. Alternatively it may take the form of persisting chronic disease. Such patients may develop acute exacerbations that settle only partially on treatment.

Patients with extensive disease are more likely to have associated extra-alimentary manifestations and are at greater risk of developing malignancy. These complications can occur in patients with disease confined to the left side of the colon but are much more frequent in extensive colitis.

Acute presentation

About 5% of patients present with acute severe colitis as the first manifestation of the disease. The patient will be ill with severe local symptoms, weight loss, anorexia, and water and sodium depletion. Intensive medical treatment has a high chance (70%) of inducing remission but when unsuccessful urgent or semi-urgent surgery will be necessary. Acute severe colitis may progress to toxic dilatation recognised by distension of the colon to a diameter greater than 6 cm on a plain radiograph. Perforation is a rare but serious occurrence with a mortality still approaching 40%. Rarely, deep ulceration (usually in the rectum) may cause severe bleeding.

Extra-alimentary manifestations

Up to one-third of patients with ulcerative colitis will develop at least one extra-alimentary manifestation during the course of the illness. These can be divided into those related or not to disease activity. Amyloid or hypertrophic osteoarthropathy are rare and are the result of long-standing chronic illness.

Arthropathy

Arthropathy is the commonest extra-alimentary manifestation. It can be divided into three broad groups.

Activity-related polyarthropathy

This occurs in up to 20% of patients and is more likely in those with extensive disease. It affects predominantly the large joints of the limbs, knees being the most common. The arthropathy is fleeting and asymmetrical and is rheumatoid factor negative. It disappears when medical treatment induces a remission or after proctocolectomy. It can develop in patients with pouchitis after restorative proctocolectomy.

Ankylosing spondylitis

This axial arthropathy involving the sacroiliac joints and one or more vertebrae occurs in up to 5% of patients. The majority of such cases are HLA-B27 positive. The disease is unrelated to the activity of colitis and does not respond to proctocolectomy. There may be a genetic basis.

Asymptomatic sacroileitis

This is an arthropathy limited to the sacroiliac joint and is HLA-B27 negative. It occurs more frequently than ankylosing spondylitis and is also unaffected by treatment for the colitis.

Liver

Associated hepatic and extrahepatic disorders occur in up to 5% of cases, predominantly in those with extensive colonic involvement. Fatty degeneration is common. It has no obvious clinical importance. Parenchymal liver disease of the chronic active hepatitis type and cirrhosis can occur. The latter may lead to portal hypertension.

Primary sclerosing cholangitis is more often seen in ulcerative colitis than in Crohn's colitis. The disease is characterised by a fibrous inflammatory reaction within the biliary tree, leading to multiple intra- and extrahepatic stenoses. The diagnosis is made on endoscopic retrograde cholangiopancreatography or magnetic resonance imaging (MRI). There is no apparent relationship between duration of disease and disease activity, although patients with primary sclerosing cholangitis undergoing restorative proctocolectomy have a higher subsequent incidence of pouchitis and dysplasia in the ileal pouch mucosa.[4,5] Treatment by steroids, colectomy or antibiotics is ineffectual. Ultimately the disease progresses to liver failure. Such patients may be considered for liver transplantation.

Cholangiocarcinoma is a rare association with ulcerative colitis. There may be an induction period of many years and the risk appears to continue even after proctocolectomy.

Skin

Erythema nodosum is the commonest cutaneous manifestation of IBD. It occurs more often in Crohn's disease. The condition is activity related. Pyoderma gangrenosum is more often associated with ulcerative colitis. It usually occurs in the lower limb as a circumscribed area of erythema with a punched-out ulcerated centre. Lesions may be multiple and occasionally are very extensive. Proctocolectomy is associated with healing in about 50%, although this may take weeks to months.

Eyes

Uveitis is rare and is not related to disease activity. The condition can lead to scarring with visual impairment, and ophthalmological management is essential. Episcleritis is activity related and occurs more often in Crohn's disease. It does not lead to chronic changes.

Cancer

The occurrence of malignant transformation has been known for years, but it was not until 1967 that dysplasia was recognised as a histopathological marker for impending or actual malignancy. Ulcerative colitis should always be considered when large-bowel cancer presents at an early age.

The incidence of cancer depends on the duration of the disease. This is estimated to be less than 1% within 10 years of onset, increasing to 10–15% in the second decade and to over 20% in the third. As a rule of thumb, after 10 years of colitis the incidence of colorectal cancer increases by 1% per year.

Colonoscopic surveillance relies on the identification of flat dysplasia or a dysplasia-associated lesion or mass (DALM). There is general agreement among pathologists on the criteria for its diagnosis. The presence of low-grade dysplasia is as likely as high-grade dysplasia (54% vs. 67%) to be associated with an already established cancer.[6]

Cancers can be missed by colonoscopy surveillance programmes. The American College of Gastroenterology Practice Parameters Committee has recommended annual colonoscopy every 2 years with multiple biopsies taken at 10-cm intervals through the colon and rectum. An experienced histopathologist is essential.[7]

Diagnosis and assessment

Diagnosis

A classification of IBD is shown in Box 9.1. In the tropics, infective causes comprise the vast majority of cases. In temperate regions infective causes may occur in hospitals and long-stay institutions. The diagnosis is made by histopathological examination of biopsy material taken during endoscopy, having excluded microbiological causes. Endoscopy will determine the extent of inflammation in the assessment of severity.

Microbiology

A specimen of stool must be sent for microbiological examination. If amoebiasis is suspected, the specimen

---

Box 9.1 • Classification of inflammatory bowel disease

Infective

Virus
- Cytomegalovirus

Bacteria
- *Campylobacter*
- *Escherichia coli*
- *Shigella*
- *Clostridium difficile*
- *Chlamydia*
- *Gonococcus*

Protozoa
- Amoebiasis
- *Cryptosporidium**
- *Giardia**

Non-infective
- Ulcerative colitis
- Crohn's disease
- Radiation enteritis
- Drug induced

---

* Especially in immunocompromised patients.

should be examined in the laboratory within a few hours. In addition, diagnosis of amoebiasis requires a biopsy to demonstrate cysts. *Shigella*, *C. difficile* and *Campylobacter* infection should be excluded. These may occur in epidemics in institutions with a significant mortality in frail elderly patients. The microbiologist should be warned on the request form that these could be present.

Proctitis can be caused by gonorrhoeal and chlamydial infection. The inflammation is catarrhal and consists of an erythematous flare associated with a purulent exudate. It rarely extends proximally beyond a few centimetres from the anal verge. When suspected, rectal, urethral and vaginal swabs should be taken. Again, the microbiologist should be forewarned. Opportunistic infection may cause proctocolitis in immunocompromised patients (e.g. those with human immunodeficiency virus infection) or those on immunosuppressive drugs. Examples include cytomegalovirus, *Mycobacterium avium-intracellulare* and cryptosporidia (see also Chapter 16).

Endoscopy

Loss of the vascular pattern (the submucosal vessels seen through the transparent mucosa) is the most sensitive sign of inflammation. This is due to oedema of the mucosa, which makes it opaque. Oedema also causes fine granularity in which there is a delicate regular stippled appearance of the mucosal surface. More severe changes include erythema, contact bleeding and frank ulceration. Where previous acute attacks have been followed by repair, mucosal regeneration nodules (coarse granularity) or pseudopolyps may be seen. Pseudopolyps represent tags of mucosa that have been partially detached during the active episode and remain as projections after healing of ulceration. Rigid rectoscopy will only visualise the rectum. Colonoscopy allows assessment of the proximal extent of the disease.

Histopathology

Histopathological examination of a mucosal biopsy is the basis of diagnosis.

Biopsy technique

A biopsy is obligatory and is most easily obtained during rigid rectoscopy. Colonoscopy used for surveil-

lance allows multiple biopsies to be taken. Perforation and bleeding are potential complications. The patient must be asked whether anticoagulants or immunosuppressive drugs are being taken before a biopsy is performed. The biopsy taken during rigid rectoscopy itself should be obtained with forceps with a circular cusp that minimises the depth of penetration. The optimal site is about 7 cm from the anal verge in the posterior quadrant of the rectum. Adequate vision during rectoscopy must be assured and the jaws of the forceps are firmly closed, taking a bite of mucosa and submucosa. After the biopsy has been taken, the site must be inspected for bleeding. If this persists a topical solution of adrenaline (epinephrine) 1 in 1000 soaked in a small swab should be applied to the biopsy site. The biopsy should be oriented onto a piece of absorbent paper and placed in formalin (10%).

Active disease

In active disease (**Fig. 9.2**) there is mucosal thickening with infiltration of the lamina propria by neutrophils, plasma cells, lymphocytes, eosinophils and mast cells. Mucin within goblet cells is discharged so that these are less evident or absent (goblet cell depletion). The degree of neutrophil infiltration is the best histopathological marker of severity. In mild disease, neutrophils are confined to the lamina propria. Extrusion of neutrophils into the crypt lumen forms a crypt abscess, the number of which correlates with the severity of disease. Mucosal ulceration is partly the result of rupture of crypt abscesses leading to mucosal destruction. Damage to the crypt basal epithelium leads to loss of crypts. Attempts at regeneration may be mistaken for dysplasia but the presence of more normal cells towards the luminal surface allows these to be distinguished. There may be branching of crypts owing to regeneration following crypt epithelial damage.

Acute severe colitis

Progression of these acute changes occurs in cases with acute severe colitis. Ulceration can be very extensive, leaving large areas of exposed muscularis propria covered with granulation tissue. This may be associated with thinning of the musculature and colonic dilatation. Inflammation may be transmural and fissure formation may be seen.

Remission

Colitis in remission may leave a distorted architectural pattern with crypt depletion. Mucosal

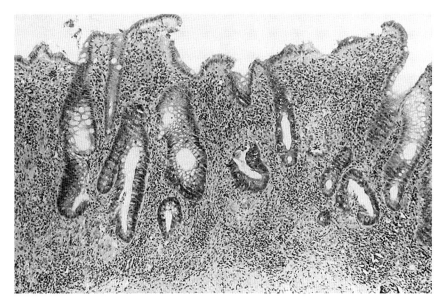

Figure 9.2 • Microscopic appearances of active colitis. Note the white cell infiltration of the lamina propria, goblet cell depletion and crypt abscess formation.

cells that remain often regain normal function and show retained mucin as identifiable goblet cells. A chronic inflammatory cell exudate in the lamina propria is likely to be present, although this may be very mild in patients in remission for long periods. Paneth cell metaplasia indicates episodes of previous colitis.

Ulcerative colitis or Crohn's disease

Diagnostic difficulties in differentiating ulcerative colitis and Crohn's disease have been recognised for many years. The pathological criteria distinguishing them are shown in Table 9.1.

Indeterminate colitis

In some patients insufficient numbers of these diagnostic attributes are present or there is considerable overlap and atypical features are seen. Thus it may be impossible for the pathologist to separate the two diseases, which may be reported as unclassified colitis or as unclassified colitis with additional indication of the possible or probable presence of Crohn's disease or ulcerative colitis. In about 10% of cases, however, the pathologist will be able to state only that the colitis is indeterminate.[8]

Indeterminate colitis is not a disease entity. It is a term which indicates that the histopathologist is unable to come to a firm diagnosis owing to the presence of features of both conditions. Usually the

dilemma arises in emergency colectomy specimens where severe inflammation may be combined with features of ulcerative colitis and Crohn's disease.

In trying to resolve the diagnostic dilemma more biopsies should be taken. If the patient has had a colectomy for acute disease, then these will come from the rectal stump which may have already developed diversion proctitis, making the histopathologist's task more difficult. The small bowel should be examined by endoscopy or radiology, which if abnormal is suggestive of Crohn's disease, as would be the presence of an anal lesion.

When histopathological, radiological and clinical features are considered together, patients with indeterminate colitis can usually be judged to incline more to Crohn's disease or ulcerative colitis. Where they cannot, the natural history tends to incline to that of ulcerative colitis.[9]

Radiology

A plain abdominal X-ray is the most useful means of identifying colonic dilatation (**Fig. 9.3**). There has been a movement away from tubular contrast radiology to computed tomography (CT). The instant barium enema is now rarely used, although it gave an excellent record of the extent of the disease in most cases.

Table 9.1 • Histopathological distinction between ulcerative colitis and Crohn's disease

	Ulcerative colitis	Crohn's disease
Macroscopic		
Distribution	Colon and rectum	Gastrointestinal tract
Rectum	Involved	Often spared
Anal disease	Rare	Common
Malignant risk	10% at 20 years	Probably similar (large bowel disease)
Intestinal fistula	Never	Common
Stricture (non-neoplastic)	Rare	Common
Microscopic		
Bowel wall involvement	Mucosa and submucosa	Full thickness
Granulomas	None	60–70%
Mucus secretion	Impaired (goblet cell depletion)	Slightly impaired
Fissuring	Absent	Common
Crypt abscess	Common	Rare

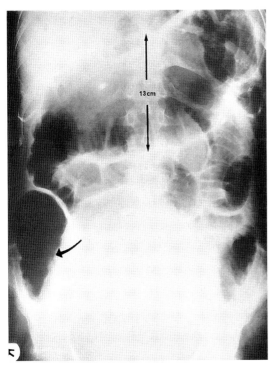

Figure 9.3 • Plain abdominal radiograph of toxic dilatation. Note the bowel diameter (>6 cm), absence of caecal faecal shadowing and widening of the bowel wall shadow (lower left arrow).

Management

The unit

Best care is likely to be achieved by a multidisciplinary team including medical staff, specialist nurses, nutritionists and stomatherapists with social and psychological support. Collaboration between gastroenterologist and surgeon is essential and should include patient sharing where appropriate, joint outpatient consultations for difficult cases, and early involvement of the surgeon in acute disease.

Treatment

Proctitis

Most patients are satisfactorily treated medically by a combination of steroids and 5-aminosalicylic acid preparations. The former are intended to induce a remission, the latter to maintain a remission once achieved. Both can be given as suppositories or as an enema, the choice depending on the proximal extent of disease. Steroid preparations such as budesonide have a lesser tendency for absorption. An oral 5-aminosalicylic acid preparation should also be prescribed from the beginning. Modern 5-aminosalicylic drugs (asacol, pentasa and balsalazide) no longer contain sulphonamide, which was responsible for some of the side-effects of salazopyrine. They are formulated to protect the aspirin from degradation before it arrives in the colon. Proctitis refractory to this treatment may respond to other preparations, including bismuth, nicotine and witch hazel. Rarely, patients with persisting severe symptoms may require surgery.

Acute severe colitis

Patients with severe acute colitis require admission to hospital. Initial treatment is medical but about 30% of patients will come to surgery. Surgery is absolutely indicated in cases with acute toxic dilatation or perforation.

Management

Management consists of monitoring and treatment.

Monitoring

Monitoring is essential to assess improvement or deterioration. The pulse rate, temperature and blood pressure are regularly recorded. The patient should be weighed on admission and twice weekly thereafter. Blood should be sent for haemoglobin, albumin and electrolyte estimations. A stool chart is essential. This should record every defecation with an assessment of volume and consistency of stool and the presence or absence of blood on each occasion. The abdomen should be examined regularly. Distension suggests the possible development of toxic megacolon. A plain radiograph will allow assessment of the colonic diameter (Fig. 9.3). Abdominal tenderness and rigidity suggest local or general peritonitis. The presence of intramural gas on the plain abdominal radiograph is a sign of imminent perforation and is therefore an indication for immediate surgery.

Medical treatment

Treatment involves bed rest and the correction of water and electrolyte depletion by intravenous infusion of Ringer lactate solution. Severely anaemic patients should be given blood. The patient should be encouraged to eat a high-protein and -calorie diet. Intravenous nutrition may be indicated in severely malnourished patients, as judged by decrease in lean body mass and serum albumin.

Intravenous prednisolone (60 mg daily) and an H_2 receptor antagonist or a proton-pump inhibitor to protect against upper gastrointestinal ulceration are given. Ciclosporin has been reported to induce remission in over 50% of patients unresponsive to steroids but early relapse may occur, resulting in the same clinical situation within a short period.[10,11]

More recently, a number of studies have reported the use of biological agents for the treatment of acute ulcerative colitis. Infliximab (Remicade® Centocor, Malvern PA) is a chimeric (75% mouse, 25% human) anti-tumour necrosis factor-α monoclonal antibody that mediates multiple proinflammatory processes central to the pathogenesis of IBD.

In a study of 30 patients with active ulcerative colitis treated with infliximab between 2000 and 2006 at Oxford, 53% of patients came to colectomy at a median time of 140 days after their first infusion (range 4–607). Of those avoiding colectomy, only 17% sustained a steroid-free remission. The role of immunotherapy in the acute setting remains to be established.[12]

Surgery

Indications

Surgery has a major role in the management of acute colitis. The need for surgery is greatest during the first year after onset of the disease (**Fig. 9.4**). The indications and their relative frequency are shown in Table 9.2.

Unresponsiveness to medical treatment

Failure to respond to medical treatment should be recognised early. The gastroenterologist and surgeon should confer at least daily to decide whether there has been improvement, stagnation or deterioration. Deterioration despite adequate medical treatment should be an indication for surgery. Stagnation over several days with no sign of improvement should also be an indication for operation.

Clinical indicators that surgery is likely to be necessary at the time of admission include a frequency of defecation of over 10 times per 24 hours with the passage of blood at every defecation attempt. A low

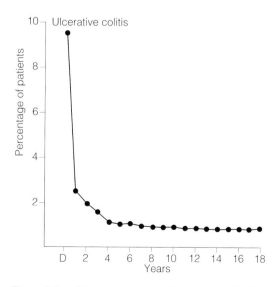

Figure 9.4 • Colectomy rates in different years after the diagnosis of ulcerative colitis.

Table 9.2 • Urgent surgery for ulcerative colitis 1976–90

Main reason for surgery	No. of patients
Unresponsiveness to medical treatment	71
Toxic dilatation	23
Perforation	9
Bleeding	2
Other	1
Total	**106**

Data from Melville DM, Ritchie JK, Nicholls RJ et al. Surgery for ulcerative colitis in the area of the pouch: the St Mark's Hospital experience. Gut 1994; 35:1076–80. With permission from BMJ Publishing Group Ltd.

albumin, low haemoglobin and a fall in lean body mass of more than 10% are other risk factors for surgery.

Previous acute attacks, poor general health and social circumstances affected by the disease should be taken into account. A significant history of chronic illness and social incapacity should sway the decision in favour of surgery.

Megacolon, perforation and bleeding

Megacolon is an indication for surgery. If signs of peritonism are present, operation should not be delayed. When surgery is performed before perforation, the reported mortality is 2–8%. Perforation is a grave development, with a mortality of around 40%. It may be silent in a patient on large doses of steroids, and may become evident only by the presence of free gas on the plain abdominal radiograph. Its occurrence without megacolon is rare and should raise the possibility of Crohn's disease. Severe bleeding usually arises from ulceration in the rectum.

Colectomy with ileostomy and preservation of the rectum

This is the operation of choice for acute severe colitis.

Operative technique

Position of the patient

For all surgery for ulcerative colitis the reversed Trelendenburg (Lloyd–Davies) position with the legs raised should be used, thereby allowing access to the rectum. The bladder is routinely catheterised. It is helpful to insert a proctoscope before starting to drain the rectum and deflate the bowel.

Ileostomy trephine

When an ileostomy forms part of the procedure, the trephine should be made before opening the abdomen.

Incision

For open colectomy this should be midline. This can be limited to 7 cm or less in a thin patient. A paramedian incision is no longer appropriate. For laparoscopic colectomy a small Pfannestiel incision is made to remove the specimen. It also allows a manual port if hand-assisted laparoscopy (HALS) is used.

On opening the abdomen, care must be taken to avoid perforation. Where adhesions have formed between the colon and the parietes, dissection should be made within the latter.

Steps in the operation

1. Mobilisation of the right colon. The surgeon stands on the patient's left side.
2. Division of the bowel. The bowel is divided at the ileocaecal junction before proceeding further. This allows control of the right colon manually to allow safe division of the ileocolic and right colic vessels, by avoiding tension.
3. Division of vessels of the transverse colon.
4. Mobilisation of the left colon. The surgeon moves to the other side of the table to do this.
5. Mobilisation of the splenic flexure. The splenic flexure is often drawn down owing to shortening of the bowel due to the disease process and may be very easy to mobilise.
6. Division of the sigmoid. The level of division should allow sufficient length of distal bowel to be able to exteriorise it through the anterior abdominal wall whether a mucous fistula is formed or not (**Fig. 9.5**). Division at the level of the peritoneal reflection leaves a distal stump that is too short to be exteriorised in the uncommon event of breakdown of the distal suture line and also makes identification of the rectum at a subsequent operation difficult. A long rectosigmoid stump should therefore be aimed for unless it is necessary to remove the rectum in the case of severe bleeding.

Mucous fistula

Although leakage of the distal closure suture line is uncommon (<5%), the creation of a mucous fistula should be considered in patients in poor condition with malnutrition and where the bowel wall is too

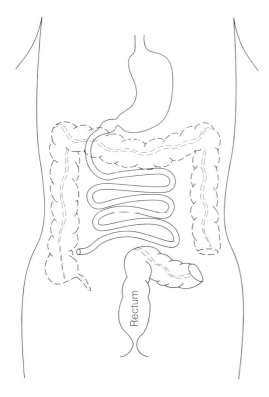

Figure 9.5 • Emergency colectomy: level of division of the sigmoid allowing adequate mobility for exteriorisation.

diseased safely to take sutures. The ileostomy and mucous fistula should be brought out sufficiently far apart to allow a stoma appliance to be placed over each without interference. Placing the mucous fistula in the contralateral iliac fossa achieves this. Some surgeons prefer to close the stump and leave it in the subcutaneous fat deep to the abdominal wound.

Postoperative outcome

In the immediate postoperative period it is advisable to drain the rectum (particularly if the stump is closed) by daily insertion of a proctoscope. Complications include intestinal obstruction and sepsis. Obstruction usually resolves spontaneously. Sepsis may be due to an intra-abdominal collection or leakage from a closed rectosigmoid stump. This will usually require re-operation and exteriorisation of the distal bowel if possible. Rarely, rectal excision preserving the anal canal will be necessary. Occasionally, persisting inflammation in the rectal stump may be so severe despite local treatment that rectal excision is required.

Recovery usually occurs within a few weeks to a couple of months, during which steroids and other medication are gradually withdrawn. Health and self-confidence are restored, allowing return to work or education. The timing of any subsequent operation is determined by the patient but should not be before 3 months.

Mortality

Mortality ranges from <1% to 5% from specialist centres in the UK, Denmark and the USA.

> Recent linkage analysis of 8245 patients with ulcerative colitis having a first hospital admission for ulcerative colitis of more than 4 days in England between 1998 and 2000 indicates that the mortality up to 2003 (3 years) is lower after an elective (2.2%) or emergency procedure (3.2%) than if no operation is carried out (7.4%).[13]

If substantiated, these data suggest that the threshold for surgery may be too high. There is evidence that mortality is higher in small, low-volume hospitals.[14]

Chronic proctocolitis

Medical treatment

Medical management includes anti-inflammatory, nutritional, symptomatic and psychological treatments.

Prednisolone is given at an initial dose of 40 mg, gradually reducing this as remission occurs over the next few weeks. Azathioprine can be tried in patients who do not respond to steroids or in those who are steroid dependent in the hope of avoiding long-term steroid treatment. Ciclosporin can be effective in inducing remission in patients suffering from acute severe colitis, but its role in chronic disease is not established. The nutritional state should be monitored. There is no specific diet that influences the activity of the disease, but a high protein and calorie intake should be encouraged. Specific replacement treatment such as iron may be necessary. Antidiarrhoeal agents including codeine phosphate and loperamide are usually effective in reducing frequency and urgency. Maximal doses are 60 mg four times daily and 8 mg four times daily respectively. Lomotil (atropine and diphenoxylate) is occasionally effective where there has been a poor response to the others. Bone densitometry should be carried out where steroid medication has been prolonged.

Indications for elective surgery

Most patients requiring surgery have extensive disease. They are more likely to have severe local symptoms and systemic illness. There is a greater risk of acute severe colitis and malignant transformation. Very occasionally, a patient with distal disease may require surgery, usually because of severe local symptoms.

The indications for elective surgery include:

1. Unresponsiveness to medical treatment.
2. Retardation of growth in the young.
3. Malignant transformation.

Unresponsiveness to medical treatment

This indication can be divided into various clinical categories.

Chronic disease

The patient continues to suffer from systemic and local symptoms despite adequate medical treatment. Chronic anaemia associated with general weakness, poor energy levels, amenorrhoea and extra-alimentary manifestations may leave the patient unable to lead a normal life. Patients may have experienced multiple hospitalisations, periods off work, disruption of family life and education, and other social effects of chronic illness. Patients who have never experienced a complete remission from medical treatment are included in this group.

Steroid dependence

A response to steroids may be maintained only by continuing the therapy with relapse on withdrawal. If alternative medication such as immunosuppression is unsuccessful, then surgery is indicated unless there are particular reasons against.

Recurrent acute exacerbations

The decision for surgery will depend on the frequency and severity of attacks. Surgery during an acute attack will usually take the form of a colectomy with ileostomy. A decision taken during remission may allow an elective definitive procedure such as restorative proctocolectomy to be performed as the first-stage procedure.

Severe symptoms

The patient may be systemically well but severely inconvenienced by frequency and urgency of defecation, particularly if associated with urge incontinence.

Extra-alimentary manifestations

Not all symptoms will respond to removal of the large bowel; liver manifestations and sacroiliitis do not. However, the activity-related polyarthropathy does respond, as will some cases of pyoderma gangrenosum, although the latter may improve only slowly over several months.

Retardation of growth

Ulcerative colitis, if extensive, has an inhibitory effect on growth and the development of secondary sexual characteristics. Steroid medication itself leads to early fusion of epiphyses, resulting in permanent stunting of growth. Patients in this category are usually under the care of a paediatrician expert in the assessment of growth. However, within the years of puberty a delay in surgery may occur, partly because of the antipathy of the paediatrician and/or of the patient (or parents) to an ileostomy.

Malignant transformation

The presence of high- or low-grade dysplasia or an established invasive tumour is an indication for surgery. The surgical technique should be as though invasion had occurred, since this can be determined only by examination of the resected specimen.

Choice of operation: general considerations

There are four surgical options:

1. colectomy with ileostomy and preservation of the rectum;
2. conventional proctocolectomy and permanent ileostomy;
3. colectomy and ileorectal anastomosis;
4. restorative proctocolectomy and ileal reservoir.

All these operations involve total removal of the colon. There is no place for partial colectomy, even in cases with a normal right colon, where experience has shown a high frequency of recurrence in the remaining colon. In patients having a permanent ileostomy, a Kock pouch (see below) may be possible in certain circumstances.

Colectomy with ileorectal anastomosis should be considered only where the rectum is minimally inflamed and distensible, and where there is no evidence of dysplasia anywhere in the large bowel. Most patients do not fulfil these criteria, leaving the alternative of conventional or restorative proctocolectomy. The latter is excluded, however, if the anal sphincter is inadequate or the anus is diseased. Much will depend on the wishes of the patient. Here, it is essential for the clinician to give detailed information on the morbidity, function, late complications and likely duration of treatment of the various options. Input from the stomatherapist and patient support groups should be obtained. The introduction of restorative proctocolectomy has resulted in this operation being the most commonly used, with over 80% of patients requiring elective surgery.

Colectomy with ileostomy and preservation of the rectum

This operation also has a place in elective treatment. For patients too unfit for a restorative proctocolectomy it may be preferable to carry out an initial colectomy. Besides the advantages of rapid return to health (see above), the experience of an end-ileostomy is useful to the patient when considering further surgery. Where the diagnosis of ulcerative colitis is in doubt, a colectomy gives the histopathologist more material to make a diagnosis. Dysplasia is extremely rare within 10 years of the onset of colitis, and there is therefore no hurry for re-operation in most cases. All of the options discussed below can then be considered.

Conventional proctocolectomy with permanent ileostomy

The introduction of the everted ileostomy established this operation as the standard procedure for ulcerative colitis until the description of restorative proctocolectomy. Ulcerative colitis is cured, with the only disadvantage being a permanent ileostomy.

Indications

The indications include:

1. Rectum and anus not suitable for restorative procedure:
   a. inadequate sphincter;
   b. cancer in the low rectum.
2. Patient preference.

The patient should appreciate the possibility of ileostomy-related complications requiring further surgery and delayed healing of the perineal wound. These are offset by those of pelvic sepsis and long-term developments such as pouchitis after restorative proctocolectomy.

Technique

Creating the ileostomy trephine before the midline incision and colectomy has already been discussed. Where a carcinoma or dysplasia is present a conventional anatomical dissection (total mesorectal excision) should be carried out. The majority of patients do not have neoplastic transformation and, in these, the rectum may be removed by close (perimuscular) dissection to minimise the incidence of pelvic nerve damage, which might cause urinary or sexual dysfunction, although there was no statistically significant difference in a non-randomised comparison of perimuscular and conventional dissection.[15] Whatever technique is used, dissection should be kept behind Denonvilliers' fascia anteriorly and close to the rectal wall laterally, where the autonomic pelvic nerves are most at risk. In the absence of carcinoma in the low anorectal region, the anal canal should be removed using the intersphincteric technique. Good ileostomy technique includes preparation of the mesentery and its fixation to the peritoneum of the anterior abdominal wall. The terminal 5 cm of ileum are perfused by the marginal vessel after division of the ileocolic artery and vein (**Fig. 9.6**). The stoma itself is completed by mucocutaneous interrupted sutures. It will evert spontaneously; a projection of 2.5 cm is ideal.

Results

Obstruction may occasionally require re-operation but usually settles spontaneously. Rarely, it is due to herniation of the small bowel into the space lateral to the ileostomy. A haematoma in the cavity left by the rectum may become infected. Drainage with resolution of the acute problem may be followed by a perineal sinus. This may require subsequent surgery with curettage and rarely in refractory cases the need for a perineal myocutaneous rectus abdominus flap. Delayed healing of the perineal wound at 6 months occurs in 10–20% of cases.

Ileostomy complications are common. Stricture formation, prolapse and retraction may cause difficulty in maintaining a watertight appliance, as may parastomal herniation. Corrective surgery is often

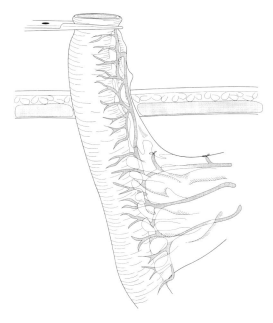

Figure 9.6 • Formation of terminal ileostomy. Division of mesenteric vessels with preservation of the 'marginal' vessels to the terminal ileum.

required, with a reported cumulative ileostomy revision rate of around 25% at 5 years. It is usually possible to carry out a local revision, but in some cases, particularly with herniation, resiting is required. This is a major undertaking.

Continent ileostomy

Kock[16] developed this operation initially for bladder replacement and then adapted it to create a continent abdominal intestinal stoma. The procedure

still has a place in patients in whom the anal sphincter has been removed. A reservoir is constructed from 30 cm of the terminal ileum and the most distal 15 cm of small bowel are invaginated into the reservoir to form a nipple valve (**Fig. 9.7**). This maintains continence and the reservoir is emptied several times per day by catherisation of the abdominal stoma using a wide bore tube.

Early complications include leakage from the reservoir, causing peritonitis or fistulation. The most important late complication is subluxation of the nipple valve. It is suggested by the onset of incontinence of the stoma and difficulty in inserting the catheter. Contrast radiology may show partial or complete prolapse of the valve. Valve slippage occurs in 17% to over 40% of cases, and is the most common cause of failure. Reported fistula rates range from 10% to 26%. Of 330 patients treated at a single institution between 1974 and 2001, pouch survival at 10 and 20 years was 87% and 77% respectively.[17] Patients with indeterminate colitis or Crohn's disease were 4.5 times more likely to lose the pouch than those without, and in one series the cumulative 10-year recurrence rate in 49 patients with Crohn's disease was 48%, with excision of the pouch required in eight.[18]

Long-term continence rates of over 90% have been reported. The cumulative 4-year incidence of pouchitis is around 40%. Dysplasia has been reported in 3 of 40 patients followed for a median of 30 years.[19] One case of carcinoma in the pouch has been reported.[20]

Continent ileostomy may be indicated in motivated patients in whom restorative proctocolectomy

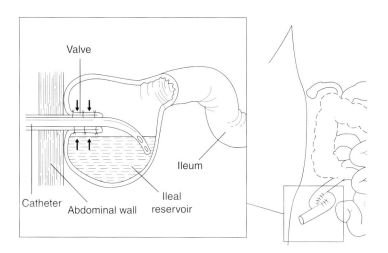

Figure 9.7 • The Kock continent ileostomy.

is not an option, and in patients who already have a permanent ileostomy and desire an improved quality of life. It has also been carried out after failure of restorative proctocolectomy.

Colectomy with ileorectal anastomosis (IRA)

Indications

Colectomy with IRA is a well-tolerated, one-stage procedure. Before the introduction of restorative proctocolectomy it was the only procedure that avoided an ileostomy, being used in 10% to over 80% of patients according to the preference of the surgeon. Since then, its usage has fallen to below 10%.

The indications are as follows:

1. a non- or mildly inflamed rectum with good compliance;
2. absence of dysplasia anywhere in the large bowel;
3. adequate anal sphincter;
4. availability of the patient for follow-up;
5. presence of disseminated colonic carcinoma with relative rectal sparing.

The patient must also be prepared to be followed by annual rectoscopy with biopsy owing to the risk of malignancy in the rectal stump, which is about 5% at 20 years. If this is not possible, then the operation should not be advised.

Technique

The technique is identical to colectomy with ileostomy up to the point of removal of the specimen. The upper rectum is very accessible for manual or stapled anastomosis.

Results

The operation is a compromise since there is potentially active disease in the rectum. This can lead to failure because of persisting inflammation causing poor function or the development of malignancy. The results demonstrate a low mortality and morbidity but considerable differences in failure requiring removal of the rectum.[21] There were 12 deaths among 22 cancers that developed during follow-up in a series of 384 patients.[22]

Patients who fail are candidates for rectal excision with permanent ileostomy or restorative proctectomy, provided that any cancer in the rectum can be adequately cleared without having to sacrifice the anal canal and provided there is no dissemination.

Restorative proctocolectomy with ileal reservoir

The strategy of complete removal of the large bowel with sphincter preservation was first described fully by Ravitch and Sabiston.[23] The 'straight' ileoanal anastomosis was adopted by a few surgeons at the time and the functional results were subsequently reviewed by Valiènte and Bacon.[24] Function was often poor, due largely to urgency and frequency.

The introduction of the continent ileostomy[16] showed that a small-bowel reservoir could function in humans, and this led Parks and Nicholls[25] to combine this with their own endoanal anastomotic technique to create the ileoanal ileal reservoir procedure. Capacitance of the neorectum is inversely related to frequency, irrespective of whether the neorectum is constructed using straight ileum or an ileal reservoir.

Indications

The only reason for the operation is to avoid a permanent ileostomy. A conventional proctocolectomy gives excellent results except for this. Where there is no medical objection, the choice lies between a restorative or conventional proctocolectomy and is almost entirely the patient's to make. This is possible only if the disadvantages are fully discussed. These include failure and complication rates, total treatment time, the possibility of pouchitis occurring and the likely functional outcome. A pouch support nurse, stomatherapist and patient support group can offer valuable advice, but in the end the patient must decide.

The indications include:

1. Ulcerative colitis.
2. Familial adenomatous polyposis (FAP).
3. Non-acute severe colitis. Any severely ill patient should have an initial colectomy.
4. Absence of low rectal cancer. Where a cancer is present, it must be possible to achieve locoregional clearance, an assessment similar to that made when considering neoadjuvant chemoradiotherapy, anterior resection or total rectal excision for 'ordinary' rectal carcinoma. The operation is not indicated in patients with disseminated disease.
5. Adequate anal sphincter. Manometry should be performed where there is clinical uncertainty of sphincter function.

Controversies

1. **Age.** Failure, complication rates and function are similar in paediatric patients to overall series.[26] General health and quality of life are similar to healthy children in those patients with a functioning pouch. There is some evidence that incontinence, usually minor, is more common in patients over 45 years of age.[27,28] There is, however, no absolute contraindication in older patients and the decision should depend on assessment of the individual patient, particularly regarding sphincter function.

2. **Female fertility.** Female infertility is increased by more than three times following restorative proctocolectomy.[29,30]

> This applies to both ulcerative colitis[31] and FAP, but more so in the former.[32] Fertility is not affected by colectomy.[32]

There is also a higher incidence of fertility treatment among patients after restorative proctocolectomy than in the normal population.[33] The pelvic dissection is one factor responsible, as well the advancing age of the patient. Fertility is of medico-legal importance when counselling females of child-bearing age. The patient may decide to have a restorative proctocolectomy accepting the risk of reduced fertility or she may decide to have a colectomy with ileostomy, allowing recovery from the disease while preserving fertility. A restorative proctectomy can then be considered at a later date convenient to the patient.

3. **Crohn's disease.** With the exception of one group,[34] patients with Crohn's disease experience a higher failure rate than the general pouch population (Table 9.3). In one series failure rates for ulcerative colitis and Crohn's disease were 10% and 50% respectively.[35]

> Over a 20-year period of follow-up, failure occurred in 55%.[36] Failure in Crohn's disease is significantly greater than in indeterminate colitis.[37]

Thus, as a general principle, Crohn's disease is a contraindication to restorative proctocolectomy.

4. **Indeterminate colitis.** Indeterminate colitis without radiological or clinical evidence of Crohn's disease tends to behave like ulcerative colitis. Failure rates in large series followed for 10 or more years are around 10%[35,38] and at

Table 9.3 • Outcome of restorative proctocolectomy in Crohn's disease

Reference	n	Failed
Galandiuk et al.[74]	16	4
Deutsch et al.[75]	9	4
Hyman et al.[76]	25	7
Grobler et al.[77]	20	8
Panis et al.[78]	31	2
Regimbeau et al.[34]	41	3
Tulchinsky et al.[35]	13	6
Hahnloser et al.[36]	44	20

20 years there was no significant difference in the failure rates among patients with ulcerative or indeterminate colitis (6% and 12%).[36] Complications and function also appear to be similar to patients having the operation for ulcerative colitis.[36,39] Exclusion of small-bowel and anal disease is obligatory.

5. **Previous anal pathology.** A history of anal disease may suggest Crohn's disease. The presence of an anal lesion increases the risk of anastomotic leakage,[40] pouch–vaginal and perineal fistula, and subsequent failure.[41]

6. **Sclerosing cholangitis.** Patients with sclerosing cholangitis have double the incidence of pouchitis after restorative proctocolectomy.[42] They are also at increased risk of dysplasia developing in the pouch, although this risk is small.[5] While not a contraindication, the patient should be carefully counselled. Liver function tests should be performed routinely preoperatively.

Technique (**Fig. 9.8**)

The steps in the operation include:

1. Mobilisation of the colon and rectum. This is identical to conventional proctocolectomy.

2. Division of the gut tube. The rectum is mobilised to the anorectal junction. If a stapled ileoanal anastomosis is intended, a transverse stapler is applied at this level. Where a manual anastomosis is to be carried out, the bowel is divided, leaving an open anal stump.

3. Mobilisation of the mesentery. Having removed the surgical specimen, the small-bowel mesentery is fully mobilised. It is useful to perform a trial descent to the anal canal of the point on the ileum selected for the ileoanal anastomosis. If it does not reach, further mobilisation is necessary.

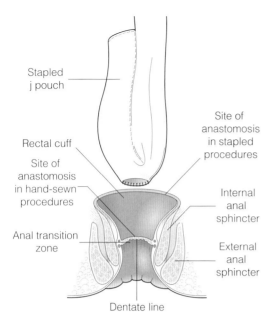

Stapled j pouch

Rectal cuff

Site of anastomosis in hand-sewn procedures

Anal transition zone

Dentate line

Site of anastomosis in stapled procedures

Internal anal sphincter

External anal sphincter

Figure 9.8 • Restorative proctocolectomy. Reproduced from McLaughlin SD, Tekkis PP, Ciclitira PJ et al. Review article: restorative proctocolectomy, indications, management of complications and follow-up: a guide for gastroenterologists. Aliment Pharmacol Ther 2008, in press. With permission from Blackwell Publishing.

This may require the division of selected vessels but care must be taken to avoid ischaemia.

4. Ileal reservoir. The two-loop (J) reservoir is easy to make by hand or by stapling. The original three-loop (S) reservoir of Parks often led to evacuation difficulty due to the short segment of ileum distal to the pouch. The four-loop (W) reservoir achieves a capacitance generally greater than that of the J reservoir and similarly has no distal segment. In general, the larger the reservoir, the lower the frequency.[43]

5. Anastomosis. (i) Manual. A mucosectomy is performed via an endoanal approach. Using suitable retraction (e.g. the Lone Star) the mucosa is removed by sharp scissor dissection after elevation by the submucosal injection of saline with adrenaline (1:300 000). The reservoir is then brought through the anal canal and sutures (12, one for each hour of the clock) are placed after removal of the retractor to minimise tension. (ii) Stapled. A transverse stapler is applied at the level of the anorectal junction and the bowel is then divided. The anvil of a circular stapling instrument is fixed

in the reservoir by a purse-string suture and the anastomosis completed on firing the instrument after insertion per anam.

The manual technique allows a precise level for the anastomosis and avoids the possibility of leaving rectal mucosa behind, while stapling may sometimes result in an anastomosis to the rectum, leaving a length of distal proctitis (**Fig. 9.9**). This may cause continuing bleeding, discomfort, urgency and evacuation difficulty. 'Strip proctitis' or 'cuffitis' has been reported in around 10–15% of cases having a stapled anastomosis,[44,45] with a small cumulative risk of dysplasia of 3% over a mean follow-up of 16 months in one study.[46] A few cases of carcinoma distal to the ileoanal anastomosis have been reported but these have occurred in patients who had either dysplasia or invasive cancer in the original operative specimen.[47]

A stapled anastomosis is easier and quicker to perform, it may cause less trauma to the anal sphincter and is preferred for patients in whom there may be tension in the mesentery on bringing the reservoir down to the anal level.

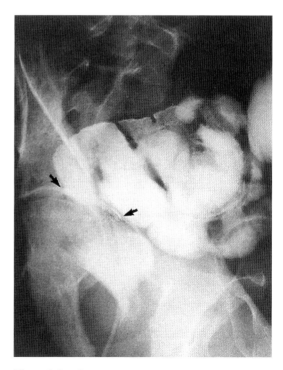

Figure 9.9 • Restorative proctocolectomy. Radiograph of pouch showing faulty technique by creation of anastomosis between ileal reservoir and rectal stump.

A recent meta-analysis of 21 comparative studies has demonstrated no significant differences in the incidence of postoperative complications between the two types of anastomosis. The incidence of nocturnal seepage and pad usage favoured the stapled anastomosis but persisting symptoms due to inflammation or dysplasia favoured the manual technique.[48]

The surgeon should be capable of using either method.

6. Defunctioning ileostomy. Most surgeons include a defunctioning ileostomy routinely. The ileostomy can cause morbidity, however, both in its formation and its closure, and this may account for 20% of complications. The operation has been carried out without ileostomy with excellent results. However, in a meta-analysis the rate of anastomotic leakage and the subsequent development of an anal lesion was double in patients not given a defunctioning ileostomy.[49]

Results
Failure

Failure is defined as the need for excision of the reservoir or indefinite diversion. The learning curve in ileal pouch surgery is related to failure, which improved following an initial training period of 23 cases in one study. Adequate results for manual anastomosis followed an initial experience of 31 procedures.[50]

Reports on failure in the early years after closure of the ileostomy gave rates ranging from around 5% to 10% (Table 9.4). Over the longer term, failure continues in a linear manner with rates approaching 15% at 15 years,[35] although in another large study a failure rate of 3.7% at 5 years had risen to only 7.9% at 20 years.[36]

The reasons for failure include pelvic sepsis (50%), poor function (30%) and pouchitis (10%).[35]

Pelvic sepsis in the early postoperative period confers a fivefold increase in the chance of subsequent failure.[51] In a series of 1965 patients treated in a single centre between 1983 and 2001, four preoperative and four postoperative factors were found to be associated with ileal pouch failure. Using a multifactorial survival analysis, each factor was assigned appropriate weights to form a scoring system (Table 9.5) for quantifying the risk of pouch failure in individual patients.[41]

Complications

Morbidity ranges from 20% to 50%. Many complications resolve spontaneously but some may require active intervention.

Pelvic sepsis due to breakdown of the ileoanal anastomosis or an infected haematoma, or both, has been reported in 5–20% of patients. A pyrexia develops within a few days and digital examination per anum may reveal an anastomotic defect or an extraluminal swelling (usually posterior) indicating the presence of a collection. The passage of fresh blood is highly suggestive of sepsis. A CT scan and examination under anaesthesia should be performed and any collection drained into the lumen.

Table 9.4 • Failure after restorative proctocolectomy: patients with ulcerative colitis only

Reference	n	Follow-up (months)*	Pouch excision	Indefinite diversion	Overall failure (%)
Gemlo et al.[79]	253	>12	–	–	9.9
Foley et al.[80]	460	–	7	9	3.5
MacRae et al.[81]	551	>30	49	9	10.5
Korsgen and Keighley[82]	180	>24	23	8	17.2
Meagher et al.[83]	1310	24–180 (77)	84	50	10
Tulchinsky et al.[35]	634	36–288 (85)	41	20	9.7
Fazio et al.[41]	1975	1–228 (49)	38	39	4.1

* Numbers in parentheses indicate mean values.

Chapter 9

Table 9.5 • Ileal pouch failure model **(a)** and conversion chart for the prediction of ileal pouch failure following restorative proctocolectomy **(b)**

(a)	Points
Preoperative risk factors	
Diagnosis	
Familial adenomatous polyposis	0
Ulcerative colitis or indeterminate colitis	1
Crohn's disease	1.5
Patient comorbidity	
No comorbid conditions	0
One comorbid condition	0.5
Two or more comorbid conditions	1.0
Prior anal pathology	
No prior anal pathology	0
Prior anal pathology	1
Anal sphincter manometry	
Normal manometry	0
Abnormal manometry	1
Postoperative risk factors	
Anastomotic separation	
No anastomotic separation	0
Anastomotic separation	1
Anastomotic stricture	
No stricture or asymptomatic stricture	0
Symptomatic stricture	1
Pelvic sepsis	
No sepsis	0
One episode of pelvic sepsis	1
Two or more episodes of pelvic sepsis	2
Fistula formation	
No fistula	0
Pouch–perineal fistula	1
Pouch–vaginal fistula	2

(b) Score	Follow-up (years)		
	1	5	10
0	0.1%	0.4%	0.8%
1	0.3%	1.1%	2.0%
2	0.8%	2.9%	5.0%
3	2.0%	7.2%	12.3%
4	5.0%	17.4%	28.5%
5	12.4%	38.7%	57.7%
6	28.7%	71.5%	89.0%

Stricture of the anastomosis requiring active intervention (either dilatation or a more major procedure) has been reported in 15% to over 30%.

Intestinal obstruction occurs in 5–20% of patients and surgery may be necessary, although most cases resolve spontaneously.

Pouch–vaginal fistula (the male equivalent is pouch–perineal fistula) occurs in 5–10% of (female) patients and is an important reason for late failure. It can occur months or years after closure of the ileostomy and is associated with an anastomotic complication in most cases. Patients with indeterminate colitis or Crohn's disease have a significantly higher incidence compared with ulcerative colitis patients (hazard ratio 1.4 and 2.2 respectively). The presence of perianal abscess or fistula-in-ano preoperatively is associated with 3.7- and 6-fold increases in the risk of developing pouch–vaginal fistula.[41]

Function

Frequency ranges from a median of 4–7 defecations per 24 hours but 20–30% have a frequency of 8 or more. This is usually regarded by the patient as acceptable, probably because urgency is present in less than 5% of patients. Nocturnal defecation is probably the most sensitive indicator of function. Frequency varies spontaneously and is also influenced by diet. Continence rates also vary but faecal incontinence is rare (5%). The need for antidiarrhoeal medication ranges from 20% to 50%.

There is a tendency for function to improve with time. In the long term, frequency of defecation has remained stable at a median of around 6 times per 24 hours and one per night in large series followed over 20 years. Minor incontinence (seepage) has increased from 4 to nearly 20% during the same period[52] (Table 9.6). Similar results for minor incontinence (3.9% at 1 year, 21% at 20 years) with a sight increase in 24-hour frequency (7.2 at 1 year, 8.4 at 20 years) have been reported by others.[36] Function is therefore well maintained over time with a small decline in continence.

Long term

General

Deficiencies of iron and vitamin B_{12} occur in less than 10% over a follow-up of 2–3 years. These may be associated with anaemia. There is a rise in the concentration of bacteria in the pouch by over a million fold from the concentration of 10^4–10^6 colony-forming units per gram of faeces found in the normal terminal ileum.

Pouchitis

The small-bowel mucosa develops a degree of villous atrophy in almost all cases (including those with FAP). The endoscopic appearances of a non-inflamed pouch are shown in **Fig. 9.10**. In some patients, however, acute inflammation occurs and when this is associated with frequency, urgency, liquid stool and extra-alimentary manifestations the condition is known as pouchitis (**Fig. 9.11**). There is evidence that pouchitis occurs early after closure of the ileostomy.[53,54] It is rare in FAP, and is more common in non-smokers[55] and in patients with sclerosing cholangitis.[4]

The cumulative incidence over 5 years approaches 50% but the prevalence of unremitting chronic pouchitis is only about 5%. The diagnosis depends on clinical, endoscopic and histopathological features, the latter being essential and must show acute inflammation. Grading systems to assess severity have been described.[56–58]

Table 9.6 • Long-term functional outcomes following restorative proctocolectomy based on the data from the Association of Coloproctology of Great Britain and Ireland (ACPGBI) Ileal Pouch Registry[52]

Functional outcome	1 year	5 years	10 years	15 years	20 years
Median stool frequency					
Per 24 hours	5	5	6	5	5
Night	0	0	1	0	1
Seepage – daytime	3.9%	3.8%	6.6%	7.2%	20.5%
Seepage – night	8.0%	8.2%	10.6%	10.1%	15.4%
Pad use – daytime	2.9%	2.5%	5.9%	5.8%	12.8%
Pad use – night	6.1%	5.0%	7.2%	8.7%	17.9%
Faecal urgency	5.1%	5.9%	9.4%	9.1%	2.9%
Antidiarrhoeal medication	38.9%	34.0%	37.2%	25.4%	38.5%

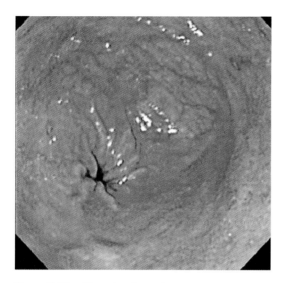

Figure 9.10 • Normal endoscopic appearances.

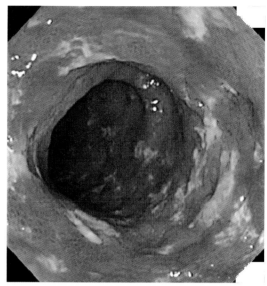

Figure 9.11 • Pouchitis.

A bacterial cause is likely to be partly responsible since pouchitis responds to antibacterials and probiotics. Antibacterial drugs, including metronidazole, ciprofloxacin and augmentin, can induce a response in over 80% of patients.[59,60]

Maintenance of remission by daily administration of the probiotic VSL3 has been shown to be effective in 85% of patients compared with controls (0%) when taken over a 9-month period.[61]

Withdrawal of treatment is followed by recurrence. Long-term metronidazole should be avoided due to the risk of peripheral neuropathy. An algorithm for the treatment of pouchitis is shown in **Fig. 9.12**.[62]

Removal of the reservoir for pouchitis accounts for only 10% of failures. Defunctioning does not affect the degree of inflammation, and excision with construction of a new reservoir is followed by pouchitis.

Neoplastic transformation

Dysplasia in the pouch mucosa is rare.[63–65] To date, over 20 case reports of carcinoma in the pouch or the distal anorectal segment have been described. Almost all of these had either dysplasia or a carcinoma in the original operative specimen and in none did the carcinoma appear within less than 10 years from the diagnosis of ulcerative colitis.[47]

These patients should be selected for surveillance by endoscopy with multiple biopsies at yearly intervals beyond 10 years from the onset of colitis. A suggested surveillance protocol is shown in **Fig. 9.13**.

Salvage surgery

Removal of the pouch has a significant morbidity, with readmissions and delayed healing of the perineal wound in 40% of patients.[66] Thus, where failure is threatened by sepsis or poor function, it may be in the patient's interest to consider a salvage procedure which may be less traumatic and offers a chance of retaining satisfactory anal function.

Such patients often have poor function and should be investigated by contrast radiology, including evacuation pouchography, anal manometry, pouch volumetry, MRI and histopathological examination of biopsy material. Action will depend on the diagnosis (**Fig. 9.14**).

Success rates for abdominal salvage for pelvic sepsis range from <30% to 80%.[51,67–69] Pouch–vaginal fistula should be treated by defunctioning followed by an attempt at repair. If low, a local approach via the endoanal or transvaginal route will be necessary and success rates of around 60% of patients have been reported,[70,71] although late recurrence can occur. If high (usually associated with a stapled ileoanal anastomosis), abdominal advancement of

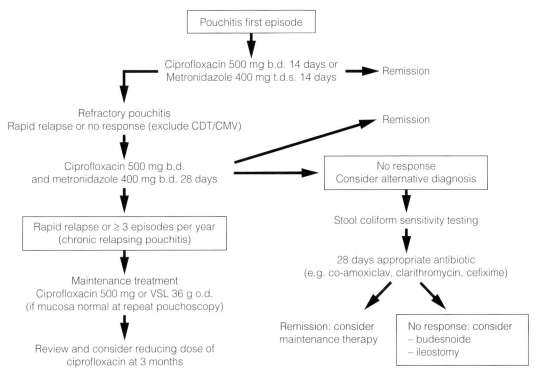

Figure 9.12 • Algorithm for the treatment of pouchitis. CDT, [definition?]; CMV, cytomegalovirus. Adapted from McLaughlin SD, Tekkis PP, Ciclitira PJ et al. Review article: restorative proctocolectomy, indications, management of complications and follow-up: a guide for gastroenterologists. Aliment Pharmacol Ther 2008, in press. With permission from Blackwell Publishing.

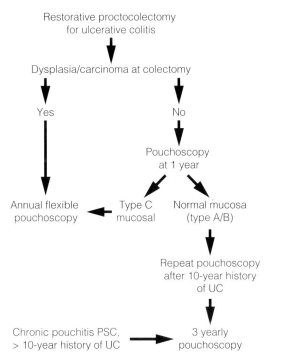

Figure 9.13 • Surveillance protocol. PSC, [definition?]; UC, ulcerative colitis. Adapted from McLaughlin SD, Tekkis PP, Ciclitira PJ et al. Review article: restorative proctocolectomy, indications, management of complications and follow-up: a guide for gastroenterologists. Aliment Pharmacol Ther 2008, in press. With permission from Blackwell Publishing.

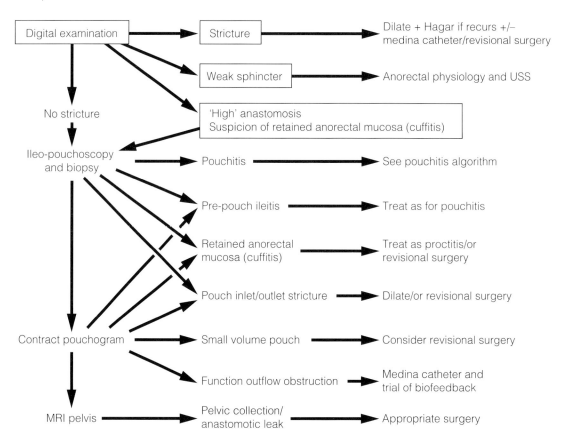

Figure 9.14 • Algorithm for the investigation of pouch dysfunction. USS, [definition?]. Adapted from McLaughlin SD, Tekkis PP, Ciclitira PJ et al. Review article: restorative proctocolectomy, indications, management of complications and follow-up: a guide for gastroenterologists. Aliment Pharmacol Ther 2008, in press. With permission from Blackwell Publishing.

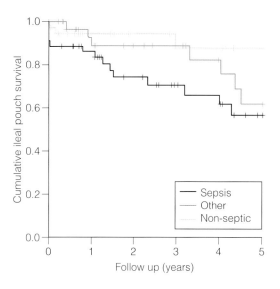

Figure 9.15 • Anal function up to 5 years following abdominal salvage surgery for septic and non-septic indications. Reproduced from Tekkis PP HA, Smith JJ, Das P et al. Long-term results of abdominal salvage surgery following restorative proctocolectomy. Br J Surg 2006; 93:231–7. With permission from Blackwell Publishing.

the anastomosis with mucosectomy has achieved success in over 70%.[72,73] Pouch–perineal fistula in males is difficult to close and managment by a long-term seton can be satisfactory.

Abdominal revision for mechanical outflow obstruction due to anastomotic stricture or a retained rectal stump is successful in 70–90%.[68,69]

 This is significantly higher than the rates achieved when sepsis is the indication for salvage (**Fig. 9.15**).

Augmentation of a small-volume reservoir may improve function.

Key points

- The prevalence of ulcerative colitis is about 160 per 100 000 population, compared with about 50 per 100 000 for Crohn's disease.
- At presentation, 50% of cases have disease confined to the rectum, in 30% this extends to the left colon and in a further 20% disease extends beyond the splenic flexure.
- About 25% of patients with ulcerative colitis will develop at least one extra-alimentary manifestation during the course of the illness, such as arthropathy, primary sclerosing cholangitis, erythema nodosum or uveitis.
- The incidence of cancer in patients is estimated to be 0% within 10 years of onset of ulcerative colitis, 10–15% in the second decade and over 20% in the third.
- Histopathological examination of a mucosal biopsy is the basis for the diagnosis of ulcerative colitis.
- The initial treatment of acute severe colitis is medical but about 30% of patients will require surgery. Surgery is absolutely indicated in cases with acute toxic dilatation or perforation.
- The operation of choice for acute severe colitis is subtotal colectomy with ileostomy and preservation of the rectal stump.
- Indications for elective surgery for chronic ulcerative colitis include failure of medical treatment, growth retardation in the young and neoplastic transformation.
- Restorative proctocolectomy is the procedure of choice for the majority of patients with chronic ulcerative colitis.
- Contraindications to restorative proctocolectomy include Crohn's disease, indeterminate colitis favouring Crohn's disease, weak sphincter and patient choice.
- The choice of ileal pouch reservoir (J vs. W) or type of anastomosis (hand-sewn vs. stapled) has similar postoperative outcomes and bowel function.
- One-third of patients undergoing restorative proctocolectomy develop at least one adverse event, which include anastomotic separation, pelvic sepsis, anastomotic stricture, fistula, small-bowel obstruction, bleeding or pouchitis.
- Ileal pouch failure is a time-dependent outcome with an estimated 5–10% pouch excision rate or indefinite diversion at 10 years following restorative proctocolectomy.
- Patients who are threatened with pouch failure may be considered for salvage surgery, with successful outcome in 80% of patients.

References

1. Tysk C, Linkberg E, Jarnesot G et al. Ulcerative colitis and Crohn's disease in an unselected population of monozygotic and dizygotic twins: a study of heritability and the influence of smoking. Gut 1988; 29:990–6.

2. Thompson NP, Driscoll R, Pounder RE et al. Genetics versus environment in inflammatory bowel disease: results of a British twin study. Br Med J 1996; 312:95–6.

3. Thompson-Fawcett MW, Mortensen NJ. Anal transitional zone and columnar cuff in restorative proctocolectomy. Br J Surg 1996; 83(8):1047–55.

4. Penna C, Dozois R, Tremaine W et al. Pouchitis after ileal pouch–anal anastomosis for ulcerative colitis occurs with increased frequency in patients with associated primary sclerosing cholangitis. Gut 1996; 38(2):234–9.

5. Stahlberg D, Veress B, Tribukait B et al. Atrophy and neoplastic transformation of the ileal pouch mucosa in patients with ulcerative colitis and primary sclerosing cholangitis: a case control study. Dis Colon Rectum 2003; 46(6):770–8.

6. Thomas T, Abrams KA, Robinson RJ et al. Meta-analysis: cancer risk of low-grade dysplasia in chronic ulcerative colitis. Aliment Pharmacol Ther 2007; 15:657–68.

7. Sachar AKaD. Ulcerative colitis practice guidelines in adults (update); American College of Gastroenterology, Practice and Parameters Committee. Am J Gastroenterol 2004; 99:1371–85.

8. Price AB. Overlap in the spectrum of non-specific inflammatory bowel disease – 'colitis indeterminate'. J Clin Pathol 1978; 31:567–77.

9. Wells AD, McMillan I, Price AB et al. Natural history of indeterminate colitis. Br J Surg 1991; 78(2):179–81.

10. Jakobovits SL, Travis SP. Management of acute severe colitis. Br Med Bull 2006; 75/76:131–44.

11. Shibolet O, Regushevskaya E, Brezis M et al. Cyclosporine A for induction of remission in severe ulcerative colitis. Cochrane Database Syst Rev 2005; 1:CD004277.

12. Jakobovits SL, Jewell DP, Travis S. Infliximab for the treatment of ulcerative colitis: outcomes in Oxford from 2000 to 2006. Aliment Pharmacol Ther 2007; 25:1055–60.

13. Roberts S, Williams JG, Yeates D et al. Mortality in patients with and without colectomy admitted to hospital for ulcerative colitis and Crohn's disease: record linkage studies. Br Med J 2007; 335:1033–41.

14. Kaplan G, McCarthy EP, Ayanian JZ et al. Impact of hospital volume on postoperative morbidity and mortality following a colectomy for ulcerative colitis. Gastroenterology 2008 (Epub ahead of print).

15. Lindsey I, George BD, Kettlewell MG et al. Impotence after mesorectal and close rectal dissection for inflammatory bowel disease. Dis Colon Rectum 2001; 44(6):831–5.

16. Kock NG. Intra-abdominal 'reservoir' in patients with permanent ileostomy. Arch Surg 1969; 99:223–31.

17. Nessar G, Fazio VW, Tekkis PP et al. Long-term outcome and quality of life after continent ileostomy. Dis Colon Rectum 2006; 49:336–44.

18. Myrvold H. The continent ileostomy. World J Surg 1987; 11:720–6.

19. Hulten L, Willen R, Nilsson O et al. Mucosal assessment for dysplasia and cancer in the ileal pouch mucosa in patients operated on for ulcerative colitis-a 30-year follow-up study. Dis Colon Rectum 2002; 45(4):448–52.

20. Cox CL, Butts DR, Roberts MP et al. Development of invasive adenocarcinoma in a long-standing Kock continent ileostomy: report of a case. Dis Colon Rectum 1997; 40(4):500–3.

21. Aylett SO. Three hundred cases of diffuse ulcerative colitis treatment by total colectomy and ileorectal anastomosis. Br Med J 1966; 1:1001–5.

22. Baker WNW, Glass RE, Ritchie JK et al. Cancer of the rectum following colectomy and ileorectal anastomosis for ulcerative colitis. Br J Surg 1978; 65:862–8.

23. Ravitch MM, Sabiston DC. Anal ileostomy with preservation of the sphincter; a proposed operation in patients requiring total colectomy for benign lesions. Surg Gynecol Obstet 1947; 84:1095–9.

24. Valiènte MA, Bacon HE. Construction of pouch using 'pantaloon' technique for pull through following colectomy. Am J Surg 1955; 90:6621–43.

25. Parks A, Nicholls RJ. Proctocolectomy without ileostomy for ulcerative colitis. Br Med J 1978; 2:85–8.

26. Alexander F, Sarigol S, Difiore J et al. Fate of the pouch in 151 pediatric patients after ileal pouch anal anastomosis. J Pediatr Surg 2003; 38(1):78–82.

27. Delaney C, Fazio VW, Remzi FH et al. Prospective, age-related analysis of surgical results, functional outcome, and quality of life after ileal pouch–anal anastomosis. Ann Surg 2003; 238:221–8.

28. Farouk R, Pemberton JH, Wolff BG et al. Functional outcomes after ileal pouch–anal anastomosis for chronic ulcerative colitis. Ann Surg 2000; 231(6):919–26.

29. Waljee A, Waljee J, Morris AM et al. Three-fold increased risk of infertility: a meta-analysis of infertility after pouch surgery in ulcerative colitis. Gut 2006; 55:1575–80.

30. Cornish JA, Tan E, Teare J et al. A systematic review. The effect of restorative proctocolectomy on sexual function, urinary function, fertility, pregnancy and delivery. Dis Colon Rectum 2007; 50:1128–38.

31. Olsen K, Juul S, Berndtsson I et al. Ulcerative colitis: female fecundity before diagnosis, during disease, and after surgery compared with a population sample. Gastroenterology 2002; 122(1):15–19.

An epidemiological study of a cohort of women of child-bearing age in which fecundability was compared with the general population before and after the onset of ulcerative colitis and following restorative proctocolectomy.

32. Olsen KO, Juul S, Bulow S et al. Female fecundity before and after operation for familial adenomatous polyposis. Br J Surg 2003; 90(2):227–31.

A similar analysis by the same group of patients with familial adenomatous polyposis showing that colectomy with ileorectal anastomosis was not associated with a fall in fecundability.

33. Lepisto A, Sarna S, Tiitinen A et al. Female fertility and childbirth after ileal pouch–anal anastomosis for ulcerative colitis. Br J Surg 2007; 94:478–82.

34. Regimbeau JM, Panis Y, Pocard M et al. Long-term results of ileal pouch–anal anastomosis for

colorectal Crohn's disease. Dis Colon Rectum 2001; 44(6):769–78.

35. Tulchinsky H, Hawley PR, Nicholls J. Long-term failure after restorative proctocolectomy for ulcerative colitis. Ann Surg 2003; 238(2):229–34.

36. Hahnloser D, Pemberton JH, Wolff BG et al. Results at up to 20 years after ileal pouch–anal anastomosis for chronic ulcerative colitis. Br J Surg 2007; 94:333–40.

A prospective long-term follow-up over 20 years in a large series of patients having restorative proctocolectomy.

37. Tekkis PP, Heriot AG, Smith O et al. Long-term outcomes of restorative proctocolectomy for Crohn's disease and indeterminate colitis. Colorectal Dis 2005; 7:218–23.

A long-term analysis of patients with Crohn's disease and indeterminate colitis after restorative proctocolectomy.

38. Yu CS, Pemberton JH, Larson D. Ileal pouch–anal anastomosis in patients with indeterminate colitis: long-term results. Dis Colon Rectum 2000; 43(11):1487–96.

39. Delaney CPR, Gramlich FH, Dadvand T et al. Equivalent function, quality of life and pouch survival rates after ileal pouch–anal anastomosis for indeterminate and ulcerative colitis. Ann Surg 2002; 236(1):43–8.

40. Richard CS, Cohen Z, Stern HS et al. Outcome of the pelvic pouch procedure in patients with prior perianal disease. Dis Colon Rectum 1997; 40(6):647–52.

41. Fazio V, Tekkis PP, Remzi F et al. Quantification for risk failure after ileal pouch anal anastomosis surgery. Ann Surg 2003; 238:605–17.

A multivariate risk analysis of factors associated with failure after restorative proctocolectomy resulting in a scoring system for failure applicable to individual patients.

42. Penna C, Dozois RR, Tremaine W et al. Pouchitis after ileal pouch anal anastomosis for ulcerative colitis occurs with increased frequency in patients with associated primary sclerosing cholangitis. Gut 1996; 38:234–9.

43. Lovegrove R, Heriot AG, Constantinides V et al. Meta-analysis of short-term and long-term outcomes of J, W and S ileal reservoirs for restorative proctocolectomy. Colorectal Dis 2007; 9:310–20.

44. Lavery IC, Sirimarco MT, Ziv Y et al. Anal canal inflammation after ileal pouch–anal anastomosis. The need for treatment. Dis Colon Rectum 1995; 38(8):803–6.

45. Thompson-Fawcett MW, Mortensen NJ, Warren BF. "Cuffitis" and inflammatory changes in the columnar cuff, anal transitional zone, and ileal reservoir after stapled pouch–anal anastomosis. Dis Colon Rectum 1999; 42(3):348–55.

46. Ziv Y, Fazio VW, Sirimarco MT et al. Incidence, risk factors, and treatment of dysplasia in the anal transitional zone after ileal pouch–anal anastomosis. Dis Colon Rectum 1994; 37(12):1281–5.

47. Das P, Johnson MW, Tekkis PP et al. Risk of dysplasia and adenocarcinoma following restorative proctocolectomy for ulcerative colitis. Colorectal Dis 2007; 9:15–27.

48. Lovegrove RE, Constantinides VA, Heriot AG et al. A comparison of hand-sewn versus stapled ileal pouch anal anastomosis (IPAA) following proctocolectomy: a meta-analysis of 4183 patients. Ann Surg 2006; 244:18–26.

A meta-analysis of 21 studies comparing manual and stapled ileoanal anastomosis.

49. Weston-Petrides G, Lovegrove RE, Tilney HS et al. Comparison of outcomes after restorative proctocolectomy with or without defunctioning ileostomy. Arch Surg 2008; 143:406–12.

50. Tekkis PPF, Remzi VW, Senagore FH et al. Evaluation of the learning curve in ileal pouch–anal anastomosis surgery. Ann Surg 2005; 241:262–8.

51. Heuschen U, Allemeyer EH, Hinz UH et al. Outcome after septic complications in J pouch procedures. Br J Surg 2002; 89:194–200.

An analysis of a prospectively maintained database in which immediate postoperative sepsis conferred a fivefold risk of subsequent failure.

52. Tekkis PLR, Tilney H, Sagar P et al. Primary and salvage ileal pouch surgery in the United Kingdom – a multicenter study of 2,491 patients. Dis Colon Rectum 2007; 50:756.

53. Apel R, Cohen Z, Andrews CW Jr et al. Prospective evaluation of early morphological changes in pelvic ileal pouches. Gastroenterology 1994; 107(2):435–43.

54. Setti-Carraro P, Talbot IC, Nicholls RJ. A long term appraisal of the histological appearances of the ileal reservoir mucosa after restorative proctocolectomy for ulcerative colitis. Gut 1994; 35:1721–7.

55. Merrett MN, Mortensen NJ, Kettlewell M et al. Smoking may prevent pouchitis in patients with restorative proctocolectomy for ulcerative colitis. Gut 1996; 38:362–4.

56. Moskowitz R, Shepherd NA, Nicholls RJ. An assessment of inflammation in the reservoir after restorative proctocolectomy with ileoanal ileal reservoir. Int J Colorectal Dis 1986; 1:167–74.

57. Sandborn WJ. Pouchitis following ileal pouch–anal anastomosis: definition, pathogenesis, and treatment. Gastroenterology 1994; 107(6):1856–60.

58. Shen B, Achkar JP, Connor JT et al. Modified pouchitis disease activity index: a simplified approach to the diagnosis of pouchitis. Dis Colon Rectum 2003; 46(6):748–53.

59. Shen B, Achkar JP, Lashner BA et al. A randomized clinical trial of ciprofloxacin and metronidazole to treat acute pouchitis. Inflamm Bowel Dis 2001; 7(4):301–5.

60. Mimura T, Rizzello F, Helwig U et al. Four-week open-label trial of metronidazole and ciprofloxacin for the treatment of recurrent or

refractory pouchitis. Aliment Pharmacol Ther 2002; 16(5):909–17.

61. Gionchetti P, Rizzello F, Venturi A et al. Oral bacteriotherapy as maintenance treatment in patients with chronic pouchitis: a double-blind, placebo-controlled trial. Gastroenterology 2000; 119(2):305–9.

A randomised controlled clinical trial of VSL3 as maintenance treatment in patients with pouchitis after an initial induction of remission by antibiotics.

62. McLaughlin SD, Tekkis PP, Ciclitira PJ et al. Review article: restorative proctocolectomy, indications, management of complications and follow-up: a guide for gastroenterologists. Aliment Pharmacol Ther 2008 (Epub ahead of print).

63. Veress B, Reinholt FP, Lindquist K et al. Long-term histomorphological surveillance of the pelvic ileal pouch: dysplasia develops in a subgroup of patients. Gastroenterology 1995; 109(4):1090–7.

64. Thompson-Fawcett MW, Marcus V, Redston M et al. Risk of dysplasia in long-term ileal pouches and pouches with chronic pouchitis. Gastroenterology 2001; 121(2):275–81.

65. Borjesson L, Willen R, Haboubi N et al. The risk of dysplasia and cancer in the ileal pouch mucosa after restorative proctocolectomy for ulcerative colitis is low: a long term follow-up study. Colorectal Dis 2004; 6:494–8.

66. Karoui M, Cohen RG, Nicholls J. Results of surgical removal of the pouch after failed restorative proctocolectomy. Dis Colon Rectum 2004; 47:869–75.

67. Fazio VW, Wu JS, Lavery IC. Repeat ileal pouch-anal anastomosis to salvage septic complications of pelvic pouches: clinical outcome and quality of life assessment. Ann Surg 1998; 228(4):588–97.

68. Dehni N, Remacle G, Dozois RR et al. Salvage reoperation for complications after ileal pouch-anal anastomosis. Br J Surg 2005; 92:748–53.

69. Tekkis PP, Heriot AG, Smith JJ et al. Long-term results of abdominal salvage surgery following restorative proctocolectomy. Br J Surg 2006; 93:231–7.

70. Shah NS, Remzi F, Massmann A et al. Management and treatment outcome of pouch–vaginal fistulas following restorative proctocolectomy. Dis Colon Rectum 2003; 46:911–17.

71. Heriot A, Tekkis PP, Smith JJ et al. Management and outcome of pouch–vaginal fistulas following restorative proctocolectomy. Dis Colon Rectum 2005; 48:451–4.

72. Cohen Z, Smith D, McLeod R. Reconstructive surgery for pelvic pouches. World J Surg 1998; 22:342–6.

73. Zinicola R, Wilkinson KH, Nicholls RJ. Ileal pouch–vaginal fistula treated by abdominoanal advancement of the ileal pouch. Br J Surg 2003; 90:1434–5.

74. Galandiuk S, Scott NA, Dozois RR et al. Ileal pouch–anal anastomosis. Reoperation for pouch-related complications. Ann Surg 1990; 212(4):446–52; discussion 452–4.

75. Deutsch AA, McLeod RS, Cullan J et al. Results of the pelvic pouch procedure in patients with Crohn's disease. Dis Colon Rectum 1991; 34:475–7.

76. Hyman NH, Fazio VW, Tuckson WB et al. Consequences of ileal pouch–anal anastomosis for Crohn's colitis. Dis Colon Rectum 1991; 34(8):653–7.

77. Grobler SP, Hosie KB, Affie E et al. Outcome of restorative proctocolectomy when the diagnosis is suggestive of Crohn's disease. Gut 1993; 34(10):1384–8.

78. Panis Y, Poupard B, Nemeth J et al. Ileal pouch/anal anastomosis for Crohn's disease. Lancet 1996; 347(9005):854–7.

79. Gemlo BT, Wong WD, Rothenberger DA et al. Ileal pouch–anal anastomosis. Patterns of failure. Arch Surg 1992; 127(7):784–6; discussion 787.

80. Foley EF, Schoetz DJ Jr, Roberts PL et al. Rediversion after ileal pouch–anal anastomosis. Causes of failures and predictors of subsequent pouch salvage. Dis Colon Rectum 1995; 38(8):793–8.

81. MacRae HM, McLeod RS, Cohen Z et al. Risk factors for pelvic pouch failure. Dis Colon Rectum 1997; 40:257–62.

82. Korsgen S, Keighley MR. Causes of failure and life expectancy of the ileoanal pouch. Int J Colorectal Dis 1997; 12:4–8.

83. Meagher AP, Farouk R, Dozois RR et al. J ileal pouch–anal anastomosis for chronic ulcerative colitis: complications and long-term outcome in 1310 patients. Br J Surg 1998; 85(6):800–3.

10

Crohn's disease

Mark W. Thompson-Fawcett
Neil J.McC. Mortensen

Introduction

Crohn's disease is a chronic transmural inflammatory process that can affect the gastrointestinal tract anywhere from mouth to anus and which may be associated with extraintestinal manifestations. The disease is commonly confined to a region of the gut. Frequent disease patterns observed include ileal, ileocolic and colonic. Perianal disease may coexist with any of these. Often there are discontinuous segments of disease with areas of normal mucosa intervening. Inflammation may cause ulceration, fissures, fistulas and fibrosis with stricturing. Histology reveals a chronic inflammatory infiltrate that is typically patchy and transmural, and may reveal classic granulomas with giant cell formation. Clinically, patients have abdominal pain and diarrhoea, and they may develop bowel obstruction or intestinal fistulas. A combination of the clinical, macroscopic, radiological and pathological features is required to make the diagnosis. It is a chronic disease with varying lengths of remission interspersed with acute episodes.

Epidemiology

Crohn's disease has a prevalence of around 0.1%. Peak age of onset is 15–25 years, with a slightly higher incidence in females. There is no association with socio-economic status or occupation, but an urban environment, cooler climate and increased standards of domestic hygiene may increase the risk.

In northern Europe, Scandinavia and North America the annual incidence of Crohn's disease is 5–6 per 100 000 population. This has steadily increased over recent decades but has now plateaued. Rates are lower but increasing in southern and eastern Europe, and Asia. Evidence of environmental effects is seen from studies of migrant populations.[1] Current thinking is that environmental factors, rather than ethnicity, are a more important explanation for regional variation in incidence.

Aetiology

Crohn's disease involves an interplay between environmental and genetic factors. The specific cause of the exaggerated inflammatory response at the mucosal level remains unclear. There are a number of areas where much investigation has been focused.

Smoking and oral contraception

Smoking increases the relative risk of Crohn's disease by 2–2.4 times, in contrast with ulcerative colitis where smoking provides a protective effect. Oral contraception may be associated with a small increase in risk, but whether this is causal or by association is not clear. Evidence suggests that oral contraceptive use has no effect on disease activity.[1]

Infection

Mycobacterium paratuberculosis causes a granulomatous inflammatory disorder in the intestine of cattle (Johne's disease) and it has been hypothesised that Crohn's is the human form of this disease. Many remain sceptical as the evidence is conflicting; the issue requires resolution.[2]

It has been controversially proposed that measles virus infection or vaccination may cause the granulomatous vasculitis observed in Crohn's disease, but current evidence does not support this.[3]

Genetic

It is likely inflammatory bowel disease (IBD) results from a genetic predisposition to an abnormal interaction between the immune system and environmental factors, especially the gut microbiota. Epidemiological studies have demonstrated familial aggregation; 2–22% of patients with Crohn's disease have a first-degree relative with IBD. There is greater concordance for IBD in monozygotic (36%) than dizygotic twins (4%). Early-onset disease has a higher familial prevalence rate, suggesting a greater genetic contribution compared with late-onset disease. Clinical patterns of IBD in affected parent–child and sibling pairs are concordant for each of disease type, extent and extraintestinal manifestations in the majority of cases. The relatives of patients with Crohn's disease also have an increased risk of developing ulcerative colitis. Crohn's disease and ulcerative colitis seem polygenetic disorders with some shared susceptibility genes.

These familial patterns have led to genome-wide scanning that has identified nine loci (IBD1–9) implicated in susceptibility to IBD. Of these, all variants of IBD1 or the caspase recruitment domain family member 15 (CARD15) gene have generated most interest in regard to Crohn's disease. CARD15 encodes the protein nucleotide-binding oligomerisation domain 2 (NOD2). It is associated with ileal disease and displays ethnic variation (less common in northern Europe and Asia). Most evidence suggests CARD15 variants impair the innate immune system at mucosal level, limiting the ability of the intestinal epithelium to deal with pathogens or components of them in the gut microbiota. It is hoped that further advances in genetics will improve phenotyping, prognosis and the development of new targeted therapies.[4]

Pathogenesis

Normally, the gut exists in a state of tolerance to the stream of microbial, dietary and other antigens in contact with the mucosa, but this tolerance and the ability to suppress an immune-mediated inflammatory response is lost in IBD. In Crohn's disease defects in immunoregulation are coupled with an increased mucosal permeability due to leaky paracellular pathways.

Defects in immunoregulation may include disturbed innate immune mechanisms at the epithelial barrier, problems with antigen recognition and processing by dentritic cells, and effects of psychosocial stress via a neuroimmunological interaction. In Crohn's disease the cell-mediated response is predominant, with excessive activation of effector T cells (Th1) that predominate over the regulatory T cells (Th3, Tr) that turn off the process. Proinflammatory cytokines released by effector T cells stimulate macrophages to release tumour necrosis factor (TNF)-α, interleukin (IL)-1 and IL-6. In addition, abnormal dendritic cell function may further drive the inflammatory response. Leucocytes then enter from the local circulation releasing further chemokines, amplifying the inflammatory process. The result is a local and systemic response, including fever, an acute-phase response, hypoalbuminaemia, weight loss, increased mucosal epithelial permeability, endothelial damage and increased collagen synthesis. Due to immune dysregulation the inflammatory response in the intestinal mucosa proceeds unchecked, producing a chronic inflammatory state.[1,5]

Pathology

Distribution

The macroscopic appearance and distribution are the first important considerations that provide key information towards differentiating Crohn's disease from other forms of IBD, particularly ulcerative colitis. Frequencies of regions involved are:

1. small bowel alone, 30–35%;
2. colon alone, 25–35%;
3. small bowel and colon, 30–50% (usually ileocolic);
4. perianal lesions, over 50%;
5. stomach and duodenum, 5% (minor subclinical mucosal abnormalities in 50%).

Skip lesions (areas of disease separated by normal bowel) strongly suggests Crohn's disease, although occasionally a periappendiceal or caecal patch of overt colitis may be observed with distal ulcerative colitis.

Macroscopic appearance

The unmistakable appearance of Crohn's disease is of a stiff, thick-walled segment of bowel with fat wrapping. There is creeping extension of mesenteric fat around the serosal surface of the bowel wall towards the antimesenteric border. This is part of the connective tissue changes that affect all layers of the bowel wall. As inflammation is full thickness, there can be fibrinous exudate and adhesions on the serosal surface. Narrow linear ulcers with intervening islands of oedematous mucosa give the mucosal surface its classic cobblestone appearance. Ulceration is discrete, and serpiginous linear ulcers usually run along the mesenteric aspect of the lumen. Deep fissuring from linear ulceration may lead to formation of fistulas through the bowel wall. Closer inspection may reveal multiple aphthous ulcers that usually develop on the surface of submucosal lymphoid nodules. Aphthous ulcers are the earliest macroscopic lesions in Crohn's disease and are seen before the classic appearances of more established disease. Inflammatory polyps are often found in the involved colon but are unusual in the small bowel. Enlarged lymph nodes may be present in the resected mesentery but are not caseated or matted together. Strictures can vary from 1 to 30 cm in length. These may be stiff like a hosepipe with turgid oedema, or tight fibrotic strictures from burnt-out inflammation. The narrowing of the lumen may be sufficient to produce obstruction and proximal dilatation, and there may be multiple dilated segments between multiple tight strictures. Fistulas, sinuses and abscesses are often present in the ileocaecal region but may arise from any segment of active disease and can communicate with other loops of bowel, stomach, bladder, vagina, skin or intra-abdominal abscess cavities.

Microscopy

Inflammation involves the full thickness of the bowel wall. Early mucosal changes show neutrophils attacking the base of crypts, causing injury and focal crypt abscesses. The formation of mucosal lymphoid aggregates followed by overlying ulceration produces aphthous ulcers. There is relative preservation of goblet cell mucin by comparison with ulcerative colitis, where there is usually mucin depletion. As the disease progresses, connective tissue changes occur in all layers of the bowel wall giving the stiff, thick-walled, macroscopic appearance. There is submucosal fibrosis and muscularisation. The muscularis mucosa and muscularis propria are thickened from increased amounts of connective tissue. Typically, the chronic inflammatory infiltrate and the architectural changes in the mucosa are patchy. Transmural inflammation is in the form of lymphoid aggregates seen throughout the bowel wall, leading to the formation of a Crohn's 'rosary' on the serosal surface. The following three features are diagnostic hallmarks of Crohn's disease:

1. deep non-caseating granulomas (excluding those that are mucosal or related to crypt rupture) are present in 60–70% of patients and are commonly located in the bowel wall but may be in the mesentery, regional lymph nodes, peritoneum, liver or contiguously involved tissue;
2. intralymphatic granulomas;
3. granulomatous vasculitis.

Pitfalls in differentiating Crohn's colitis from ulcerative colitis

Sometimes it is difficult even for an experienced gastrointestinal pathologist to differentiate between Crohn's colitis and ulcerative colitis on histology, and considerable interobserver variation is reported among pathologists. There can be overlap between the diseases and this can lead to the diagnosis of indeterminate colitis in 5–10% of patients with colonic involvement alone. During the course of the disease subsequent disease behaviour may change, leading to a change in diagnosis, usually towards Crohn's disease. For difficult cases, consideration of the macroscopic, microscopic, radiological and endoscopic features and the history and clinical picture is essential, for it is often the cumulative evidence that makes the diagnosis. A definitive diagnosis is more likely if the resected colon is available for assessment as opposed to mucosal biopsies. If only endoscopic biopsies are available, the endoscopic findings are important and must be discussed with, or shown to, the pathologist.

Rectal sparing may be seen in ulcerative colitis, especially if topical preparations have been used. Patchy inflammation is a feature of Crohn's disease, but treated ulcerative colitis can itself show patchy mucosal inflammation. Perianal disease is very suggestive of Crohn's, although patients with ulcerative colitis can develop cryptoglandular fistulas and abscesses. Lymphoid follicles may be seen in the base of the mucosa in severe ulcerative colitis, but they are a prominent feature of Crohn's disease, where they are transmural. In Crohn's disease there is relative preservation of goblet cell mucin, whereas mucin depletion is a feature of ulcerative colitis (with the exception of fulminant ulcerative colitis, where there may be surprisingly little mucin depletion). In established diversion proctitis or pouchitis it is difficult to exclude Crohn's disease as both these conditions may mimic Crohn's disease.

Clinical

Gastrointestinal symptoms

The clinical presentation varies depending on the site of disease. Acute first presentations of disease are uncommon, but ileal disease can mimic acute appendicitis and colonic disease may present as a fulminating colitis.

The majority of patients complain of diarrhoea (70–90%), abdominal pain (45–65%), rectal bleeding (30%) and perianal disease (10%). The symptom profile will reflect the disease location. Diarrhoea may result from mucosal inflammation, fistulation between loops of bowel, a short bowel from previous resections, bacterial overgrowth from obstructed segments, or bile salt malabsorption from terminal ileal disease. These latter two also produce steatorrhoea. Distal colitis and proctitis, and decreased rectal compliance, produce tenesmus and frequent bowel motions. Abdominal pain may be colicky from obstructing lesions or more continual from peritoneal irritation caused by acute inflammation. Terminal ileal disease is the most common site for obstructive lesions. Rectal bleeding is uncommon from terminal ileal disease, but does occur in 50% of patients with colonic disease. Massive bleeding occurs in 1–2%, though the site is often difficult to identify. When perianal disease is present, patients often complain of purulent discharge and minor leakage of faecal material with local discomfort. Fissures may be large, indolent

and painless. Significant perianal pain suggests undrained sepsis. Fistulas extending to the bladder can produce pneumaturia and recurrent urinary tract infection, while those extending to the vagina may cause wind or faeces vaginally.

Systemic symptoms

Weight loss is reported by 65–75% of patients. This is usually of the order of 10–20% of body weight and is the result of anorexia, food fear, diarrhoea and, less often, malabsorption. The latter may be caused by inflammatory disease but more commonly is due to bacterial overgrowth as a result of coloenteric fistulas, blind loops or stasis from chronic obstruction. If there is extensive small-bowel disease, there may be poor absorption of fat-soluble vitamins leading to symptoms and signs of osteomalacia (vitamin D) or a bleeding tendency (vitamin K). Other deficiencies are uncommon, usually resulting from inadequate intake rather than increased losses, but may include deficiencies of magnesium, zinc, ascorbic acid and the B vitamins. Symptoms of anaemia are common and usually result from iron deficiency due to intestinal blood loss and, less commonly, from vitamin B_{12} or folate deficiency. After resection of more than 50 cm of terminal ileum, vitamin B_{12} absorption falls below normal. Malabsorption of bile salts and fats, which can cause diarrhoea, usually only follows an ileal resection of greater than 100 cm. The inflammatory process produces a low-grade fever in 30–49% of patients; where high and spiking, or the patient reports rigors, it is likely that there is a suppurative intra-abdominal complication.[1]

Extraintestinal manifestations

These are outlined in Box 10.1 and are more common in association with Crohn's colitis than isolated small-bowel disease. They are similar to those that occur in ulcerative colitis, and may precede, be independent of or accompany active IBD, and can cause significant morbidity. Gallstones are said to be common due to malabsorption of bile salts in the terminal ileum; however, symptomatic problems are not increased compared with the general population. Steatorrhoea promotes increased absorption of oxalate, thereby increasing the incidence of oxalate renal stones. Patients may have a fatty liver as a result of malnutrition or from receiving total

Box 10.1 • Extraintestinal manifestations of Crohn's disease

Related to disease activity

- Aphthous ulceration (10%)
- Erythema nodosum (5–10%)
- Pyoderma gangrenosum (0.5%)
- Acute arthropathy (6–12%)
- Eye complications (conjunctivitis, etc.) (3–10%)
- Amyloidosis (1%)

Unrelated to disease activity

- Sacroiliitis (often minimal symptoms) (10–15%)
- Ankylosing spondylitis (1–2%)
- Primary sclerosing cholangitis (rare)
- Chronic active hepatitis (2–3%)
- Cirrhosis (2–3%)
- Gallstones (15–30%)
- Renal calculi (5–10%)

parenteral nutrition. Mild abnormalities of liver function are common with active disease, so this does not imply significant liver disease.

Thromboembolic complications occur with IBD and are usually associated with severe active colonic disease. Common sites are the lower extremities and pelvic veins, but cerebrovascular accidents have also been reported. Metastatic Crohn's disease is an unusual complication in which nodular ulcerating skin lesions occur at distant sites including the vulva, submammary areas and extremities. Biopsies of these show non-caseating granulomas. Clubbing is seen in some cases of extensive small-bowel disease.

Amyloidosis is reported in 25% of patients with Crohn's disease at post-mortem but only 1% have clinical manifestations. It can occur in the bowel or within other organs, including the liver, spleen and kidneys. If renal function is affected, resection of the diseased bowel will result in regression of amyloid and improvement of renal function.[1]

Physical signs

Patients may appear well and have a normal physical examination. With more severe disease there may be evidence of weight loss, anaemia, iron deficiency, clubbing, cachexia, proximal myopathy, easy bruising, elevated temperature, tachycardia and peripheral oedema. Signs of extraintestinal manifestations may be present.

Abdominal examination can be normal but tenderness in the right iliac fossa is common. Thickened loops of bowel may be palpable and if matted

together can produce an abdominal mass. A psoas or intra-abdominal abscess produces signs and occasionally there is free peritonitis. Enterocutaneous fistulas are most common when there has been previous surgery and usually presents through a scar. Acute or chronic strictures or carcinoma may produce signs of obstruction. There is a 3–5% risk of adenocarcinoma complicating Crohn's colitis and also an increased risk of small-bowel carcinoma. Perianal disease varies from an asymptomatic fissure or inflamed skin tag to severe disease that may look like a 'forest fire', with erythema, large fleshy skin tags, deep chronic fissures with bridges of skin and multiple fistulas creating the so-called 'watering-can perineum'. Fibrosis from chronic inflammation may have produced a woody, stiff anal canal or an anal or rectal stenosis.

Paediatric age group

In children and adolescents the gastrointestinal manifestations are similar but extraintestinal and systemic manifestations of disease become more important. About 15% have arthralgia and arthritis that often precedes bowel symptoms by months or years. Diagnosis may be delayed by a non-specific presentation with systemic symptoms of weight loss, growth failure and unexplained anaemia and fever. If active disease is dealt with promptly by medical or surgical treatment and adequate nutrition is maintained, retardation of growth and sexual development can usually be reversed.[1]

Pregnancy

This issue is often of concern as the disease frequently affects young adults. For the majority of patients with IBD fertility is normal but in some subgroups fertility rates are slightly reduced. In the absence of active disease, the outcome of pregnancy equals that of matched controls. With active disease at conception, there is an increase in spontaneous abortions and premature delivery, and a greater than 50% chance of relapsing disease during pregnancy. The risk of relapse is only 20–25% if disease is inactive at conception. It is therefore advisable to avoid conception during an acute phase of disease. Pregnancy probably does not affect the long-term course of the disease. Aminosalicylates, steroids and azathioprine are safe in pregnancy, but the use of methotrexate is contraindicated.[1]

Investigations

Laboratory

Anti-*Saccharomyces cervisiae* antibodies (ASCAs) and perinuclear antineutrophil cytoplasmic antibody (p-ANCA) can be useful to discriminate ulcerative colitis from Crohn's. ASCAs are positive in 35–50% of patients with Crohn's compared to less than 1% in ulcerative colitis. The specificity is around 90%. On the other hand, p-ANCA is often raised in ulcerative colitis with a sensitivity of 55% and specificity of about 90%. If p-ANCA is elevated in Crohn's, it is only with colitis.[6]

In more severe or established disease, magnesium, zinc and selenium levels should be checked. Serum albumin is often low in active disease due to downregulation of albumin synthesis by cytokines (IL-1, IL-2, TNF). Mild episodic elevations of liver function tests are common but persistent abnormalities require further investigation. Evidence of anaemia should be sought, and if present investigated. A neutrophil leucocytosis usually indicates active disease or septic complications. Of the serum protein markers for inflammation, C-reactive protein and orosomucoid most closely match clinical disease activity. Erythrocyte sedimentation rate is useful in Crohn's colitis but not in small-bowel disease. Faecal fat excretion may be increased if malabsorption is present. Severe ileocaecal involvement can cause right hydronephrosis or sterile pyuria, and an enterovesical fistula will lead to bacteria in the urine.

Radiology

A small-bowel barium study has traditionally been the key to confirming the presence of small-bowel disease. Now good results can also be achieved with computed tomography (CT), magnetic resonance enteroclysis and high-resolution ultrasound. The technique that is used tends to be governed by local preference, local expertise and availability. A small-bowel barium follow-though remains most commonly used and widely available. This is usually done at diagnosis to determine disease extent in the small bowel. It is debated whether this is best done by barium meal and follow-through techniques or by a small-bowel enema with a nasoduodenal tube; probably most important is a radiologist committed to producing good-quality images. More subtle features of small-bowel Crohn's include thickening of the valvulae coniventes, a granular mucosal pattern and aphthous ulcers. As disease progresses features include wall thickening, cobblestoning and fissure-like ulcers, sinus tracts and fistulas. There may be stenosis causing obstructive symptoms, commonly in the terminal ileum (**Fig. 10.1**). Multiple tight stenoses with intervening dilated segments produce a 'chain of lakes' appearance (**Fig. 10.2**).

With frequent use of CT to investigate acute abdominal pain, thickened small-bowel loops, especially terminal ileum, may strongly suggest a diagnosis of Crohn's disease (**Fig. 10.3**). CT is effective at detecting intra-abdominal abscesses and dilated segments of small bowel. High-resolution magnetic resonance imaging (MRI) can produce good images in comparison to CT. MRI is as good as a small-bowel barium study to identify stenosis but in addition can discriminate areas of inflammation from fibrosis. MRI is free of ionising radiation and not limited by poor renal function, but is more costly. MRI is the investigation of choice for complicated perianal sepsis. High-resolution ultrasound is popular in Europe and effective at detecting inflamed bowel, although operator dependent.

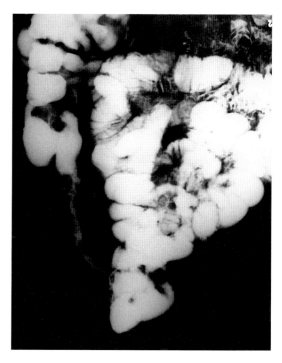

Figure 10.1 • Small-bowel enema with classic terminal ileal disease showing narrowing, cobblestone mucosa and fissures.

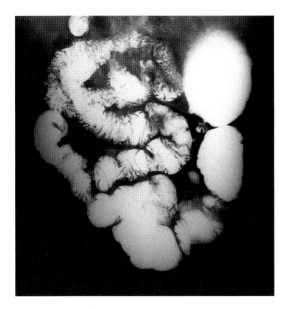

Figure 10.2 • Small-bowel barium enema showing multiple stenoses with intervening dilatation.

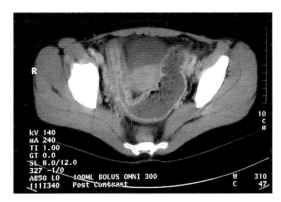

Figure 10.3 • CT scan showing thick-walled terminal ileum with proximal dilatation.

A double-contrast barium enema of the colon provides an overall picture of disease extent and severity, and a record for future comparison. It is probably being used less now in favour of colonoscopy. Changes in the colon are similar to those seen in the small bowel. Fistulas are uncommon and there is frequently rectal sparing. Strictures, which must be differentiated from carcinoma, are seen in 25% of patients and half of these are multiple. Chronic disease leads to shortening and loss of haustral folds. In severe cases plain abdominal films should be made initially to look for evidence of obstruction, mucosal oedema or dilatation.

Endoscopy

Colonoscopy provides a macroscopic view that can be recorded, allows biopsies to aid in the differential diagnosis, can assess and biopsy strictures, and can clarify the situation where significant symptoms are not backed up by clinical evidence of disease. Intubation of the ileocaecal valve allows examination and biopsy of the terminal ileum. Small aphthous ulcers are the early features of Crohn's disease, in contrast with the erythema and loss of vascular pattern in ulcerative colitis. In more severe disease the oedematous mucosa is penetrated by deep fissuring ulceration to give a cobblestone appearance. Multiple biopsies should be taken even if the mucosa appears normal as granulomas may be present that can confirm the diagnosis. There is not usually a role for routine follow-up endoscopy and endoscopic findings correlate poorly with clinical remission. There is a cancer risk in long-standing Crohn's colitis and most apply the same colonoscopic surveillance as they do in cases of extensive ulcerative colitis, despite various objections and limitations.

Endoscopy of the oesophagus, stomach and duodenum is necessary if there are appropriate symptoms, or abnormalities on a barium meal. Findings may include rugal hypertrophy, deep longitudinal ulcers and a cobblestone mucosa, the latter being the main differentiating feature from peptic ulcer disease. Biopsies should be taken but granulomas are often absent.[1]

Very occasionally the diagnosis of Crohn's disease is made by capsule endoscopy; this is usually in the context of investigating obscure chronic gastrointestinal bleeding when other investigations have been negative. One of the technical problems is that the capsule may be held up by strictures and cause small-bowel obstruction. If there is any significant concern that this may happen, a dummy dissolvable capsule can be used first.

Disease activity assessment and quality of life

For clinical purposes, disease activity is best assessed by clinical features and the investigations outlined above. It is usually categorised as mild, moderate or severe. If patients are asymptomatic (and off steroids) and/or have no obvious residual disease they are considered in remission. A number of indices of disease activity have been developed for Crohn's disease, including the Crohn's Disease Activity Index and the Harvey–Bradshaw index, but their role is largely confined to clinical trials for standardisation and comparison of patient groups.

Health-related quality of life (HRQOL) is a quantitative measurement of the subjective perception a person has of their health state, including emotional and social aspects. If treatments are being compared, use of HRQOL instruments is essential for providing a valid and objective measure of a real change in health state.

Phenotyping

Different phenotypes of Crohn's disease are recognised as the clinical picture varies with the site of disease and the behaviour of the disease (i.e. stricturing or fistulating). To date it seems that the location of disease tends to be stable over time. However, the behaviour of Crohn's disease according to the Vienna classification varies dramatically over the course of the disease. At 10 years, 46% of patients exhibit different disease behaviour than at diagnosis. Phenotype is important for genetic studies as differing phenotypes may correlate with particular genetic variations. Phenotype is also relevant for studying the outcome of therapy, medical or surgical. The Vienna classification was developed in 1998. At the time of diagnosis the following are recorded: age <40 years or ≥40 years, location of disease (terminal ileum, colon, ileocolon, upper gastrointestinal tract), behaviour (non-stricturing/non-penetrating, stricturing, penetrating), as well as data on sex, ethnicity, whether Jewish, family history of IBD, and extraintestinal manifestations.

Differential diagnosis

Small-bowel Crohn's disease

In most cases, after an appropriate work-up involving history and clinical, laboratory, radiological, endoscopic and pathological findings, the diagnosis will be fairly clear-cut. Box 10.2 shows the differential diagnoses of small-bowel Crohn's disease; perhaps the two that cause most difficulty are *Yersinia* and tuberculosis.

Box 10.2 • Differential diagnosis of small-bowel Crohn's disease

Differential diagnosis

Appendicitis
Appendix abscess
Caecal diverticulitis
Pelvic inflammatory disease
Ovarian cyst or tumour
Caecal carcinoma
Ileal carcinoid
Behçet's disease
Systemic vasculitis affecting the small bowel
Radiation enteritis
Ileocaecal tuberculosis
Yersinia enterocolitica ileitis
Eosinophilic gastroenteritis
Amyloidosis
Small-bowel lymphoma
Actinomycosis
Chronic non-granulomatous jejunoileitis

Useful discriminating features

History, CT scan
History, ultrasound/CT scan
Older age, barium enema
History
Ultrasound
Barium enema/colonoscopy
Small-bowel enema
Painful ulceration of the mouth and genitalia
Underlying systemic connective tissue disorder
History of radiotherapy
History of tuberculosis, circulating antibodies to *Mycobacterium*, stool cultures
Self-limiting, stool cultures, serology
Gastric involvement, peripheral eosinophilia
Biopsy
Radiological appearance
Microscopy of fine-needle aspirate
Clinical picture and histology

Large-bowel Crohn's disease

When there is no small-bowel or perineal involvement, there are two areas where the diagnosis may be difficult. An isolated segment of disease, especially if it is a short segment, has to be differentiated from carcinoma, ischaemia, tuberculosis and lymphoma; occasionally, severe diverticular disease can appear as or disguise a segment of Crohn's disease. Inflamed diverticular disease can mimic Crohn's disease, with the presence of granulomas, transmural inflammation and fissuring ulceration. Isolated involvement of the sigmoid colon is not common in Crohn's disease, so care should be taken before making this diagnosis in the presence of diverticular disease. Differentiating Crohn's disease from ulcerative colitis has been discussed earlier.

Medical treatment

A summary of first-line medical treatment options for Crohn's disease is given in Box 10.3. The concept of treating Crohn's disease is to induce remission and then to maintain it. The most effective agents for inducing remission are corticosteroids and more recently in selected cases infliximab. Budesonide may also have a role in ileocolic disease or right-sided colitis. For moderate to severe disease, steroids are commenced and at the same time immunosuppression, usually with azathioprine, is commenced. After some weeks or months, when the therapeutic benefit of immunosuppression commences, steroids can be removed. Aminosalicylates possibly have a role as induction therapy for less severe disease in the colon. Rather than gradually building up therapy for response, the current favoured concept is 'top-down therapy', using more powerful agents upfront.

Aminosalicylates

Sulfasalazine and 5-aminosalicylic acid (5-ASA; also known as mesalazine or mesalamine) are used to treat disease of mild to moderate severity in the colon. Sulfasalazine consists of a sulfapyridine

Box 10.3 • Summary of medical treatment options for Crohn's disease

Induction of remission

Mild to moderate disease

- Prednisone 20–40 mg daily for 2–3 weeks then tapering
- Ileal and/or right colon: budesonide 9 mg per day
- Crohn's colitis: appropriate salicylate compound (oral and/or enema)
- Perianal disease: metronidazole 400 mg t.d.s. or ciprofloxacin 500 mg b.d.

Severe disease

- Intravenous prednisone 60–80 mg per day
- Infliximab or other biological

Maintenance of remission

- Azathioprine, 6-mercaptopurine, methotrexate, budesonide 6 mg per day (ileal and/or right colon)

carrier linked to the active 5-ASA. In the colon bacteria cleave off the active 5-ASA, of which about 20% is absorbed. If 5-ASA is taken orally by itself, it is completely absorbed in the proximal small bowel. Although 5-ASA is the main active drug, the sulfapyridine produces most of the adverse effects, including nausea, vomiting, heartburn, headache, oligospermia and low-level haemolysis. These adverse effects are dose related. There are also a number of hypersensitivity reactions unrelated to drug levels, including worsening colitis. Adverse effects occur in 30% of people taking 4 g daily of sulfasalazine. Newer 5-ASA preparations use different carriers, or use pH- or time-dependent protective coatings that allow release to start in the jejunum, ileum or colon, thereby giving a much lower adverse effect profile.

Aminosalicylates have historically had a significant place in the management of Crohn's disease, but this is now being questioned. They have been used to treat ileal and colonic disease and to prevent recurrence after surgery, but their therapeutic benefit is now considered to be very limited and alternative treatments are usually more effective.[7,8] If preferred they may have a role for mild to moderate colonic disease and for preventing recurrence after small-bowel resection.[9]

Steroids

Systemically absorbed corticosteroids are the most effective and commonly used drugs for moderate to severe Crohn's disease and will induce remission in 70–80% of cases. They are less effective if only the colon is involved. Doses of prednisone range from 20–40 mg/day orally for moderate disease to 60–80 mg/day intravenously for severe disease. Steroids should be used in short courses and must be tapered when a clinical response is achieved. They can be useful in resolving the obstructive symptoms in early disease caused by narrowing due to inflammatory oedema. Steroids will not help with obstructive symptoms caused by established fibrotic stenosis. Steroids are useful for maintaining a steroid-induced remission in the short term, which implies steroid-dependent disease, but they do not have a role in maintenance beyond this. There is no advantage in combining salicylate therapy with steroids.

Rectal administration of steroid is effective for left-sided colonic disease, but steroid is still absorbed systemically, and prolonged therapy can cause adrenal suppression. 5-Aminosalicylic acid foam enemas are equally effective and can be used in combination with oral steroids in an exacerbation of disease.

To avoid systemic adverse effects, topically active corticosteroids have been developed. Budesonide, formulated as a slow-release oral preparation, acts in the small bowel and colon or can be given as an enema. The systemic bioavailability of budesonide is only 10–15% because of rapid first-pass metabolism in the liver, but it can still produce some suppression of plasma cortisol levels.

In active Crohn's disease, budesonide produced remission in 51–60% of patients compared with 60–73% on systemic steroids, but with a halving of reported adverse effects from 60% to 30%. When budesonide 9 mg daily was compared with mesalamine 4 g daily for ileal and/or ascending colon disease, remission in the budesonide group at 16 weeks was 62% vs. 36% for mesalamine, and budesonide was better tolerated. Budesonide appears to have a limited role in maintenance therapy.[10] Budesonide was compared to placebo in a double-blind randomised controlled trial of endoscopic recurrence (at 3 and 12 months) after an ileal or ileocolic resection, with no overall benefit.[11]

Antibiotics

Metronidazole and ciprofloxacin are used to treat perianal disease. Metronidazole is the most frequently used. Its mechanism of action is unclear, but may be by a variety of antibacterial effects or by its ability to suppress cell-mediated immunity. These antibiotics are widely used and recommended for perianal disease, although there is little evidence to support this practice. Long-term use of metronidazole in doses >10 mg/kg is contraindicated because of the risk of peripheral neuropathy.

Nutrition for therapy

The rationale for nutritional therapy is that intraluminal dietary antigens may drive the inflammatory response and that removal of these and bowel rest will bring remission.

Total parenteral nutrition is effective in inducing remission in 60–80% of patients, which matches the effect of steroids, but combining both these therapies gives no added benefit over using only one. Relapse rates are high after cessation. Total enteral nutrition is equally as effective and has a similar relapse rate after cessation. Polymeric diets seem as effective as elemental and peptide-based diets, but polymeric diets are cheaper and more palatable and are therefore preferred.[12]

Immunomodulatory therapy

This is used to reduce and eliminate steroid requirements, particularly after a remission has been achieved, and in refractory disease. Azathioprine and 6-mercaptopurine are purine analogues, azathioprine being quickly metabolised to 6-mercaptopurine. They inhibit cell proliferation and suppress cell-mediated events by inhibiting the activity of cytotoxic T cells and natural killer cells. The onset of a therapeutic effect takes 3–6 months. Toxicity is not uncommon and 3–15% of patients will develop pancreatitis, which will resolve on stopping the drug.

Fever, rash, arthralgias and hepatitis may occur and marrow suppression is dose related. In trials to improve disease or to decrease steroid requirements, there is a success rate of about 70–80%, and this applies equally to all disease sites, including perianal disease. Methotrexate is used occasionally for treating Crohn's disease. Limited data suggest it is as effective as azathioprine or 6-mercaptopurine and it is prescribed for patients who do not tolerate or respond to the latter two drugs.[12]

Clinical trials are ongoing with a number of monoclonal antibodies directed at specific mediators of the inflammatory response.

The initial placebo-controlled trial with a mouse–human chimeric monoclonal antibody to TNF-α (infliximab) addressed induction of remission after a single dose. At 4 weeks after a single dose, an initial treatment response was seen in 65% (54 of 83) who received infliximab and 17% (4 of 24) in the placebo group; at 12 weeks this was 41% and 12% respectively.[13] The ACCENT I study followed and addressed the maintenance of remission with a year of treatment with infliximab; 573 patients were recruited. After an initial infusion, 58% responded. The responders were then randomised to placebo or infliximab at 2 and 6 weeks and then 8-weekly up to 54 weeks. At week 54, of initial responders, about 15% in the placebo group and 35% in the treatment group were in clinical remission.[14]

Similar results with initial moderate efficacy have been demonstrated using infliximab to treat fistulas. The ACCENT II study recruited patients with perianal and enterocutaneous draining fistulas. The primary end-point of the study was a reduction in the number of fistulas by 50% or more. After three infusions at 0, 2 and 6 weeks, the study randomised responders at week 14 to placebo or infliximab infusions 8-weekly to week 54. The primary end-point was loss of response, with fistulas reactivating or reappearing. Of 306 patients enrolled, 195 (64%) responders were randomised at week 14. At week 54, 23 of 98 patients receiving placebo maintained a response compared with 42 of 91 receiving infliximab. This means that of all 306 patients entered into the study, about 30% of patients treated with infliximab will maintain a response at 1 year, 22% having a complete response. In the placebo group after initial infliximab response, 19% (19 of 98) had a complete response.[15] The efficacy at 1 year judged by complete response is therefore modest.

Infliximab therapy is costly, can have adverse effects and long-term safety data are not available. In clinical practice it is best used short term as an agent to induce remission when conventional modalities have been ineffective, with a view to following on with conventional immunosuppression. Infliximab should only be used in the context of an experienced multidisciplinary team. Recently adalimumab (a human anti-TNF monoclonal antibody) has been evaluated in the CLASSIC I and II and the CHARM studies, and has similar efficacy to infliximab. There are a number of other antibodies against mediators of the inflammatory response under investigation. In the modest proportion of patients who remain in remission on these expensive agents, continuing length of treatment is unknown.

Surgery and immunosuppression

With increasing use of immunosuppressive therapies there is concern about the impact of these treatments on perioperative morbidity. Fortunately there seems to be no evidence of problems with surgery following infliximab therapy, and azathioprine does not cause problems in the perioperative period. Use of greater than 20 mg prednisone for more than 6 weeks probably does have an impact and steroids should be reduced before surgery if possible.[9]

Prophylaxis against recurrent disease after surgery

After surgery medical treatment can be used to prevent recurrence. There was a phase of excitement for using mesalazine a decade ago. With more data the efficacy of this was questioned.

 However, after a series of updated meta-analysis there is probably a 15% difference in clinical recurrence. Therapy recommended after small-bowel resection at a dose of >2 g/day should continue for 2 years starting 2 weeks after surgery.[9]

There has been a trend to use azathioprine for 'higher risk patients' but there are no data to support this.[7,8]

Other drugs

Antidiarrhoeal medication and anticholinergic agents to relieve colicky pain are useful in mild to moderate disease but should be avoided in severe exacerbations. Non-steroidal anti-inflammatory drugs should also be avoided as they may make the disease worse, and opioids can increase bowel spasm. Cholestyramine is useful for treating bile salt diarrhoea.

Surgery

Development of surgery

Crohn and colleagues initially described radical resection of involved segments of bowel, but high recurrence rates led to a vogue for bypassing affected segments. Frequent complications with the bypassed segments caused a return to resectional surgery. Modern surgery for Crohn's disease involves resecting the least amount of bowel to re-establish satisfactory intestinal function.

This is based on the concept that Crohn's is a gut-wide disease and that microscopic disease at the resection margin does not influence recurrence of disease.[16,17]

Furthermore, one small study has shown that asymptomatic endoscopic small-bowel lesions remaining after ileocolic resection did not correlate with clinical recurrence.[18] Although the term 'recurrence of disease' is widely used, a better term is 'recrudescence', implying a new outbreak of already present disease.

It is important to avoid any unnecessary sacrifice of gut as these patients may need resections of further segments for future disease recrudescence. In the move to conservatism, however, it is important not to procrastinate when there is an indication for surgery. When patients were questioned on the timing of their surgery, most would have preferred to have had the procedure 12 months earlier because of the benefits it gave.[19] Low quality-of-life scores with active disease improve to normal when remission is obtained, whether by surgery or medical treatment.[20] When medical treatment does not induce remission or the adverse effects of therapy are unacceptable, in most cases the best course of action for the patient is to proceed to surgery.

Laparoscopic surgery is feasible and safe and is increasingly being used for more complicated cases. Most surgeons would favour an extracorporeal anastomosis and, where possible, extracorporeal ligation of the mesentery. For ileocolic resections this can usually be accomplished with relative ease, giving the patient a small 3–5 cm midline incision through the umbilicus. A meta-analysis has shown quicker short-term recovery after laparoscopic ileocolic resection.[21] However, equivalent early discharge can be achieved with fast-track open surgery.[22] As for laparoscopic colorectal surgery in general, patients usually prefer a laparoscopic approach, with its cosmetic advantage. Perioperative care, as for open surgery, should incorporate the principles of accelerated recovery pathways to optimise the benefits of smaller wounds.

Risk of operation and re-operation

Accurate population figures about patterns of disease and complications are not easy to obtain. Many of the data presented in this chapter are from specialist centres and these figures may not always apply to the Crohn's population at large. In perhaps the largest population-based cohort reported of 1936 patients from Sweden, the cumulative rate of intestinal resection was 44%, 61% and 71% at 1, 5 and 10 years respectively after diagnosis; the subsequent risk of recurrence was 33% and 44% at 5 and 10 years respectively.[23] In another population-based study involving 210 patients with Crohn's disease at a mean of 11 years from disease onset, 56% required surgery; by life-table analysis the re-operation rate was 25% at 10 years and 56% at 20 years.[24]

In a tertiary referral centre experience of 592 patients with Crohn's disease, 74% required surgery at a median of 13 years' follow-up. The chance of surgery varied with the site of disease and was 65% in those with small-bowel involvement, 58% in those with colonic or anorectal disease, and 91% in those with ileocolic disease.[25] Half of the patients in a tertiary referral centre who have had one operation will require re-operation for further disease with follow-up of more than 10 years.[26,27] Most studies report the annual rate of symptomatic recurrence to be 5–15% and the annual re-operation rate 2–10%. Recurrence is at the site of previous disease in the majority, but may be at a new site.[28] For patients presenting to a surgical service, the cumulative chance of a permanent stoma at 20 years is 14% and of a temporary stoma 40%.[29]

Risk factors for recurrence

Many studies have looked at risk factors for recurrence. Recurrence (or recrudescence) can be defined by radiological findings, endoscopic findings, the return of symptoms or the need for further surgery. Most studies have been retrospective, and although some claim to identify risk factors, others report no association for the same risk factor. There is no consistently robust evidence that age of onset of disease, gender, site of disease, number of resections, length of small-bowel resection, proximal margin length, microscopic disease at the resection margin, fistulising vs. obstructive disease, number of sites of disease, presence of granulomas or blood transfusion have an important impact on recurrence.[30]

Although a recurrence frequently occurs immediately proximal to the previous anastomosis, there is no consistent or high-quality evidence to date that anastomotic technique (side-to-side, end-to-end,

end-to-side, hand-sewn or stapled) affects recurrence. Many consider a wider anastomosis may be preferable as achieved with side-to-side stapling, and further randomised studies are in progress.

 However, it is now clear that continuing to smoke after a surgical resection doubles the risk of recurrence and patients must be urged to stop smoking.[31–33] Prophylactic use of 5-ASA has a modest effect to reduce recurrence (as discussed above) by 15%, giving a number needed to treat of 8.

Principles of surgery for Crohn's disease

Perioperative considerations

Excellent perioperative care is essential for a good outcome in patients with Crohn's disease. As there is always potential for colonic involvement with small-bowel disease, in all elective cases adequate bowel preparation of the colon should be considered. Deep vein thrombosis prophylaxis is mandatory because patients with IBD are at increased risk of thrombotic complications.[34] Usually, low-molecular-weight heparin (at higher risk doses) and compression stockings suffice, but these measures are not necessarily adequate if there is a history of thrombosis. Patients will often be at risk of adrenal suppression and the need for intravenous steroid cover should be considered every time. Before elective surgery, significant malnutrition should be restored by either enteral or parenteral nutrition, all potential electrolyte problems corrected and sepsis controlled. If this is not possible, consideration should be given to a temporary stoma rather than an anastomosis. Joint management with a gastroenterologist is an essential principle in the decision-making and hospital care, and psychological well-being needs to be addressed.

Technique

Patients with Crohn's disease can be among the most technically difficult cases a surgeon will face. Compromise of good technique can be unforgiving. Any part of the bowel can be affected or involved with Crohn's disease, so in most cases the patient should be placed in a modified lithotomy or Lloyd–Davies position. For open surgery a midline infraumbilical incision gives good access, is more easily reopened

in the future and will not interfere with stomas that may be needed on either side of the abdomen. At each operation a full laparotomy should be carried out to stage the disease and the length of remaining and resected bowel measured. In the event of recurrence it is helpful to have marked anastomotic sites with a metal clip. At the first abdominal operation for Crohn's disease, consideration should be given to removing the appendix to prevent future diagnostic problems and confusion.

Thick oedematous vascular mesenteric pedicles require special mention. A standard tie may allow a vessel to retract into the mesentery, resulting in a mesenteric haematoma with potential to compromise the blood supply to large segments of bowel. Thick pedicles should be dealt with by a fail-safe technique and some recommend double-suture ligation. Spillage of gastrointestinal contents must be minimised and controlled, and meticulous haemostasis is important as there may be inevitable loss from oozing, inflamed, raw surfaces. Great care should be taken not to damage or perforate other loops of bowel or other organs in the presence of difficult adhesions and inflammation.

 Hyaluronidase-impregnated methylcellulose membranes have been developed to reduce adhesions. Membranes have been effective in reducing adhesions between midline wounds and abdominal contents, and may have particular application to this group of patients who have a high rate of re-operation.[35]

There are a number of similar products available, including spray-on application and membranes that are easier to use than the above, with claimed similar efficacy. In addition, one of the benefits of laparoscopic surgery may be a decrease in adhesion formation.

Surgery for small-bowel and ileocolic Crohn's disease

Indications

Surgery for small-bowel Crohn's disease is aimed at treating complications not amenable to medical therapy. Surgical interventions are required for:

1. stenosis causing obstructive symptoms;
2. enterocutaneous or intra-abdominal fistulas to other organs;

3. draining intra-abdominal or retroperitoneal abscesses;
4. controlling acute or chronic bleeding;
5. free perforation.

Of these, obstruction is the most frequent indication.

Gastroduodenal disease

Symptomatic gastroduodenal disease is present in 0.5–4% of patients and is usually associated with disease in other sites. The first and second parts of the duodenum are most commonly involved and the disease often extends into the gastric antrum. Most patients who require surgery require it for problems of stenosis or occasionally bleeding. Often it is difficult at endoscopy to differentiate Crohn's from peptic ulcer disease but a trial of medical ulcer therapy may help. Gastrojejunostomy is the standard procedure for duodenal or pyloric stenosis. Historically vagotomy was often added to reduce stomal ulceration. Proton-pump inhibitors can now be effective in this role and the potential side-effects of vagotomy avoided.

In selected cases pyloric or duodenal strictureplasty may be considered, and produce better function. Results of a duodenal strictureplasty are variable and complications can be significant.[36,37] Massive acute upper gastrointestinal bleeding is rare, but if endoscopic methods are unsuccessful, bleeding should be controlled by under-running the bleeding vessel with a suture. Balloon dilatation of benign upper gastrointestinal tract strictures is safe, but the limited experience in Crohn's disease suggests dilatation has little long-term benefit. Fistulas involving the duodenum occur in 0.5% of patients with Crohn's disease and generally arise from other diseased segments fistulating into the duodenum. Surgical therapy for these is usually successful and prognosis relates to the severity of disease in the primary segment. Closure of secondary duodenal defects with a jejunal serosal patch or Roux-en-Y limb may be preferable to primary suture.

Ileocolic disease

The cumulative operation rate for patients with distal ileal disease at 5 years from the time of diagnosis is up to 80%. Ileocaecal disease is treated with a limited ileocaecal resection, including a few centimetres of macroscopically normal bowel at each end. The anastomotic technique that gives the best results is still debated but most favour a technique producing a widely patent lumen.

After a first operation the re-operation rate at 5 years is 20–25% and at 10 years 35–40%. Re-operation rates for second and subsequent operations are the same. Further disease is usually on the ileal side of the anastomosis and it is important to stress that this is new disease and does not relate to an inadequate resection margin. Although recurrent disease rates are high and on average a patient will need an operation every 10 years, surgery is highly successful at relieving symptoms and restoring health when disease is refractory to medical treatment.

Balloon dilatation of selected symptomatic ileocolic strictures, usually short anastomotic strictures, is a treatment option with at least short-term benefit in 60–80% (with a risk of perforation of 2–11%) and with longer-term benefit in 40–60%.[38]

Ileal and jejunal multisite disease

If there is isolated small-bowel disease, it is almost invariably in the terminal ileum and is usually suited to a limited resection. More extensive disease can produce obstructive strictures throughout the small bowel. In the past, these patients requiring surgery had multiple resections, with a risk of short-bowel syndrome. In an endeavour to maximise conservation of bowel length the concept of strictureplasty was introduced, and this technique is now preferred for all suitable lesions. It is ideally suited to short fibrotic strictures but it may be used for strictures up to 10–15 cm long. Long strictures with active inflammation are usually better managed with resection unless there is concern about bowel length. In most series half the patients having a strictureplasty will also have a segmental resection.

Strictureplasty is carried out using the same methods as used for pyloroplasty. The Heineke–Mikulicz technique is usually used. In a small number of cases with longer strictures where bowel conservation is required, a Finney or a Jaboulay strictureplasty may be used. For even longer narrowed segments a side-to-side isoperistaltic technique described by Michelassi et al. may be used.[39] The diseased bowel is divided at its midpoint and the proximal and distal ends advanced so that the diseased segments lie side by side, where they are anastomosed to each other, trying to ensure stenotic segments are complemented with dilated segments. Despite often long suture lines, results are similar to other strictureplasty techniques. Most candidates for strictureplasty have three or four strictureplasties but in some cases there may be 10–15. To ensure no significant strictures have been missed a Foley catheter should be passed along the small bowel through an enterotomy. The balloon is then inflated to a diameter of 25 mm and pulled back through the bowel, and strictures not easily seen externally will be identified. Alternatively, a marble, steel or wooden ball with a diameter of 25 mm can be traced through the bowel to identify strictures.

Results of strictureplasty have proved it to be a safe and effective technique. Overall morbidity is 10–20%. Postoperative abdominal septic complications occur in 5–10%, and overall 98–99% have symptomatic relief. Postoperative bleeding from a strictureplasty site occurs in about 3% of patients, but this usually resolves with conservative measures. Recurrence requiring re-operation is about 30% at 5 years. Re-operation rates after a stricture-plasty are similar whether or not a limited resection is included in the operation. The re-operation rates are similar after first, second and third recurrences requiring surgery. Less than 10% of the stricture-plasties themselves restricture, so most of the recurrent disease occurs at new sites.[40–44]

Fistulas and abscesses

Enteric fistulas may affect up to 30% of patients with Crohn's disease and in a referral centre about 40% are internal, 40% external and 20% mixed. Internal fistulas are usually spontaneous and external ones postoperative. Fistula tracts have an associated abscess, at least initially, in most cases. In expert hands surgical repair is successful in closing the fistula in more than 95% of cases, but failure after an attempt at definitive surgery can result in a high mortality rate.

Enterocutaneous fistulas and intra-abdominal abscess

Enterocutaneous fistulas in Crohn's disease are a common cause of intestinal failure and patients who develop intestinal failure are best managed in a specialised unit with a multidisciplinary team. Intra-abdominal abscesses that are drained externally will usually result in a fistula. When abscesses complicate existing fistulas it is necessary to convert these fistula/abscess complexes into a well-draining fistula. Fistulas, whether postoperative or sponta-

neous, will drain along the line of least resistance, which is often previous scar tissue from incisions or drain sites.

Management principles

Although spontaneous and postoperative fistulas behave differently, the same management principles apply. The steps are outlined below.

1. Resuscitate the patient, correcting electrolytes and restoring haemoglobin levels. Control sepsis by open or percutaneous drainage and antibiotics; occasionally, exteriorisation of the bowel ends will be required. Attempts at repair and anastomosis should never be made in a patient with significant nutritional compromise or sepsis. Protect the skin from the fistula output by expert application of stoma appliances.

 There has been a vogue for using somatostatin analogues to decrease fistula output but it has shown no benefit.[45]

2. Establish nutrition by either enteral feeding or total parenteral nutrition.
3. Support morale as these patients are often emotionally very fragile. They are upset and angry about what has happened to them and often demoralised and frightened as well. The surgeon should at all times recognise this and be prepared directly to address these issues with the patient.
4. Mobilise the patient. If it is reasonable to anticipate closure with conservative measures, or the fistula is postoperative, wait for at least 6 weeks. If a fistula has not closed by 12 weeks, it probably never will. However, a fistula will generally close spontaneously by 6 weeks unless it:
   (a) originates from a diseased segment of bowel;
   (b) arises from an anastomotic breakdown greater than 50% of the circumference of the bowel;
   (c) has a very short tract or communication between skin and mucosa;
   (d) has bowel obstruction distal to it.
5. Plan a definitive operation with:
   (a) complete enterolysis;
   (b) en bloc resection of the diseased or damaged bowel and the fistula tract with primary anastomosis.

The work-up includes radiological imaging to (i) define the extent of intestinal disease, (ii) exclude any obstructing lesions and (iii) delineate the fistula tracts. Avoid the temptation to carry out earlier and repetitive imaging unless the results will alter management. There are reports of vacuum-assisted dressings and gelfoam embolisation of the fistula tract achieving closure; whether the closure is simply accelerated or whether surgery can be avoided is unknown.

Spontaneous enterocutaneous fistulas

In Crohn's disease this implies that there is a segment of diseased bowel that will require resection. This group generally benefits from earlier surgery for the following reasons:

1. The fistula will not heal spontaneously.
2. There is no concern about a more recent laparotomy making surgery difficult.
3. The bowel perforation occurs slowly and abdominal sepsis is usually localised, lessening the initial systemic insult.
4. Although the aim is to optimise the patient's general and nutritional state before surgery, active Crohn's disease will limit what is achievable.

Postoperative fistulas

In contrast to spontaneous fistulas, these will usually close with conservative measures if there is no downstream obstruction because the previously diseased bowel has been removed. However, the patient is often very ill and can have extensive abdominal contamination, which will usually drain by the incision or a drain site but may require added open or percutaneous drainage. On occasions the abdominal wound may be better left open initially and managed with a vacuum-assisted dressing, although there are some concerns that enterocutaneous fistulas can be induced in this way.

Intra-abdominal fistulas

These fistulas are usually spontaneous. The primary defect may arise from any segment of diseased bowel but is most commonly from the ileocaecal region. Similar management principles apply to these fistulas as to those described above, but the patients are generally in better health and less symptomatic. About half of the fistulas are diagnosed clinically, the remainder being asymptomatic and discovered at surgery. A fistula should always be suspected between two loops of adherent bowel. The secondary defect can occur in the stomach, duodenum, vagina, fallopian tube, ureter or urethra, but the sigmoid colon, small bowel and bladder are the most common sites. Most high vaginal fistulas are from the rectum but some are from the ileum.

Surgery involves en bloc resection of the primary defect and fistula with primary anastomosis and often only simple closure of the secondary defect, but with the exception of the duodenum.

Spontaneous free perforation in the small bowel or colon

Free perforation occurs in about 1% of patients with Crohn's disease and involves the small bowel and colon with similar frequency. Best results are from operation within 24 hours, with resection of the diseased segment and exteriorisation of the bowel ends.

Surgery for colonic and rectal Crohn's disease

Indications

The most common indication for colonic surgery is intractable disease that is not well controlled with medical therapy. The need for surgery and the choice of operation will depend on the extent of the disease. About one-third will have segmental disease, a third left-sided disease and a third total colitis. Overall a third will have associated perianal disease. After 10 years about half will have had surgery and a quarter will have an ileostomy.[46] Of those with severe colitis many will settle with medical treatment, but of those who do over half will require colectomy within 1–2 years.[47]

Emergency colectomy and colectomy and ileostomy

Acute colectomy for Crohn's disease constitutes a small portion of operations for acute Crohn's disease. The indications for this include toxic dilatation, haemorrhage, perforation and severe colitis not responding to medical therapy. If medical treatment brings a response in 48–72 hours and urgent surgery is avoided, early elective colectomy should be considered as the chance of recurrent toxic colitis in the following years is significant and symptomatic control is often poor. Severe haemorrhage and perforation both occur in about 1% of patients with colitis. Urgent surgery is usually a total colectomy and ileostomy.

Completion proctectomy, if possible, is usually left until the patient is in good health, but severe haemorrhage can be a problem. The rectal stump, if left initially, will usually need to be removed to control residual symptoms. If the rectum is retained long term there is a risk of cancer and surveillance is required. In selected cases a loop ileostomy can be used to defunction moderately severe colitis. This will allow clinical improvement in over 80%. Half will be able to have the stoma closed initially, but only 20% continue without relapse after medium-term follow-up.[48]

Other than an urgent colectomy or a high-risk patient, colectomy and ileostomy may be used in the presence of substantial anorectal disease when there is concern about perineal wound healing. After colectomy with a period of maximal medical therapy the perianal disease may settle, facilitating better results with proctectomy, but doubt remains as to whether this is effective.

Segmental colectomy

Segmental colectomy has become more popular in recent years, and the usual indication is a symptomatic stricture. In some cases it may be required to exclude cancer. The pattern of recurrence is similar to that seen with segmental small-bowel disease (Table 10.1). A meta-analysis of case series has compared segmental colectomy to colectomy and ileorectal anastomosis. If there were multiple colonic segments involved recurrence was earlier with segmental resections, but there was no difference in permanent stoma rates. Treatment choices should be guided by the extent of colonic disease.[49]

Total colectomy and ileorectal anastomosis

In patients needing a colectomy for Crohn's colitis, 25% have rectal sparing, with a normally functioning rectum and sphincter mechanism. These patients are suitable for an ileorectal anastomosis. Some patients with a mild proctitis and/or mild perianal disease may even achieve reasonable function. With more severe disease colectomy and ileorectal anastomosis may be done in two stages.

Clinical recurrence is reported in 50% at 10 years. Of those who lose their ileorectal anastomosis, many will still have obtained 4–5 years of useful function, and this can be particularly important if a stoma is deferred for teenage and young adult years. At 10 years over half will retain their rectum. The development of perianal disease usually leads to proctectomy.

Panproctocolectomy

This operation is the gold standard for treating colorectal disease and is associated with the lowest recurrence rate, albeit at the price of a stoma. Recurrence usually involves small-bowel disease, but it can be from perineal Crohn's after removal of the anorectum. Recurrence rates after panproctocolectomy are of the order of 15–25% at 10 years. Patients report a good quality of life after colectomy and ileostomy for disease confined to the colon.[26] In addition, a portion will need revisional surgery for ileostomy complications.[29]

Removal of the rectum requires particular care not to damage the pelvic nerves, and a technique of intersphincteric and perimuscular dissection of the rectum has been used. As there is no natural anatomical plane, the dissection is more vascular and time-consuming than dissection in the mesorectal plane. It is probably safe for the specialist to carry out most of the dissection in the mesorectal plane, perhaps coming inside the mesorectal plane at the critical points, anteriorly and laterally in relation to the parasympathetic nerves. Whichever technique is preferred, the surgeon has to be prepared to modify this to take account of severe perineal or perirectal disease that can make the dissection very

Table 10.1 • Long-term outcome of patients with segmental colonic Crohn's disease who have a segmental resection

Reference	n	Mean follow-up (years)	Clinical recurrence (%)	Re-operation rate at 10 years (%)	Permanent stoma avoided (%)
Allan et al.[70]	36	–	–	66	–
Makoweic et al.[71]	142	12	60	32	88
Prabhakar et al.[72]	48	14	77	33	86
Polle et al.[73]	91	8.3	–	33 (at mean 8.3 years)	56*

The series by Prabhakar et al. includes 10 patients who had the majority of their colon removed.
*Some patients had a stoma formed after segmental resection.

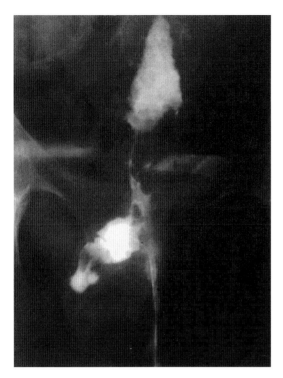

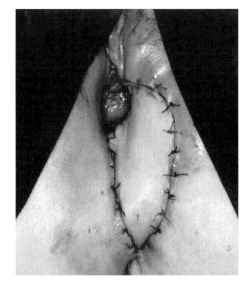

Figure 10.5 • A rectus abdominis myocutaneous flap used to reconstruct a severely diseased perineum complicated by a squamous carcinoma arising in a fistula tract (vagina at the top end of flap).

Figure 10.4 • Sinogram examination demonstrating an enteroperineal fistula.

difficult. The perineal wound is best treated with primary closure and suction drainage (if desired) from above. Delayed wound healing is frequently a problem, although 60–80% will have uncomplicated healing. Up to 30% will traditionally take 4–6 months to heal completely, but vacuum-assisted closure systems can now reduce this in many cases. About 10% will have longer-term problems with perineal sinuses, most of which settle with further surgical procedures. These may include several attempts at scraping the sinus tract to remove necrotic tissue and freshen the walls, and excluding an enteroperineal fistula (**Fig. 10.4**) and cutaneous Crohn's disease. In troublesome cases of active perineal disease after proctectomy, there is a role for wide excision and a vertical rectus abdominis transpelvic musculocutaneous flap reconstruction (**Fig. 10.5**). Disappointingly, in a small number the flap of normal skin can also develop granulomatous cutaneous Crohn's disease.

Restorative proctocolectomy

Crohn's disease has traditionally been regarded as a contraindication for an ileal pouch because of the risk of developing small-bowel or perianal dis-

ease that will lead to pouch excision. Now some surgeons are prepared to offer an ileal pouch to a well-informed patient who has isolated colonic Crohn's and requires a proctocolectomy. Other surgeons still regard Crohn's as an absolute contraindication.[9] The risk of pouch failure (and excision) is in the range of 10–45%, and is higher than for ulcerative colitis. However, for Crohn's disease at other sites re-operation rates of 50% at 10 years are acceptable, and small-bowel recurrence probably involves a similar sacrifice of bowel to that of excising a pouch.[50,51] The group in Paris who controversially promoted pouches in selected patients with colorectal Crohn's disease have reported 10-year follow-up documenting Crohn's-related events in 35%, with 10% requiring pouch excision.[52]

Crohn's colitis and cancer

With extensive Crohn's colitis an 8% risk of developing colon cancer at 22 years after disease onset has been reported, which is the same as the cancer risk with ulcerative colitis.[53] In another tertiary centre series for patients requiring colonic resection there was a 5% risk of cancer or dysplasia.[54] Field change in the colonic mucosa with areas of dysplasia is observed as in ulcerative colitis.[55] The absolute numbers for surveillance are small because many patients with Crohn's colitis will have had colectomies, but surveillance colonoscopy should be offered to patients with Crohn's colitis. Particular care is needed in the presence of colonic strictures, which should always be regarded as malignant until proven otherwise; this may entail a resection to make the diagnosis.

Perianal disease

Some 30–70% of patients with Crohn's disease will have a degree of involvement of the anal canal, ranging from minor skin tags to severe disease.[1] However, only a much smaller proportion will need surgical intervention for anal disease.[56] It is more frequent in association with colonic and, particularly, rectal disease.[57] A small percentage of patients have their initial presentation with anal disease, but over time half of these will develop disease at other intestinal sites. The activity of anal disease is unrelated to more proximal disease activity.

Generally, the prognosis is good, with only 5–10% of patients with perianal Crohn's requiring a proctectomy. If rectal disease is also present, proctectomy will be needed in up to twice this number. Fissures or fistulas may be asymptomatic, and after some years about half will have healed spontaneously and a further 20–30% will heal after a surgical procedure. Carcinoma is a rare but recognised complication, and hidradenitis suppurativa may coexist. The benign course of most perianal lesions caused by an incurable disease has led many (but not all surgeons) to a general policy of conservative treatment. Carefully selected cases without active disease can benefit from active surgical management. Preserving a functioning sphincter must remain a paramount concern in these patients. Box 10.4 outlines a useful classification of lesions described by Hughes and Taylor.[58] Surgery is most frequently indicated for secondary and incidental lesions.

Investigation

Careful examination, often under anaesthesia, is the most useful investigation and often an essential part of the work-up. In complicated cases, MRI and/or endoanal ultrasound in combination with examination under anaesthesia allow accurate identification of obscure tracts and collections.[59]

Medical treatment

Metronidazole, azathioprine and infliximab are probably effective at controlling or improving peri-

Box 10.4 • Hughes' classification of perianal lesions in Crohn's disease

Primary lesions
- Anal fissure
- Ulcerated oedematous pile
- Cavitating ulcer
- Aggressive ulceration

Secondary lesions
- Skin tags
- Anal/rectal stricture
- Perianal abscess/fistula
- Anovaginal/rectovaginal fistula
- Carcinoma

Incidental lesions
- Piles
- Perianal abscess or fistula
- Skin tags
- Cryptitis
- Hidradenitis suppurativa

From Hughes LE, Taylor BA. Perianal lesions in Crohn's disease. In: Allan R, Keighley M, Alexander-Williams J et al. (eds) Inflammatory bowel disease, 2nd edn. Edinburgh: Churchill Livingstone, 1990; pp. 351–61. With permission from Churchill Livingstone.

anal disease (see above), but most of the claims in the literature are anecdotal and the impact of medical therapy on reducing complications or the need for surgery is not known. Case series suggest that while the initial response rate is reasonable, the long-term closure rate is little improved by adding infliximab to established medical and surgical treatment.[60] In those with active disease, however, it seems reasonable to employ any measure that is likely to help the symptomatic patient and avert proctectomy. Metronidazole is often used for septic problems and should be the first-line medical treatment, but be wary of the neurological adverse effects. Ciprofloxacin is also regarded as effective and is generally better tolerated but more expensive.

Anal fissure

Most fissures are in the midline posteriorly, one-third are multiple and two-thirds are asymptomatic. Anal canal pressures are similar to those in controls and 50–70% heal with conservative or concurrent medical therapy.[61] Initially a conservative approach should be adopted for chronic fissures. Treatment options include topical glyceryl trinitrate and diltiazem, and botulinum toxin injection. All efforts should be made to conserve the internal anal sphincter in Crohn's disease. However, if all else fails and the patient has significant symptoms, the fissure will usually heal after a lateral anal sphincterotomy without compromising continence. This should probably not be done in the presence of active proctitis. Healing the fissure may prevent future abscesses and fistulas arising from its base.[62]

Abscesses

Abscesses may arise from deep cavitating ulcers or distorted anal glands (**Fig. 10.6**). The first sign of an abscess is often increasing perianal pain. An MRI can confirm clinical suspicion if little is obvious on initial examination. Occasionally, abscesses may be above the levator muscles. Examination under anaesthesia will identify the problem (in combination with MRI for difficult cases) and collections should be drained by removing a small area of overlying skin to allow drainage. In larger cavities it may be useful to insert a mushroom catheter to facilitate drainage and irrigation. It is usually inadvisable to lay open a primary tract at this stage.

Anal fistulas

Fistulous disease may range from an incidental fistula to a 'watering-can' perineum. If a fistula has been judged incidental or there is no active inflammation in the perianal region or rectum, it can be treated by standard techniques that preserve the sphincter muscle: identification of the track and preliminary seton drainage followed by lay open (if superficial), or a rectal advancement flap, giving a success rate as high as 50–70% at 2–3 years.[56,63] There may be a role for recently introduced bovine collagen plugs to close fistula tracts, which if used seem to be more successful with single tracts rather than complex fitulas.[64] A covering stoma is probably not of benefit for the majority of cases. In complicated fistulas or in the presence of active inflammation, the aim is to establish adequate drainage and this is best done

with a loose seton, which may be left long term with a good functional result. Supralevator fistulas are a difficult problem and usually involve perforating disease from the rectum or even more proximal bowel. Again, the primary aim is drainage and identification of the internal origin, but these cases are more likely to need a proctectomy. Fistulas arising from deep cavitating ulcers are difficult to manage and proctectomy is often unavoidable in the long term.

Rectovaginal fistulas

The distressing problem of passing faeces or wind per vaginam means that these fistulas usually require surgical therapy. They occur in 10% of women presenting to specialist centres with Crohn's disease. In one series 37% had a proctectomy, but only one-third of these were primarily for the rectovaginal fistula.[65] They are more frequently associated with colon rather than small-bowel disease. The fistula, if low, will usually be identified on examination that may need to be done under anaesthesia with initial insertion of a seton and control of sepsis. An MRI will give information about surrounding sepsis and may identify the fistula. For difficult high fistulas a vaginogram may be used.

Medical therapy should be optimised. It is doubtful whether infliximab is helpful. If the disease is quiescent a variety of surgical approaches can be employed. Depending on the condition of local tissues, options include a rectal advancement flap, anocutaneous advancement flaps, vaginal flaps, a Martius graft, a gracilis interposition or sphincteroplasty.[66,67] With persistence and possibly more than one procedure, closure rates of over 50% may be a reasonable expectation. A temporary stoma may be considered for complex repairs.

Defunctioning ileostomy for perianal disease

A temporary ileostomy has a role in providing symptomatic relief to the desperate patient while more definitive treatment options are discussed or tried. In this situation, the majority will experience symptomatic improvement but with longer follow-up only a small number have intestinal continuity restored and following this an even smaller number remain in clinical remission.[48]

Long-term complications of perianal disease

Longer-term complications of perianal Crohn's disease may include rectal or anal strictures and

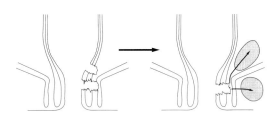

Figure 10.6 • Pathogenesis of anal suppurative disease. Deep cavitating ulcers give rise to extrasphincteric and supralevator abscesses.

incontinence due to fibrosis and sphincter damage. Symptomatic strictures should be gently dilated to not more than 20 mm, remembering that with an impaired sphincter there is a risk of precipitating or worsening incontinence. About half the patients who develop an anal or rectal stricture will require proctectomy.[68]

Prognosis

It has often been said that patients can anticipate a normal life expectancy and that they do not die of Crohn's disease. However, standardised mortality rates are high for patients who have the onset of their disease before the age of 20 years and are particularly high early in the course of the disease, although the absolute numbers dying remain small. Causes of death include sepsis, perioperative complications, electrolyte disturbances and gastrointestinal tract cancers.

Quality-of-life issues are important to these patients and they express concerns over energy levels, fear of surgery and body image. Often, loss of energy and malaise contribute more to functional disability than specific gastrointestinal symptoms. In terms of academic success and advancement, patients are not hampered by the disease, and employment rates are the same as for matched healthy controls. However, patients frequently express impairment of employment, recreation, interpersonal and sexual relationships. Most patients continue to function optimistically and adapt successfully, but disease relapses produce considerable stress, and psychological support from counsellors, psychiatrists, non-medical and patient support groups should be utilised.[69]

Key points

- Patients with Crohn's disease usually enjoy reasonable health punctuated by periods of increased disease activity, initially managed medically.
- Many patients will require surgery at some stage and a multidisciplinary team is key to optimise management.
- Surgery is restricted to dealing with troublesome segments that cannot be managed medically.
- Surgery for small-bowel disease is usually necessary because of complications of disease such as strictures and fistulas.
- Surgery for large-bowel disease is usually necessary because of inability of medical treatment to control symptoms.

References

1. Satsangi J, Sutherland LR. Inflammatory bowel diseases. Elsevier, 2003.

2. Sartor RB. Does *Mycobacterium avium* subspecies *paratuberculosis* cause Crohn's disease? Gut 2005; 54:896–8.

3. Bernstein CN, Rawsthorne P, Blanchard JF. Population-based case–control study of measles, mumps, and rubella and inflammatory bowel disease. Inflamm Bowel Dis 2007; 13:759–62.

4. Gaya DR, Russell RK, Nimmo ER et al. New genes in inflammatory bowel disease: lessons for complex diseases? Lancet 2006; 367:1271–84.

5. Baumgart DC, Carding SR. Inflammatory bowel disease: cause and immunobiology. Lancet 2007; 369:1627–40.

6. Nikolaus S, Schreiber S. Diagnostics of inflammatory bowel disease. Gastroenterology 2007; 133:1670–89.

7. Baumgart DC, Sandborn WJ. Inflammatory bowel disease: clinical aspects and established and evolving therapies. Lancet 2007; 369:1641–57.

8. Bergman R, Parkes M. Systematic review: the use of mesalazine in inflammatory bowel disease. Aliment Pharmacol Ther 2006; 23:841–55.

9. Travis SP, Stange EF, Lemann M et al. European evidence based consensus on the diagnosis and management of Crohn's disease: current management. Gut 2006; 55(Suppl 1):i16–35.

   European Crohn's and Colitis Organisation Consensus Development Conference series. Evidence-based consensus statements that include opinions of experts both for and against the various recommendations.

10. Thomsen O, Cortot A, Jewell D et al. A comparison of budesonide and mesalamine for active Crohn's disease. N Eng J Med 1998; 339:370–4.

Budesonide is twice as effective as mesalamine in treating active Crohn's with the benefit of less side-effects than systemic steroids.

11. Hellers G, Cortot A, Jewell D et al. Oral budesonide for prevention of postsurgical recurrence in Crohn's disease. Gastroenterology 1999; 116:294–300.

Budesonide does not have a role in prophylaxis after surgery.

12. Elton EHS. Review article: the medical management of Crohn's disease. Aliment Pharmacol Ther 1996; 10:1–22.

A review article that includes data on the effect of parenteral and enteral nutrition that are as effective as steroids at inducing remission, but the effect ends as soon as normal diet is reintroduced.

13. Targan SR, Hanauer SB, van Deventer SJ et al. A short-term study of chimeric monoclonal antibody cA2 to tumor necrosis factor alpha for Crohn's disease. Crohn's Disease cA2 Study Group. N Engl J Med 1997; 337:1029–35.

The first randomised controlled trial of biological agents in Crohn's disease demonstrating moderate efficacy in inducing remission.

14. Hanauer SB, Feagan BG, Lichtenstein GR et al. Maintenance infliximab for Crohn's disease: the ACCENT I randomised trial. Lancet 2002; 359:1541–9.

Many centres took part with small numbers in each. There is drug company representation on the writing committee. Infliximab is moderately effective at inducing remission but at 12 months is only a little better than placebo. The data need to be interpreted carefully; infliximab is very expensive, has a poor cost–benefit ratio, and there are concerns about serious long-term side-effects. On the other hand, there are many anecdotes of dramatic clinical responses when other measures have failed. It has a role to induce remission in refractory cases.

15. Sands BE, Anderson FH, Bernstein CN et al. Infliximab maintenance therapy for fistulizing Crohn's disease. N Engl J Med 2004; 350:876–85.

This study looks at the role of infliximab for fistulating Crohn's disease and is a similar design to ACCENT I. Similar comments apply as for ACCENT I above.

16. Fazio VW, Marchetti F, Church M et al. Effect of resection margins on the recurrence of Crohn's disease in the small bowel. A randomized controlled trial. Ann Surg 1996; 224:563–71.

From restrospective reviews and now a small randomised trial it seems highly likely that microscopic involvement of resection margin does not increase recurrence rates.

17. McLeod RS. Resection margins and recurrent Crohn's disease. Hepatogastroenterology 1990; 37:63–6.

18. Klein O, Colombel JF, Lescut D et al. Remaining small bowel endoscopic lesions at surgery have no influence on early anastomotic recurrences in Crohn's disease. Am J Gastroenterol 1995; 90:1949–52.

19. Scott NA, Hughes LE. Timing of ileocolonic resection for symptomatic Crohn's disease – the patient's view. Gut 1994; 35:656–7.

20. Thirlby RC, Land JC, Fenster LF et al. Effect of surgery on health related quality of life in patients with inflammatory bowel disease: a prospective study. Arch Surg 1998; 133:826–32.

21. Tilney HS, Constantinides VA, Heriot AG et al. Comparison of laparoscopic and open ileocecal resection for Crohn's disease: a meta-analysis. Surg Endosc 2006; 20:1036–44.

22. Andersen J, Kehlet H. Fast track open ileo-colic resections for Crohn's disease. Colorectal Dis 2005; 7:394–7.

23. Bernell O, Lapidus A, Hellers G. Risk factors for surgery and postoperative recurrence in Crohn's disease. Ann Surg 2000; 231:38–45.

24. Shivananda S, Hordijk ML, Pena AS et al. Crohn's disease: risk of recurrence and reoperation in a defined population. Gut 1989; 30:990–5.

25. Farmer RG, Whelan G, Fazio VW. Long-term follow-up of patients with Crohn's disease. Relationship between the clinical pattern and prognosis. Gastroenterology 1985; 88:1818–25.

26. Halme LE. Results of surgical treatment of patients with Crohn's disease. Ann Chir Gynaecol 1992; 81:277–83.

27. Nordgren SR, Fasth SB, Oresland TO et al. Long-term follow-up in Crohn's disease. Mortality, morbidity, and functional status. Scand J Gastroenterol 1994; 29:1122–8.

28. Fichera A, Lovadina S, Rubin M et al. Patterns and operative treatment of recurrent Crohn's disease: a prospective longitudinal study. Surgery 2006; 140:649–54.

29. Post S, Herfarth CH, Schumacher H et al. Experience with ileostomy and colostomy in Crohn's disease. Br J Surg 1995; 82:1629–33.

30. Borley NR, Mortensen NJ, Jewell DP. Preventing postoperative recurrence of Crohn's disease. Br J Surg 1997; 84:1493–502.

31. Cottone M, Rosselli M, Orlando A et al. Smoking habits and recurrence in Crohn's disease. Gastroenterology 1994; 106:643–8.

A study of 182 patients looking for risk factors for recurrence of Crohn's after surgical resection. The study found that smoking doubles the risk of recurrence of Crohn's disease.

32. Moskovitz D, McLeod RS, Greenberg GR et al. Operative and environmental risk factors for recurrence of Crohn's disease. Int J Colorectal Dis 1999; 14:224–6.

A retrospective study of 92 patients that confirms the findings of other studies that showed a doubling of recurrence rate for those who continue to smoke after surgical resection.

33. Sutherland LR, Ramcharan S, Bryant H et al. Effect of cigarette smoking on recurrence of Crohn's disease. Gastroenterology 1990; 98:1123–8.

The first of a number of papers that have shown the powerful effect of smoking on recurrence. Evidence is probably level III but the strength of the effect is such that there is little doubt.

34. Hudson M, Chitolie A, Hutton RA et al. Thrombotic vascular risk factors in inflammatory bowel disease. Gut 1996; 38:733–7.

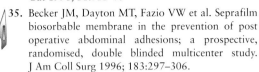

35. Becker JM, Dayton MT, Fazio VW et al. Seprafilm biosorbable membrane in the prevention of post operative abdominal adhesions; a prospective, randomised, double blinded multicenter study. J Am Coll Surg 1996; 183:297–306.

Robust evidence that adhesion formation is reduced, particularly beneath the wound.

36. Worsey MJ, Hull T, Ryland L et al. Stricturoplasty is an effective operation in the operative management of duodenal Crohn's. Dis Colon Rectum 1999; 42:596–600.

37. Yamamoto T, Bain IM, Connolly AB et al. Outcome of stricturoplasty for duodenal Crohn's disease. Br J Surg 1999; 86:259–62.

38. Sabate JM, Villarejo J, Bouhnik Y et al. Hydrostatic balloon dilatation of Crohn's strictures. Aliment Pharmacol Ther 2003; 18:409–13.

39. Michelassi F, Taschieri A, Tonelli F et al. An international, multicenter, prospective, observational study of the side-to-side isoperistaltic strictureplasty in Crohn's disease. Dis Colon Rectum 2007; 50:277–84.

40. Fearnhead NS, Chowdhury R, Box B et al. Long-term follow-up of strictureplasty for Crohn's disease. Br J Surg 2006; 93:475–82.

41. Ozuner G, Fazio VW, Lavery IC et al. How safe is strictureplasty in the management of Crohn's disease? Am J Surg 1996; 171:57–60.

42. Serra J, Cohen Z, McLeod RS. Natural history of strictureplasty in Crohn's disease: 9-year experience. Can J Surg 1995; 38:481–5.

43. Yamamoto T, Bain IM, Allan RN et al. An audit of strictureplasty for small-bowel Crohn's disease. Dis Colon Rectum 1999; 42:797–803.

44. Yamamoto T, Fazio VW, Tekkis PP. Safety and efficacy of strictureplasty for Crohn's disease: a systematic review and meta-analysis. Dis Colon Rectum 2007; 50:1968–86.

45. Scott NA, Finnegan S, Irving MH. Octreotide and postoperative enterocutaneous fistulae: a controlled prospective study. Acta Gastroenterol Belg 1993; 56:266–70.

46. Lapidus A, Bernell O, Hellers G et al. Clinical course of colorectal Crohn's disease, a 35 year follow-up study of 507 patients. Gastroenterology 1998; 114:1151–60.

47. Kornbluth A, Marion JF, Salomon P et al. How effective is current medical therapy for severe ulcerative and Crohn's colitis? An analytic review of selected trials. J Clin Gastroenterol 1995; 20:280–4.

48. Edwards CM, George BD, Jewell DP et al. Role of a defunctioning stoma in the management of large bowel Crohn's disease. Br J Surg 2000; 87:1063–6.

49. Tekkis PP, Purkayastha S, Lanitis S et al. A comparison of segmental vs subtotal/total colectomy for colonic Crohn's disease: a meta-analysis. Colorectal Dis 2006; 8:82–90.

50. Panis P, Poupard B, Neneth J et al. Ileal pouch–anal anastomosis for Crohn's disease. Lancet 1996; 347:854–7.

51. Phillips RKS. Ileal pouch–anal anastomosis for Crohn's disease. Gut 1998; 43:303–8.

52. Regimbeau JM, Panis Y, Pocard M et al. Long-term results of ileal pouch–anal anastomosis for colorectal Crohn's disease. Dis Colon Rectum 2001; 44:769–78.

53. Gillen CD, Walmsley RS, Prior P et al. Ulcerative colitis and Crohn's disease: a comparison of the colorectal cancer risk in extensive colitis. Gut 1994; 35:1590–2.

54. Maykel JA, Hagerman G, Mellgren AF et al. Crohn's colitis: the incidence of dysplasia and adenocarcinoma in surgical patients. Dis Colon Rectum 2006; 49:950–7.

55. Sigel JE, Petras RE, Lashner BA et al. Intestinal adenocarcinoma in Crohn's disease: a report of 30 cases with a focus on coexisting dysplasia. Am J Surg Pathol 1999; 23:651–5.

56. Sangwan YP, Schoetz DJ Jr, Murray JJ et al. Perianal Crohn's disease. Results of local surgical treatment. Dis Colon Rectum 1996; 39:529–35.

57. Halme LA, Sainio P. Factors related to frequency, type and outcome of anal fistulas in Crohn's disease. Dis Colon Rectum 1995; 38:55–9.

58. Hughes LE, Taylor BA. Perianal lesions in Crohn's disease. In: Allan R, Keighley M, Alexander-Williams J et al. (eds) Inflammatory bowel disease, 2nd edn. Edinburgh: Churchill Livingstone, 1990; pp. 351–61.

59. Schwartz DA, Wiersema MJ, Dudiak KM et al. A comparison of endoscopic ultrasound, magnetic resonance imaging, and exam under anesthesia for evaluation of Crohn's perianal fistulas. Gastroenterology 2001; 121:1064–72.

60. Hyder SA, Travis SP, Jewell DP et al. Fistulating anal Crohn's disease: results of combined surgical and infliximab treatment. Dis Colon Rectum 2006; 49:1837–41.

61. Sweeney JL, Ritchie JK, Nicholls RJ. Anal fissure in Crohn's disease. Br J Surg 1988; 75:56–7.

62. Fleshner PR, Schoetz DJ Jr, Roberts PL et al. Anal fissure in Crohn's disease: a plea for aggressive management. Dis Colon Rectum 1995; 38:1137–43.

63. Sonoda T, Hull T, Piedmonte MR et al. Outcomes of primary repair of anorectal and rectovaginal fistulas using the endorectal advancement flap. Dis Colon Rectum 2002; 45:1622–8.

64. O'Connor L, Champagne BJ, Ferguson MA et al. Efficacy of anal fistula plug in closure of Crohn's anorectal fistulas. Dis Colon Rectum 2006; 49:1569–73.

65. Radcliffe AG, Ritchie JK, Hawley PR et al. Anovaginal and rectovaginal fistulas in Crohn's disease. Dis Colon Rectum 1988; 31:94–9.

66. Songne K, Scotte M, Lubrano J et al. Treatment of anovaginal or rectovaginal fistulas with modified Martius graft. Colorectal Dis 2007; 9:653–6.

67. Andreani SM, Dang HH, Grondona P et al. Rectovaginal fistula in Crohn's disease. Dis Colon Rectum 2007; 50:2215–22.

68. Linares L, Moreira LF, Andrews H et al. Natural history and treatment of anorectal strictures complicating Crohn's disease. Br J Surg 1988; 75:653–5.

69. Kornbluth A, Salomon P, Sachar D. Crohn's disease. In: Feldman M, Scharschmidt BF, Sleisenger MH (eds) Sleisenger and Fordtran's gastrointestinal and liver disease, 6th edn. Philadelphia: WB Saunders, 1998; Vol. 2, pp. 1708–34.

70. Allan A, Andrews H, Hilton CJ et al. Segmental colonic resection is an appropriate operation for short skip lesions due to Crohn's disease in the colon. World J Surg 1989; 13:611–14.

71. Makowiec F, Paczulla D, Schmidtke C et al. Crohn's colitis: segmental resection or colectomy. Gastroenterology 1996; 110:A1402.

72. Prabhakar LP, Laramee C, Nelson H et al. Avoiding a stoma; the role of segmental colectomy in Crohn's colitis. Dis Colon Rectum 1997; 40:71–8.

73. Polle SW, Slors JF, Weverling GJ et al. Recurrence after segmental resection for colonic Crohn's disease. Br J Surg 2005; 92:1143–9.

11

Incontinence

Paul Durdey

Introduction

Faecal incontinence is socially disabling. The true incidence in the general population is grossly underestimated but may be up to 1–2%. This is largely due to embarrassment, with patients may be unwilling to discuss the problem with their family or their doctor. Urinary incontinence appears to carry less of a social stigma, with women in particular more willing to discuss their problems. Awareness is improving among both patients and the medical profession, and therefore the number of patients who seek treatment for this condition is likely to increase in the future. Faecal incontinence is more common in women and the peak incidence occurs in the elderly.

Aetiology

The aetiology of faecal incontinence is multifactorial. The ability to retain faeces within the rectum depends on a number of factors, including stool consistency, the capacity and compliance of the rectum, a normal rectoanal inhibitory reflex, normal internal and external sphincter function, and normal sensation in the anal canal. Failure in any component can lead to incontinence. The major aetiological factors in faecal incontinence are listed in Box 11.1. The majority of patients with the condition who present in surgical practice have an obstetric injury, damage

to the pudendal nerves (neuropathic or idiopathic faecal incontinence) or iatrogenic injuries due to previous injudicious anal surgery: iatrogenic incontinence following anal surgery is underestimated. Surgery for fistula in ano accounts for the majority of cases. Patients likely to present with incontinence after fistula surgery are those treated for high

Box 11.1 • Aetiology of faecal incontinence

Trauma
- Obstetric
- Surgical
- Accidental/war injury

Colorectal disease
- Haemorrhoids
- Rectal prolapse
- Inflammatory bowel disease
- Tumours

Congenital
- Spina bifida
- Operations for imperforate anus
- Hirschsprung's disease

Neurological
- Cerebral
- Spinal
- Peripheral

Miscellaneous
- Behavioural
- Impaction
- Encopresis

fistulas or individuals who have undergone multiple operations for recurrent or persistent fistula. A surprising number of patients after haemorrhoidectomy present with minor degrees of soiling. This may be due to loss of the normal anal cushions associated with a degree of sensory impairment in the anal canal. The majority of these patients do not require surgical intervention.

Treatment for anal fissure has been associated with faecal incontinence. Manual dilatation of the anus, which was a popular treatment for a variety of anorectal conditions, can lead to some incontinence in up to 20% of patients.[1] The more recent procedure of sphincterotomy has a much lower incidence of incontinence postoperatively; however, this is argued to be the case only if the sphincterotomy is performed in the lateral position and not through the base of the fissure. The latter procedure is claimed to be worse through formation of a keyhole deformity.

Minor degrees of incontinence can follow rectal resection such as low anterior resection and coloanal anastomoses. The aetiology of this is probably twofold. First, there is a reduction in the reservoir capacity of the neorectum, which can be addressed by the formation of a small J-shaped colonic pouch. The second factor probably relates to interference with the intramural nerve pathways to the internal anal sphincter.

Traumatic damage to the perineum can result from accidental injuries such as impalement or from acts of aggression, for example war injury or gunshot wounds. Occasionally, socially acquired injuries will present to the surgeon. The majority of patients who present with severe sphincter injury are those who suffer major pelvic trauma following road traffic accidents. These injuries are often associated with damage to the urinary tract.

The vast majority of patients who present to the surgeon with faecal incontinence are women who have suffered an obstetric injury. Many women presenting with faecal incontinence give a history of prolonged labour or traumatic vaginal deliveries. In a series of studies, Snooks et al.[2,3] demonstrated objective damage to the anal sphincter mechanism in women who had undergone a vaginal delivery, including a fall in resting and squeeze pressures associated with increase in perineal descent and prolonged pudendal nerve terminal motor latencies. Although many of these parameters improved by 6 months after delivery, some patients who had

undergone a forceps delivery developed a persistent conduction defect of the pudendal nerves.

The risk of faecal incontinence increases with the number of vaginal deliveries, delivery of large babies, prolonged second stage of labour and use of forceps. Severe injuries to the perineum, such as a third-degree tear, can lead to immediate problems with continence. A third/fourth-degree tear occurs in 0.5–2% of vaginal deliveries, and although obvious disruption of the sphincter mechanism sustained in a tear is usually repaired immediately by the obstetrician, there is evidence that many women (up to 85%) following such a repair have a persistent defect of the sphincter that can be defined on anal endosonography. Many of these women remain symptomatic.[4,5] Occult sphincter injuries may occur in up to one-third of women who undergo vaginal delivery[6] and in up to 80% following forceps delivery.[4]

In elderly women who present with faecal incontinence the precise aetiology is often unclear. In many cases there is a history of multiparity and prolonged or difficult vaginal delivery. Histochemical analysis of the pelvic floor muscles demonstrates abnormalities compatible with neuropathic damage to the sphincter with subsequent reinnervation. These changes can be seen in the external anal sphincter, puborectalis and levator ani.[7,8] The changes of denervation and reinnervation can be confirmed by electromyography of the pelvic floor striated muscles.

Pudendal neuropathy is present in the majority of patients with idiopathic faecal incontinence.[9–11] Damage to the pudendal nerves leads to low squeeze pressures in the anal canal, evidence of delayed pudendal nerve terminal motor latency, an increase in mean fibre density and decreased anal canal sensation. Further damage to the pudendal nerves may result from chronic straining and perineal descent.

Abnormal descent of the perineum was first described by Parks et al. in 1966.[12] The anorectal junction normally lies above a line drawn between the lower margin of the symphysis pubis and the tip of the coccyx defined on a lateral pelvic radiograph. In patients with the descending perineum syndrome the anorectal junction lies below this and on straining there is further descent of the perineum. Perineal descent also appears to be related to the number of vaginal deliveries and in itself may lead to further trauma to the pudendal nerves. However, the precise relationship between perineal descent and neuropathic damage to the pelvic floor is unclear and recent studies have failed to demonstrate a direct link.[13] It would therefore appear that the majority of cases of faecal incontinence secondary to obstetric damage are due to a combination of traumatic injury to the pelvic floor during delivery associated with trauma to its nerve supply.

Presentation

History

It is essential to take an accurate history from patients who present with faecal incontinence. Frequency and severity of incontinence should be documented. It is important to know whether the patient is incontinent to liquids, solids, flatus or all three. Often the history will give some indication as to whether the problem lies primarily within the rectum or sphincter apparatus. A proportion of patients with abnormalities purely of anal canal sensation demonstrate seepage of faeces due to sensory inattention. Specific features in the history may point to the underlying aetiology. Data from our unit in Bristol have suggested that patients in whom the primary presenting complaint is one of urgency of defecation – in other words they are aware of the need to defecate but are unable to retain stool for more than a few moments – will have deficiency of external anal sphincter function.[14] However, a history of coexisting urinary incontinence would suggest a neuropathic aetiology. Many older patients who present with neurogenic incontinence give a history of insensible faecal loss.

A general history should be taken with particular reference to anorectal surgery or trauma. Specifically, the patient should be asked about any neurological problems and a careful obstetric history is essential. In order to quantify the degree of incontinence it is helpful to use some type of standardised scoring system, of which there are many. My personal preference is the Cleveland Clinic scoring system[15] (Table 11.1).

Examination

A full examination of the patient's abdomen should be undertaken and neurological assessment made. On inspection of the perineum the patient should be asked to strain in order to assess perineal descent and also to exclude rectal prolapse. The perianal area should be inspected for evidence of previous surgery or the presence of minor anorectal conditions. The anus itself should be assessed at rest to see whether it is closed or patulous.

Digital rectal examination can provide some information. An assessment can be made of resting anal tone, although the correlation between clinical examination and physiological evaluation is controversial. The patient should be asked to contract the external anal sphincter voluntarily. It is possible to assess movement of the external sphincter and puborectalis separately. Patients who have a deficiency in the anterior part of the sphincter can be recognised. An assessment should be made for the presence or absence of a rectocele, and proctoscopy and sigmoidoscopy are mandatory to exclude other significant pathology.

Special investigations

Physiological assessment of the anorectum has been comprehensively addressed in Chapter 1. My practice is to assess all patients who present with symptomatic incontinence in the anorectal physiology

Table 11.1 • Cleveland Clinic scoring system for assessment of faecal incontinence

	Never	Rarely	Sometimes	Usually	Always
Solids	0	1	2	3	4
Liquids	0	1	2	3	4
Flatus	0	1	2	3	4
Use of pad	0	1	2	3	4
Lifestyle alteration	0	1	2	3	4

Definitions
Rarely: less than once a month. Sometimes: more than once a month but less than once a week. Usually: more than once a week but less than once a day. Always: more than once a day.

laboratory. The tests that are performed routinely include three-dimensional manometry examining resting and squeeze pressures. This method allows a pressure profile of the anal sphincter mechanism to be constructed, which is particularly useful when searching for defects in the sphincter mechanism and can be correlated with the anatomical appearances on anorectal ultrasound. Assessment of the sphincters by endoanal ultrasound is an extremely useful method of identifying specific anatomical defects in the internal and external anal sphincter and for monitoring the results of surgery. Patients also undergo assessment of anal mucosal electrosensitivity and rectal compliance. We do not routinely perform measurement of pudendal nerve terminal motor latency.

We also do not routinely use defaecography in the assessment of patients with faecal incontinence unless an overt rectal prolapse that is not apparent clinically or an intrarectal intussusception is suspected.

Treatment of faecal incontinence

The treatment of faecal incontinence depends on its aetiology. Minor degrees of perianal soiling may require nothing more than careful perianal hygiene, but for patients with established and troublesome faecal incontinence the choice lies between conservative measures or surgical repair of the sphincter apparatus. The majority of patients who have a specific sphincter defect following obstetric or direct injury identified by three-dimensional manometry or endoanal ultrasound are best served by surgical repair. However, those in whom the incontinence is thought to be neurological in origin may benefit from a conservative approach, at least initially.

Conservative treatment

There is a proportion of patients in whom incontinence is related to fluidity of the bowel action. These patients may be continent if their stool remains solid. In such patients it is appropriate to try antidiarrhoeal medication and sometimes even bulking agents in order to improve stool consistency. A simple regimen of bulking agents and loperamide may succeed in controlling diarrhoea and avoid the necessity of invasive treatment, as may an opposite approach of avoiding fibre in the diet.

Similarly, many patients report troublesome faecal leakage after defecation. This can be improved if the rectum can be fully evacuated. Glycerin or bisacodyl suppositories may be helpful, or alternatively the patient may require a daily phosphate enema. Isolated internal sphincter dysfunction may respond to topical application of 10% phenylephrine gel.[16]

Physiotherapy and pelvic floor retraining (biofeedback) can be helpful in a proportion of patients with incontinence. Biofeedback is particularly useful in patients who have primarily a sensory problem in the anal canal leading to insensible loss of faeces. Patients can be trained using either electromyographic or manometric feedback to improve the strength of their anal sphincters and, if coupled with an intrarectal balloon, may improve their rectal sensory awareness. Biofeedback training can be undertaken as an inpatient; however, the best results are often obtained when patients are allowed to take the biofeedback apparatus home and practise for 2–3 months.

Simple pelvic floor exercises, such as those recommended after delivery, can be beneficial in some patients. However, I have found that more specific physiotherapy using either interferential treatment of the pelvic floor and, in particular, trophic stimulation via an anal plug electrode can be extremely successful. The latter technique uses electrical impulses designed to mimic the train of signals along the pudendal nerve. The precise role of electrical stimulation of the pelvic floor is unclear.[17,18] In our hands the results of intensive physiotherapy are almost equivalent to those obtained by postanal repair in patients with neurogenic incontinence. Enthusiasts of biofeedback training have reported improvement in up to 70% of patients.[19] Biofeedback can certainly improve patients with structural defects of the anal sphincter, although long-term results are unclear.[20] There are few randomised trials.[21,22]

 A recent review of published series confirms the benefit of biofeedback.[22]

The most recent National Institute for Clinical Excellence (NICE) guidelines recommend that all patients with faecal incontinence undergo a trial of conservative treatment prior to consideration of a surgical procedure.

Surgical treatment

Surgical treatment of faecal incontinence can be divided into procedures designed to repair sphincter defects, such as have occurred after direct injury or obstetric trauma, and plication procedures, where the primary problem appears to be of neurogenic origin. In cases where the sphincter cannot be repaired further or where direct repair of the sphincter has failed, there are various techniques for augmenting or replacing the anal musculature. Such methods include gracilis muscle transposition, placement of a silastic sling around the anus, the use of an artificial anal sphincter, and sacral nerve stimulation.

The choice of operation is largely determined by the preoperative physiological and radiological findings. If the primary problem appears to be a specific sphincter defect identified manometrically or ultrasonographically, then this should be repaired directly. For patients in whom an anterior sphincter deficit is apparent clinically or on investigation, and usually following an obstetric injury, my preference is to perform an anterior sphincter repair with levatorplasty. Many of these patients will have a degree of coexisting neuropathic damage to the pelvic floor, particularly if they have undergone multiple vaginal deliveries. Such patients are still suitable for an anterior repair.[23]

For patients in whom the primary aetiology appears to be neurogenic and in whom preoperative investigations have failed to reveal a sphincter defect, my own preference is to offer a trial of sacral nerve stimulation.

Sphincter repair procedures
Preoperative preparation

Few surgeons now use a stoma as an adjunct to sphincter repair in the elective case, unless a complex sphincter reconstruction is being undertaken, as for example in a patient with Crohn's disease, for a cloacal defect, or when there is an associated anovaginal or rectovaginal fistula.

Some surgeons use full mechanical bowel preparation prior to sphincter repair. My preference is to use a phosphate enema on the morning of surgery. The rationale for this is that a failed full mechanical bowel preparation may be worse than no bowel preparation at all, with liquid faeces running over the operation site.

All patients undergoing sphincter repair are routinely administered three perioperative doses of antibiotics, such as cefuroxime and metronidazole.

Anterior sphincter repair and levatorplasty

This is the operation of choice for patients with an anterior injury. Classically, the majority of surgeons in the UK perform this operation with the patient in the lithotomy position. My practice for a number of years has been to use the prone jack-knife position, as used by the majority of surgeons in the USA. The patients are not routinely catheterised.

The intersphincteric plane is approached through a curvilinear incision close to the vaginal introitus and extending laterally around the anal margin. In a small number of women with severe obstetric injuries there may be little skin between the vagina and anal orifice, with mucosa-to-mucosa apposition. In such cases a Z-plasty is required (**Fig. 11.1**). The skin flap is dissected towards the anal margin to expose the fibres of the external sphincter. In severe cases of obstetric injury the external sphincter may have been completely divided and replaced by scar tissue.

The intersphincteric plane between internal and external sphincter is dissected. This is a relatively avascular plane. The anterior border of the external sphincter is identified by sharp dissection close to the vaginal wall. The external sphincter may be tethered by surrounding fibrosis. This dissection can be technically demanding. By dissecting laterally, normal external anal sphincter is identified. Great care must be taken in not extending the exploration too far laterally as there is a danger of damaging the neurovascular bundles to the external sphincter, which may result in a poor postoperative result.

Once the external sphincter has been mobilised from surrounding fibrosis, it is retracted caudally and dissection continued in the rectovaginal septum. The septum, particularly in young women, can be vascular and troublesome bleeding may be encountered. Great care must be taken not to enter the rectum. The vagina is carefully separated through its entire length from the anterior rectal wall. The levator muscles can then be identified in the base of the wound running anteriorly and superiorly.

An anterior levatorplasty is performed by suturing together the two sides of the levator using two or three interrupted sutures (**Fig. 11.2**). My preference is to use 2/0 PDS (polydioxanone suture; Ethicon Limited, UK). If the external sphincter has been completely divided and continuity maintained by scar tissue, the external sphincter is divided through the scar tissue. An overlapping repair is performed (**Fig. 11.3**) using two layers of horizontal mattress

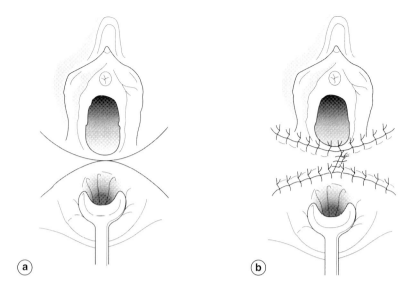

Figure 11.1 • Double Z-plasty for sphincter repair: **(a)** a cruciate incision is made over the perineal body, which is grossly deficient; **(b)** the completed operation with elongation of the skin over the perineal body. Reproduced from Keighley MRB, Williams NS. Surgery of the anus, rectum and colon. Philadelphia: WB Saunders, 1993. With permission from Elsevier.

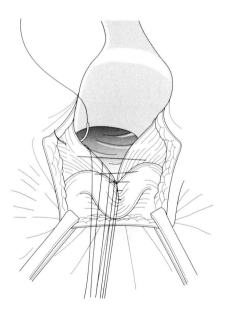

Figure 11.2 • Anterior levatorplasty. By rotation of the anterior retractor the anterior fibres of the puborectalis can be identified and then plicated so as to oppose the pelvic floor in the midline anteriorly. Reproduced from Keighley MRB, Williams NS. Surgery of the anus, rectum and colon. Philadelphia: WB Saunders, 1993. With permission from Elsevier.

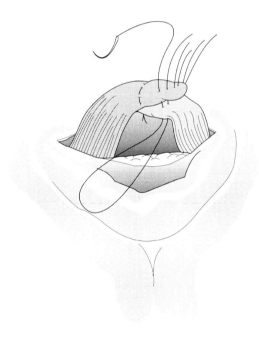

Figure 11.3 • A two-layer flap-over repair is formed. Reproduced from Keighley MRB, Williams NS. Surgery of the anus, rectum and colon. Philadelphia: WB Saunders, 1993. With permission from Elsevier.

sutures of 2/0 PDS. For each layer all the sutures should be placed prior to tying them. Some surgeons prefer not to overlap the muscle but perform an end-to-end apposition. Results appear similar.

Obstetric injuries are often associated with damage to the perineal body and distal rectovaginal septum, but attempts to correct these defects by imbrication of the rectal wall above the sphincter and internal sphincter imbrication appear to confer little benefit over simple overlapping repair of the external anal sphincter, and they are associated with more complications.[24]

It is often the case that after anterior sphincter repair and levatorplasty the skin wound, which was semicircular, has now become almost longitudinal. The skin is closed using an absorbable suture such as Vicryl. A small defect is left in the wound to facilitate drainage of any haematoma.

Postoperatively, some surgeons place the patient on fluids only and constipating agents for 48–72 hours, whereas others use laxatives and a normal diet and encourage early defecation.

Recent evidence suggests that bowel confinement may be unnecessary.[25]

In our unit, postoperative physiotherapy after wound healing at approximately 6–8 weeks using trophic stimulation has been found to be a useful adjunct to all types of sphincter repair.

A similar technique is used for patients in whom a traumatic injury to the external sphincter apparatus has been sustained. Having identified the site of injury, the tissues are dissected back to healthy muscle. The sphincter is divided through the scar tissue and an overlapping repair performed. Often the wound is left open to granulate.

Postanal repair

Postanal repair was developed in 1975 by Parks.[26] The operation was devised to restore the normal anorectal angle, which Parks had discovered was obtuse in many patients with idiopathic faecal incontinence. In my opinion there is now no indication for this procedure.

Total pelvic floor repair

The operation of total pelvic floor repair was devised in response to disappointing long-term results following postanal repair for neurogenic incontinence, and in response to the fact that many such patients have anatomical defects such as rectocele and abnormal perineal descent.[27] However, since the advent of sacral nerve stimulation this operation has become obsolete.

The question of whether to plicate the internal anal sphincter is conjectural, evidence from a recent randomised trial of longitudinal plication suggesting that it adds nothing to a standard pelvic floor repair.[28]

Isolated injuries to the internal anal sphincter can be treated by injection of silicone, collagen or a variety of implantable materials. Results are variable and any improvement in symptoms appear short term.

Plication procedures

Simple reefing procedures for the anal sphincter have been described in the literature for over 100 years. However, in my opinion the role for simple reefing of the external sphincter is extremely limited. Occasionally, in patients who appear to have an anterior deficit secondary to obstetric trauma, the external sphincter is not divided but merely thinned, sitting loosely around the anal canal. Simple plication without division of the muscle can be combined with a formal reconstruction of the perineal body via levatorplasty. I think there are now very few indications for simple reefing of the external sphincter posteriorly, but there are isolated cases of unexplained male incontinence where the procedure can be surprisingly effective.

Sphincter augmentation procedures

In a minority of patients direct sphincter repair is not possible due to insufficient residual sphincter, major neurological deficit or previous failed repairs. In such patients, consideration should be given to some form of sphincter augmentation. Various muscles have been used, including gluteus maximus, sartorius, adductor longus and, most commonly, gracilis.

Gracilis muscle transposition

The gracilis muscle has been used for anal sphincter supplementation since 1952; however, it was Corman[29] in 1978 who popularised the technique. The advantage of the gracilis muscle is that it is the most superficial muscle in the medial aspect of the thigh. It is approximately the right size and the blood and nerve supply enter proximally. Thus distal division of the muscle does not necessarily compromise the blood supply. The operation has been superseded by the electrically stimulated gracilis neosphincter.

Electrically stimulated gracilis neosphincter

One problem with transposition of muscles around the anal canal is the difference in physiology between the external anal sphincter and other adjacent skeletal muscles. The external sphincter has resting tone and a preponderance of slow twitch fibres. None of the other skeletal muscles used to augment the sphincter has these properties. This led several groups to explore the possibility of electrical stimulation of the gracilis muscle to determine whether this provided a better physiological replacement for the external sphincter.[30-32] The principle of the procedure is to provide continuous electrical stimulation to the gracilis via its nerve supply or directly into the muscle. Stimulation is achieved via an implanted stimulator. This technique has been used not only to augment an existing anal sphincter, but also in patients with anorectal agenesis. The method has also been applied to patients who have undergone abdominoperineal excision of the rectum who cannot tolerate a permanent stoma for religious or social reasons. The procedure is contraindicated in patients in whom the gracilis muscle is damaged for any reason or where perineal sepsis is likely to be problematic.

The technique is not suitable for elderly or infirm patients nor for those who cannot manage control of the stimulator. Due to the complexity of the procedure, initial studies included a covering stoma, to be fashioned before embarking on the transposition and sited on the opposite side to the proposed gracilis muscle transfer. However, more recent series have suggested that a stoma is not always necessary, that it may not prevent perineal sepsis and that it has a morbidity of its own.[33,34]

Following mobilisation of the gracilis muscle proximally the neurovascular bundle is identified. The main nerve to the gracilis muscle lies above the main vascular pedicle and this is confirmed using a nerve stimulator. The main branch of the nerve lies on the adductor brevis muscle.

There are two techniques for muscle stimulation. In the procedure devised by Williams et al.,[30] the electrodes are placed directly over the nerve to gracilis. Having identified the nerve, the stimulator and electrodes are attached. The stimulator lies in a pocket overlying the lower ribs. The lead is tunnelled subcutaneously via a small incision in the suprainguinal region and the electrode brought down to the appropriate nerve. The electrode plate is sutured over the main nerve bundle in a longitudinal fashion (**Fig. 11.4**). The electrode plate is placed in the most appropriate position to ensure an en-masse contraction of the gracilis, and once in an ideal position is sutured in place using fine silk sutures.

The alternative technique[31] utilises insertion of electrodes into the gracilis muscle adjacent to the supplying nerve (Medtronic, Minneapolis, USA).

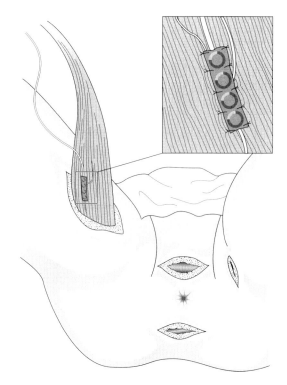

Figure 11.4 • Continuous electrical stimulation of the gracilis. An electrode for electrical stimulation is sutured to the proximal gracilis muscle near the neurovascular bundle. Reproduced from Keighley MRB, Williams NS. Surgery of the anus, rectum and colon. Philadelphia: WB Saunders, 1993. With permission from Elsevier.

This technique has become more widely adopted due to complications associated with applying the electrode directly on to the nerve.

The connection to the stimulator can be assessed using an external telemetry programmer. The gracilis muscle is then transposed around the anal canal in a tunnel in the extrasphincteric plane. Two lateral incisions placed well away from the anal canal are recommended in order to achieve this. It is also recommended that the muscle is taken around the anal canal in a gamma configuration (**Fig. 11.5**) and sutured to the periosteum of the contralateral ischial tuberosity. It is essential that the anal canal is surrounded by the muscle and not its tendon for optimal function.

Postoperatively, the patient is nursed with legs bandaged loosely together. Electrical stimulation of the muscle commences at day 10, provided the wounds are healed satisfactorily. The stimulator is programmed using a standard training protocol. Once

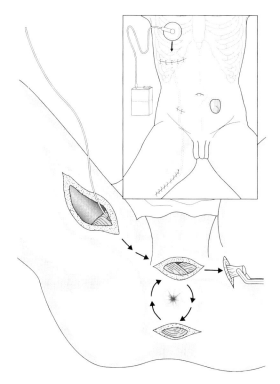

Figure 11.5 • The gracilis muscle is re-routed around the anal canal. Stimulation is triggered by an external pulse generator, which activates a receiving device under the costal margin. Reproduced from Keighley MRB, Williams NS. Surgery of the anus, rectum and colon. Philadelphia: WB Saunders, 1993. With permission from Elsevier.

the muscle is trained, the patient can be admitted for closure of the covering stoma. The stimulator can be switched on or off by passing a magnet over it.

Gluteus maximus transposition

In many respects the gluteus maximus muscle is in an ideal position to augment anal sphincter function, and recent reports of this technique have proved encouraging.[35,36] It is also possible to use a stimulator for gluteal transposition.[36] The procedure is now uncommon and is possibly obsolete.

Implants and artificial anal sphincters

Dacron-impregnated silastic sling

The use of an artificial sling to encircle the anal canal as an adjunct to continence has gained little popularity in the UK, but in the USA is used more

frequently.[37] Two incisions are made 3 cm lateral to either side of the anal verge. The ischiorectal fossae are then entered and a tunnel developed around the anal canal. A 1.5-cm strip of silastic sheet is cut. The strip is placed around the anal canal using two clamps and the adequacy of the anal lumen assessed. Once the position of the mesh is correctly identified, the ends are secured using a 30-mm linear stapler. The suture line can be reinforced with interrupted non-absorbable suture if required.

Artificial sphincter for faecal incontinence

The artificial bowel sphincter for faecal incontinence (**Fig. 11.6**) has not proved as successful as artificial sphincters for urinary incontinence. Indeed, in 1989 Christiansen and Lorentzem reported five cases using an AMS 800 artificial urinary sphincter.[38] The cuff of the sphincter was inserted around the anal canal and the pump placed in the left side of the scrotum or the left labium majus. The pressure-regulating balloon was placed extraperitoneally to the left of the bladder.

A modified artificial bowel sphincter has now been evaluated.[39,40] Indications for use of an artificial bowel sphincter include congenital anorectal abnormalities, traumatic injuries, neurological dysfunction or failure of previous sphincter repair. This device is specifically designed with different-sized cuffs to encircle the anal canal. Similar to the urinary sphincter the device has a reservoir implanted in the abdominal wall with a control pump placed in the scrotum or labium. The occlusive cuff containing a fluid-filled inflatable shell is implanted around a segment of the anal canal using multiple incisions. A tunnel is created around the anal canal by blunt dissection, with care taken to avoid injury to the rectal wall of the vagina. It is important to ensure that the cuff is inserted deeply into the tissues to avoid postoperative skin erosion. The pressure-regulating balloon is implanted in the prevesical space using a Pfannenstiel incision. The control pump is implanted into the soft tissue of the labium or scrotum. The control pump is a soft bulb that the patient squeezes and releases to transfer fluid into or out of the cuff. The technique is associated with considerable morbidity. Results of a multicentre trial suggest that the majority of patients who underwent the procedure had a device-related complication. The commonest complications reported are infection, erosion of

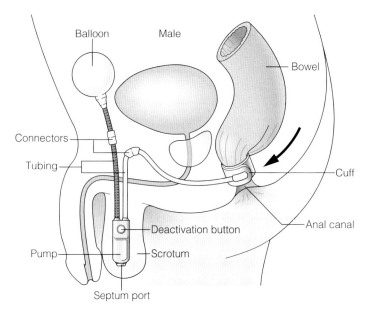

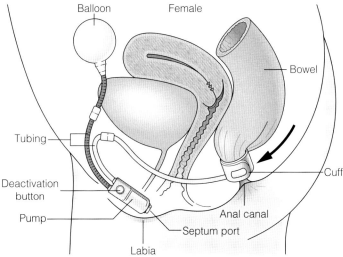

Figure 11.6 • The Acticon artificial bowel sphincter for use in male and female patients.

the device, malfunction and migration. Over one-third of the patients required explant of the device due to postoperative complications. Data from a multicentre study in the USA revealed that after 1 year two-thirds of patients retained a functioning device. Lessons from the larger studies suggest that a single perianal incision is preferable and that the cuff should be placed at least 3 cm deep at its lower border. Selection of the pressure-regulating balloon appears to be important. It is not considered that a diverting stoma is necessary in the majority of patients. A more recent device implanted trans-abdominally has been described. Long-term results are not available.

Alternative procedures

Sacral nerve stimulation

Sacral nerve stimulation (**Fig. 11.7**) has been used in the treatment of urinary incontinence. A similar technique has been utilised for faecal incontinence with promising initial results.[41,42] An initial trial stimulation is undertaken. A percutaneous wire is inserted under general or local anaesthesia into the second, third or fourth sacral foramen. Successful position is indicated by contraction of the pelvic floor and flexion of the ipsilateral great toe. The wire is connected to an external stimulator and the

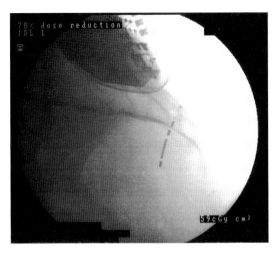

Figure 11.7 • Sacral nerve stimulation: radiograph of a percutaneously introduced tined permanent electrode with implanted stimulator.

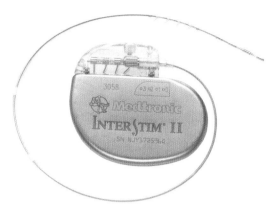

Figure 11.8 • Implanted pulse generator (IPG) and tined lead for permanent sacral nerve stimulation.

results monitored for a period of 2–3 weeks. If successful, a permanent indwelling stimulator can be inserted. A permanent tined electrode is implanted via a percutaneous approach. The implanted pulse generator (IPG; **Fig 11.8**) is connected and inserted into a subcutaneous pocket created in the ipsilateral buttock. The settings can be altered transcutaneously by the clinician or patient. The technique appears to benefit patients who have an intact anal sphincter on ultrasound and some preservation of pudendal nerve function.

Anal plug

One simple technique suggested for control of faecal incontinence is the anal continence plug.[43] This may have a role to play in some patients' treatment.

Stoma formation

When all else fails, consideration should be given to a defunctioning stoma, which can be performed laparoscopically. Generally, an end-colostomy is preferable to a loop. However, if the rectal stump remains, patients can be troubled by incontinence of mucus, and on occasions this will require a formal proctectomy. An alternative procedure is to form a continent colonic conduit in sigmoid or transverse colon to allow antegrade colonic lavage.[44]

Results of treatment

Direct sphincter repair

Direct repair of the anal sphincter following ano-rectal trauma or iatrogenic injuries has achieved good results. Browning and Motson[45] reported on 97 patients who had undergone direct sphincter repair, the vast majority of whom were in one of the above two categories. These authors reported a 78% success rate, with patients being rendered completely continent of liquids and solids. (It is noteworthy, though, that the results of the minority of patients in this series with obstetric damage were poor when treated by this approach.) Similar results of direct repair have been obtained by other authors (Table 11.2).

Table 11.2 • Results of direct sphincter repair

Reference	n	Patients with complete continence (%)
Manning and Pratt[46]	102	74
Fang et al.[47]	79	58
Corman[48]	28	100
Cterceko et al.[49]	44	54

Anterior sphincter repair

The results for anterior sphincter repair with or without levatorplasty are shown in Table 11.3, and overall can be expected to be good in approximately three-quarters of patients. It would appear that the patients who fail to derive benefit from the operation are those in whom there is coexisting pudendal neuropathy.[54,55] A proportion of patients who have poor postoperative function have persistent defects in the anal sphincter, demonstrable on post-operative anal endosonography.[54] It is of note that age in itself does not adversely influence outcome.[53] Physiological changes seen after anterior sphincter repair include restoration of mean resting pressure and increased length of the anal canal. However, the most important improved physiological parameter appears to be an increase in the maximum squeeze pressure.[56] However, not all authors report such a direct correlation between improvement in function and measurable parameters.[54]

 On longer-term follow-up, initial studies suggested that the success rate is maintained.[57] Unfortunately, more recent studies have demonstrated that the long-term success rates of anterior sphincter repair after obstetric trauma may not be maintained. In the long term, only about 40% of patients remain satisfactorily continent.[58,59]

Postanal repair

The early results of postanal repair were encouraging (Table 11.4). Unfortunately, long-term follow-up of patients has revealed that postoperative function deteriorates over time. A frank appraisal of data from patients who had undergone postanal repair from the Birmingham group demonstrated that 3 years after surgery only 34% were completely continent of liquids, solids and flatus.[60–62] This operation is no longer performed.

Summary

Physiological changes after sphincter repair are difficult to document. The Birmingham series of postanal repair reported no significant improvement in resting or squeeze pressures within the anal canal and, significantly, no improvement in the anorectal angle, the parameter which Sir Alan Parks designed the operation to correct. Preoperative physiological factors that correlate with a failure to improve after postanal repair include low resting and squeeze anal canal pressures, severe neuropathy of the pelvic floor, perineal descent and the presence of rectal prolapse. Electrophysiological investigations surprisingly reveal increased neurogenic damage to striated sphincteric muscle after postanal repair, even in some patients whose function improves postoperatively.[63] When patients deteriorate after surgery, a significant increase in neurogenic abnormality can be demonstrated. Thus it would appear that patients who do badly after postanal repair

Table 11.3 • Results of published series of anterior sphincteroplasty

Reference	n	Good/excellent results (%)
Laurberg et al.[50]	19	47
Yoshioka and Keighley[51]	27	74
Orrom et al.[23]	16	62
Wexner et al.[52]	16	74
Fleshman et al.[53]	28	75
Engel et al.[54]	55	76
Oliveira et al.[55]	55	71

Table 11.4 • Results of major series of postanal repair

Reference	n	Good/excellent results (%)
Browning and Parks[60]	140	86
Henry and Simson[61]	129	70
Yoshioka and Keighley[62]	116	57

have progressive denervation. Further evidence for this comes from our own studies, which have demonstrated an abnormal degree of neuromuscular jitter in the external anal sphincter of patients who have poor functional results after postanal repair for faecal incontinence. The aetiology of this progressive denervation remains conjectural.

Results from total pelvic floor repair were initially encouraging, with 90% of patients either being fully continent or with improved continence. However, long-term follow-up of a group of 57 patients revealed that only 14% were rendered completely continent and social activity remained compromised in 76%.[64] Careful clinical and physiological evaluation of the pelvic floor can identify patients with a specific sphincter defect in the absence of neuropathic damage, or who have primarily a neuropathic sphincter injury with no obvious anatomical defect, or in whom the injuries are combined.

The introduction of sacral nerve stimulation has meant that sphincter repair or reefing procedures for neuropathic incontinence are now obsolete.

The optimum treatment that we offer to patients is currently to repair the sphincter directly by anterior sphincteroplasty or overlapping repair of the traumatic sphincter defect in those patients in whom such a defect is demonstrated. The presence of neuropathic damage in these patients does not in my view alter the initial surgical management but does influence prognosis.

Patients with severe neuropathic incontinence are best treated by intensive conservative management with control of stool consistency and physiotherapy or biofeedback. Indeed, the current NICE guidelines consider that such a period of conservative treatment is mandatory before surgical treatment is considered. Surgical options are limited. Many of these patients do not have any sphincter defect on ultrasonography amenable to repair, and sphincter procedures, postanal repair and total pelvic floor repair have proved ineffective.

The advent of sacral nerve stimulation, however, provides an alternative avenue to explore in patients with a neuropathic faecal incontinence. Initial results were encouraging and more recent studies[65] have demonstrated that in the medium term sacral nerve stimulation is an effective option of patients with neuropathic incontinence. In my opinion, patients with neuropathic incontinence who have failed their conservative treatment and in whom incontinence is severely disabling and whose only viable alternative

option would be a stoma should be offered a trial of sacral nerve stimulation.

For young patients who have severe sphincter injuries or where there has been a failed sphincter repair, consideration should be given to either sacral nerve stimulation or some form of sphincter augmentation. One might even consider dynamic gracilo-plasty or artificial bowel sphincter.

In the elderly, who have poor prognostic factors, one must be realistic and advise patients what can be achieved. It may be in the patient's best interest not to attempt major reconstructive surgery but offer a permanent colostomy, which may well restore quality of life in the least traumatic way.

Sphincter augmentation

Dynamic graciloplasty

Unstimulated gracilis transposition has proved disappointing in the long term. There have been studies on bilateral unstimulated gracilis muscle transposition; however, the majority of data now available are on the results of the electrically stimulated gracilis neosphincter over the medium to long term.[66]

The technique has evolved, with most authorities now using intramuscular electrodes rather than direct stimulation of the nerve to gracilis. The latter is associated with significantly greater mechanical problems, particularly perineural fibrosis and electrode migration, which require revisional surgery.[33,35]

 Results of recent studies including multicentre trials have demonstrated a success rate for graciloplasty of 60–80%. There remains significant morbidity, with approximately one-third of patients developing wound complications.[35,67,68,69]

Recent third-party prospective evaluation of dynamic graciloplasty has demonstrated a significant improvement in quality of life in patients who underwent this procedure, but did confirm the higher level of morbidity. Recent studies looking at cost-effectiveness of modalities for severe faecal incontinence not amenable to direct repair concluded that graciloplasty could be considered as an alternative procedure to artificial bowel sphincter or end-colostomy, but only in specialist centres.

Artificial bowel sphincter

There are few units in this country with extensive experience of the artificial bowel sphincter. There have been two recent reports of large series giving detailed results.[40,68] The procedure is associated with significant complications, as outlined previously. Short-term follow-up would indicate that over two-thirds of patients retain a functioning artificial sphincter, and in these patients the results are good with approximately 80% of patients achieving improvement of incontinence, particularly to solid stool. A longer-term study with 7 years follow-up in a small group of patients would suggest that these results are not maintained, with less than 50% of patients retaining a functioning neosphincter at the end of follow-up, with an overall clinical success rate of 47%.[70,71]

A report of a multicentre cohort study[71] demonstrated that this procedure is associated with significant complications: 45% of patients required revisional surgery and 37% required removal of the device. In those patients who retained their device, continence was satisfactory in over 80%.

In specialist centres who have particular experience in the technique, artificial bowel sphincter does appear to be a viable alternative for patients, but even these centres report very high incidents of infective complications.[72]

 Experience of the anterior bowel sphincter is limited in this country.

Failed sphincter repair

A patient in whom a previous repair has failed can be a dilemma for the treating surgeon. There is evidence that patients in whom previous anterior repairs failed can undergo a repeat sphincter repair, with a good outcome in 50–60% of patients.[73,74]

Patients unsuitable for a repeat sphincter repair could be considered for dynamic graciloplasty, artificial bowel sphincter or sacral nerve stimulation.

Sacral nerve stimulation

Several studies have now reported on the safety and efficacy of sacral nerve stimulation.[41,42,75,76] A recent review of sacral nerve stimulation for the treatment of faecal incontinence[77] has demonstrated that the trial stimulation is associated with a very low level of complications, and a complication rate of 5–10% for insertion of a permanent implant. Initial reports suggested that sacral nerve stimulation appears to improve continence in approximately 70–80% of patients who are permanently implanted.[41,42] The mechanism of action of sacral nerve stimulation remains unknown. Longer-term studies published in larger numbers of patients with reasonable follow-up have confirmed the effectiveness of sacral nerve stimulation.[65] Other studies[77,78] demonstrated that sacral nerve stimulation is a successful cost-effective treatment for neurogenic faecal incontinence.

The role of sacral nerve stimulation in patients suffering with faecal incontinence is likely to expand. Early studies[79] have demonstrated the benefit of sacral neuromodulation in patients with partial spinal cord injuries. In my experience I have found this of value in selected patients. It would also appear that an intact anal sphincter is not necessary for success with sacral nerve stimulation in patients with faecal incontinence.[80] It is the author's view that the role of sacral nerve stimulation will increase significantly in the future.

The future

Increased awareness among patients and doctors that faecal incontinence can be successfully treated in the majority will lead to an increase in referrals. Similarly, greater awareness of injury at the time of vaginal delivery may improve obstetric practice and obviate the necessity for many of the surgical procedures listed. However, prevention of obstetric trauma altogether is unlikely, although obstetricians are becoming aware of the need to recognise injuries at the time of delivery and of the requirement that these injuries be repaired by appropriately skilled personnel.

It is well recognised that even a normal vaginal delivery is associated with a degree of damage to the nerve supply to the pelvic floor. There has been considerable interest recently in the field of nerve growth factors. It is possible in the future that use of such growth factors in the immediate postnatal period may optimise the reinnervation process in the pelvic floor. Similarly, newer electrophysiological tests and improvement in endoanal imaging could improve the selection of patients and the overall long-term outlook.

Sacral nerve stimulation is an exciting new procedure that appears to benefit the majority of patients with faecal incontinence, particularly those with neuropathic damage of the pelvic floor. It is likely that the use of sacral nerve stimulation will increase in the future. The indications for stimulated neosphincter formation are expanding and the number of patients suitable for this procedure will undoubtedly increase. The use of the artificial bowel sphincter remains controversial. Its use in the future is speculative.

Key points

- Faecal incontinence is a relatively common condition.
- The commonest cause for faecal incontinence in women is obstetric trauma.
- Following careful assessment and investigation, the majority of patients may benefit from conservative treatment.
- The majority of patients with obstetric trauma who have an identified defect on anal ultrasound will benefit from anterior sphincter repair in the short term.
- The long-term results of anterior sphincter repair suggest that only 40% of women will remain fully continent.
- Sphincter augmentation procedures can be used for patients who are not suitable for direct repair or in whom a previous repair has failed.
- Sacral nerve stimulation appears to be a promising innovation and will probably become the treatment of choice for neuropathic faecal incontinence and following failed sphincter repair.

References

1. MacIntyre IMC, Balfour TW. Results of the Lord non-operative treatment for haemorrhoids. Lancet 1977; i:1094.

2. Snooks SJ, Swash M, Henry MM et al. Risk factors in childbirth causing damage to the pelvic floor innervation. Int J Colorectal Dis 1986; 1:20–4.

3. Snooks SJ, Swash M, Mathers SE et al. Effect of vaginal delivery on the pelvic floor: a 5 year follow-up. Br J Surg 1990; 77:1358–60.

4. Sultan AH, Kamm MA, Bartram CI et al. Third degree obstetric anal sphincter tears: risk factors and outcome of primary repair. Br Med J 1994; 308:887–91.

5. Gjessing H, Backe B, Sahlin Y. Third degree obstetric tears: outcome after primary repair. Acta Obstet Gynaecol Scand 1998; 77:736–40.

6. Cook TA, Mortensen NJ. Management of faecal incontinence following obstetric injury. Br J Surg 1998; 85:293–9.

7. Perry RE, Blatchford GJ, Christensen MA et al. Manometric diagnosis of anal sphincter injuries. Am J Surg 1990; 159:112.

8. Parks AG, Swash M. Denervation of the anal sphincter causing idiopathic anorectal incontinence. J R Coll Surg Edinb 1979; 24:94–6.

9. Neill ME, Parks AG, Swash M. Physiological studies of the pelvic floor in idiopathic faecal incontinence and rectal prolapse. Br J Surg 1981; 68:531–6.

10. Kiff ES, Swash M. Slowed conduction in the pudendal nerves in idiopathic (neurogenic) faecal incontinence. Br J Surg 1984; 71:614–16.

11. Rogers J, Henry MM, Misiewicz JJ. Combined sensory and motor deficit in primary neuropathic faecal incontinence. Gut 1988; 29:5–9.

12. Parks AG, Porter NH, Hardcastle JD. The syndrome of the descending perineum. Proc R Soc Med 1966; 59:477–82.

13. Jorge JMN, Wexner SD, Ehrenpreis E et al. Does perianal descent correlate with pudendal neuropathy? Dis Colon Rectum 1992; 35:11–12.

14. Gee AS, Durdey P. Urge incontinence of faeces is a mark of severe anal sphincter dysfunction. Br J Surg 1995; 82:1179–82.

15. Jorge JM, Wexner SD. Etiology and management of fecal incontinence. Dis Colon Rectum 1993; 36:77–97.

16. Carapeti EA, Kamm MA, Evans BK et al. Topical phenylephrine increases anal sphincter resting pressure. Br J Surg 1999; 86:267–70.

17. Fynes MM, Marshall K, Cassidy M et al. A prospective randomized study comparing the effect of augmented biofeedback with sensory biofeedback alone on faecal incontinence after obstetric trauma. Dis Colon Rectum 1999; 42:753–61.

18. Osterberg A, Graf W, Eeg-Olofsson K et al. Is electrostimulation of the pelvic floor an effective

treatment for neurogenic faecal incontinence? Scand J Gastroenterol 1999; 34:319–24.

19. Norton C, Kamm MA. Outcome of biofeedback for incontinence training. Br J Surg 1999; 86:1159–63.

20. Macleod JH. Biofeedback in the management of partial anal incontinence. Dis Colon Rectum 1983; 26:244–6.

21. Heyman S, Jones KR, Ringel Y et al. Biofeedback treatment of fecal incontinence. Dis Colon Rectum 2001; 44:728–36.

22. Norton C, Chelvanayagam S, Wilson-Barnet J et al. Randomised controlled trial of biofeedback for fecal incontinence. Gastroenterology 2003; 125:1320–9.

23. Orrom WJ, Miller R, Cornes H et al. Comparison of anterior sphincteroplasty and postanal repair in the treatment of idiopathic fecal incontinence. Dis Colon Rectum 1991; 34:305–10.

24. Briel JW, De Boer LM, Hop CJ et al. Clinical outcome of anterior overlapping external anal sphincter repair with internal sphincter imbrication. Dis Colon Rectum 1998; 41:209–14.

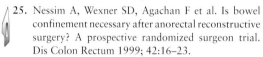

25. Nessim A, Wexner SD, Agachan F et al. Is bowel confinement necessary after anorectal reconstructive surgery? A prospective randomized surgeon trial. Dis Colon Rectum 1999; 42:16–23.

This trial has demonstrated that it is unnecessary to restrict oral intake following reconstructive surgery of the anorectum.

26. Parks AG. Anorectal incontinence. Proc R Soc Med 1975; 68:681–90.

27. Pinho M, Ortiz J, Oya M et al. Total pelvic floor repair for the treatment of neuropathic fecal incontinence. Am J Surg 1992; 163:340–3.

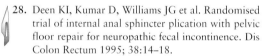

28. Deen KI, Kumar D, Williams JG et al. Randomised trial of internal anal sphincter plication with pelvic floor repair for neuropathic fecal incontinence. Dis Colon Rectum 1995; 38:14–18.

This trial demonstrated that there is no value in plicating the internal sphincter during pelvic floor repair. In this study, however, the internal sphincter was plicated longitudinally.

29. Corman ML. Gracilis muscle transposition. Contemp Surg 1978; 13:9–16.

30. Williams NS, Patel J, George BD et al. Development of an electrically stimulated neoanal sphincter. Lancet 1991; 338:1166–9.

31. Baeten CGMI, Konsten J, Spaans F et al. Dynamic graciloplasty for treatment of faecal incontinence. Lancet 1991; 338:1163–5.

32. Sielezneff I, Malouf AJ, Bartolo DCC et al. Dynamic graciloplasty in the treatment of patients with faecal incontinence. Br J Surg 1999; 86:61–5.

33. Navrantonis C, Wexner SD. Stimulated graciloplasty for treatment of intractable fecal incontinence. Dis Colon Rectum 1999; 42:497–504.

34. Cavina E, Seccia M, Evangelista G et al. Perineal colostomy and electrostimulated gracilis neosphincter after abdominoperineal resection of the colon and anorectum: a surgical experience and follow-up study in 47 cases. Int J Colorectal Dis 1990; 5:6–11.

35. Madoff RD, Rosen HR, Baeten CG et al. Safety and efficacy of dynamic muscle plasty for anal incontinence: lessons from a prospective multicenter trial. Gastroenterology 1999; 116:549–56.

36. Devesa JM, Vincente E, Enriquez JM et al. Total fecal incontinence. A new method of gluteus maximus transposition: preliminary results and report of previous experience. Dis Colon Rectum 1992; 35:339–49.

37. Corman ML. The management of anal incontinence. Surg Clin North Am 1983; 63:177–92.

38. Christiansen J, Lorentzem M. Implantation of artificial sphincter for anal incontinence. Report of five cases. Dis Colon Rectum 1989; 32:432–6.

39. Wong WD, Jensen LL, Bartolo DCC et al. Artificial anal sphincter. Dis Colon Rectum 1996; 39:1345–51.

40. Christiansen J, Rasmussen OO, Lindorf-Larsen K. Long term results of artificial anal sphincter implantation for severe anal incontinence. Ann Surg 1999; 230:45–8.

41. Ganio E, Lue AR, Clerico G et al. Sacral nerve stimulation for treatment of fecal incontinence. A novel approach for intractable fecal incontinence. Dis Colon Rectum 2001; 44:619–31.

42. Matzel KE, Stadelmaier U, Hohenfellner M et al. Electrical stimulation of sacral spinal nerves for treatment of faecal incontinence. Lancet 1995; 346:1124–7.

43. Mortensen N, Smilgin Humphreys M. The anal continence plug: a disposable device for patients with anorectal incontinence. Lancet 1991; 338: 295–7.

44. Hughes SF, Williams NS. Continent conduit for the treatment of faecal incontinence associated with disordered evacuation. Br J Surg 1995; 82:1318–20.

45. Browning GGP, Motson RW. Anal sphincter injury. Management and results of Parks sphincter repair. Ann Surg 1984; 199:351–6.

46. Manning PC, Pratt JH. Faecal incontinence caused by laceration of the perineum. Arch Surg 1964; 88:569–76.

47. Fang DT, Nivatvongs S, Vermeulen FD et al. Overlapping sphincteroplasty for acquired anal incontinence. Dis Colon Rectum 1984; 27:720–2.

48. Corman ML. Anal incontinence following obstetric injury. Dis Colon Rectum 1985; 28:86–9.

49. Cterceko GC, Fazio VW, Jagelman DG et al. Anal sphincter repair: a report of 66 cases and review of the literature. Aust NZ J Surg 1988; 58:703–10.

50. Laurberg S, Swash M, Henry MM. Delayed external sphincter repair for obstetric tear. Br J Surg 1988; 75:786–8.

51. Yoshioka K, Keighley MRB. Sphincter repair for faecal incontinence. Dis Colon Rectum 1989; 32:39–42.

52. Wexner SD, Marchetti F, Jagelman JD. The role of sphincteroplasty for faecal incontinence re-evaluated. A prospective physiologic and functional review. Dis Colon Rectum 1991; 34:22–30.

53. Fleshman JW, Dreznik Z, Fry RD et al. Anal sphincter repair for obstetric injury: manometric evaluation of functional results. Dis Colon Rectum 1991; 34:1061–7.

54. Engel AF, Kamm MA, Sultan AH et al. Anterior anal sphincter repair in patients with obstetric trauma. Br J Surg 1994; 81:1231–4.

55. Oliveira L, Pfeifer J, Wexner SD. Physiological and clinical outcome of anterior sphincteroplasty. Br J Surg 1996; 83:502–5.

56. Simmans C, Birnbaum EH, Kodner IJ et al. Anal sphincter reconstruction in the elderly: does advancing age affect outcome? Dis Colon Rectum 1994; 37:1065–9.

57. Engel AF, van Baal SJ, Brummeckamp WH. Late results of anterior sphincter plication for traumatic faecal incontinence. Eur J Surg 1994; 160:633–6.

58. Malouf AJ, Norton CS, Engel AF et al. Long term results of overlapping anterior anal sphincter repair for obstetric trauma. Lancet 2000; 355:260–5.

59. Halverson AL, Hull TL. Long term outcome of overlapping anal sphincter repair. Dis Colon Rectum 2002; 45:345–8.

60. Browning GGP, Parks AG. Postanal repair for neuropathic faecal incontinence: correlation of clinical results and anal cancer pressures. Br J Surg 1983; 70:101–4.

61. Henry MM, Simson JNL. Results of postanal repair: a retrospective study. Br J Surg 1985; 72(Suppl):517–19.

62. Yoshioka K, Keighley MRB. Critical assessment of quality of continence after postanal repair for faecal incontinence. Br J Surg 1989; 76:1054–7.

63. Laurberg S, Swash M, Henry MM. Effect of postanal repair on the progress of neurogenic damage to the pelvic floor. Br J Surg 1990; 77:519–22.

64. Pinho M, Keighley MRB. Results of surgery in idiopathic faecal incontinence. Ann Med 1990; 22:425–33.

65. Melenhorst J, Koch SM, Uludag O et al. Sacral neuromodulation in patients with faecal incontinence: results of the first 100 permanent implantations. Colorectal Dis 2007; 9:725–30.

66. Wexner SD, Baeten C, Bailey R et al. Long term efficacy of dynamic graciloplasty for fecal incontinence. Dis Colon Rectum 2002; 45:809–18.

67. Rongen MGM, Uludas O, El Naggar K et al. Long term follow up of dynamic gracioplasty for fecal incontinence. Dis Colon Rectum 2003; 46:716–21.

68. Devesa JM, Rey A, Hervas PL et al. Artificial anal sphincters: complications and functional results of a large personal series. Dis Colon Rectum 2002; 45:1154–63.

69. Tillin T, Gannon K, Fieldman RA et al. Third party prospective evaluation of patient outcomes after dynamic gracioplasty. Br J Surg 2006; 93:1402–10.

70. Wong WD, Congliosi SM, Spencer MP et al. The safety and efficacy of the artificial bowel sphincter for faecal incontinence: the results from a multicentre cohort study. Dis Colon Rectum 2002; 45:1139–53.

71. Mundy L, Merlin TL, Maddern GJ et al. Systematic review of safety and effectiveness of an artificial bowel sphincter for faecal incontinence. Br J Surg 2004; 91:665–72.

72. Melenhorst J, Koch SM, Van Gement WG et al. The artificial bowel sphincter for faecal incontinence: single centre study. Int J Colorectal Dis 2008; 23:107–11.

73. Pinedo G, Vaizey CJ, Nicholls RJ et al. Results of repeat anal sphincter repair. Br J Surg 1999; 86:66–9.

74. Giordano P, Renzi A, Efron J et al. Previous sphincter repair does not affect the outcome of a previous repair. Dis Colon Rectum 2002; 45:635–40.

75. Malouf AJ, Vaizey CJ, Nicholls RJ et al. Permanent sacral nerve stimulation for fecal incontinence. Ann Surg 2000; 232:143–8.

76. Kenefick NJ, Christiansen J. A review of sacral nerve stimulation for the treatment of faecal incontinence. Colorectal Dis 2004; 6:75–80.

77. Holtzer B, Rosen HR, Novi G et el. Sacral nerve stimulation for neurogenic faecal incontinence. Br J Surg 2007; 94:749–53.

78. Hetzer FH, Bieler A, Hahnloser D et al. Outcome and analysis of sacal nerve stimulator for faecal incontinence. Br J Surg 2006; 93:1411–7.

79. Jarrett ME, Matzel KE, Christiansen J et al. Sacral nerve stimulation of faecal incontinence in patients with previous partial spinal injury including disc prolapse. Br J Surg 2005; 92:734–9.

80. Melenhorst J, Koch SM, Uludag O et al. Is morphologically intact anal sphincter necessary for success with sacral nerve modulation in patients with faecal incontinence. Colorectal Dis 2007 (abstr).

12

Functional problems and their surgical management

Nicola S. Fearnhead

Introduction

Pelvic floor pathology tends to be complex and crosses several disciplines. Treatment of urogynaecological pathology in isolation is likely to have an adverse impact on defecatory function and vice versa.[1] Ideal care of women with pelvic floor disorders involves input from specialist urologists, gynaecologists and colorectal surgeons, together with allied specialties including radiology, physiotherapy, specialist nursing expertise, physiology, gastroenterology, psychiatry and chronic pain clinics. Preoperative assessment may include questionnaires on obstetric and urogynaecological history, constipation and incontinence scoring, visual analogues for pain, quality-of-life questionnaires, careful clinical examination, proctoscopy with or without colonoscopy, defecography, transit studies, anorectal physiology and endoanal ultrasound. Increased understanding of the anatomical and functional aspects of pelvic floor problems has led to the establishment of Multidisciplinary Pelvic Floor Clinics and Teams.[2,3]

Rectal prolapse

Rectal prolapse or procidentia refers to protrusion of the rectum through the anus. Prolapse is either mucosal, where only the mucosal layer prolapses through the anorectum, or full thickness, with circumferential protrusion through the anus of all linings of the rectal wall. Rectal prolapse occurs occasionally in young children but is most common in elderly women.

Risk factors for developing rectal prolapse include connective tissue disorders, for example the Marfan and Ehler–Danlos syndromes,[4] and a history of anorexia nervosa.[5] The latter patients may present some years after resolution of the psychiatric disorder, the prolapse resulting from poor cross-linking of collagen fibres in the pelvic floor musculature during adolescent years. Other risk factors for developing pelvic organ prolapse include high body mass index and high birth weight during vaginal deliveries.[6,7]

Mucosal prolapse

Mucosal prolapse may occur in isolation but is commonly seen in association with obstructive defecation syndrome (ODS) and solitary rectal ulcer syndrome (SRUS), which are discussed below. It may cause symptoms of perianal discomfort, passage of mucus or blood per rectum, constipation and straining at stool. The treatment of mucosal prolapse initially involves bulking laxatives and increased fibre intake. If surgical intervention is required, outpatient procedures such as suction banding or sclerotherapy of the prolapse or day case procedures such as surgical excision or plication of the prolapse and radiofrequency ablation[8–10] are commonly used. More recently some patients with mucosal prolapse and obstructive defecation have been treated with the procedure for prolapse and haemorrhoids (PPH) or stapled trans-anal rectal resection (STARR)[11–14] (see below).

Full-thickness rectal prolapse
(see Table 12.1)

Although conservative treatment with increased fibre intake and the use of bulking laxatives may improve symptoms to some extent, the definitive treatment for full-thickness rectal prolapse is almost exclusively surgical. Indeed, the Cochrane Library's review on prolapse surgery failed to identify any trials comparing surgery to non-operative management.[15] Surgical repair may be undertaken either from an abdominal or perineal approach. There is also the option of concurrent resection being undertaken either by the abdominal (resection rectopexy) or the perineal (Altemeier's procedure) approaches.

Choice of surgical approach

The choice of approach is largely influenced by the preference of the surgeon as well as patient factors including comorbidity, age, gender and sexual activity. As a general rule, most surgeons tend to prefer perineal procedures in elderly or frail patients and abdominal approaches in fit patients irrespective of age.[16] The choice of procedure should also take into account the presence of concurrent genital prolapse, preoperative constipation, evacuatory difficulties, faecal incontinence and any history of pelvic floor injury.[17] Resection rectopexy has traditionally been recommended for patients who have both constipation and rectal prolapse, although there is little evidence to support this practice (see below). Men tend to be offered perineal procedures in view of the potential for erectile dysfunction from rectal mobilisation during abdominal approaches.

A meta-analysis of randomised controlled trials in prolapse surgery was undertaken by the Cochrane Library in 2000 but only identified eight trials with 264 patients.[15] The reviewers had set out to address the issues of abdominal vs. perineal approaches, rectopexy methods, open vs. laparoscopic approaches, and no resection vs. resection. The paucity of data, small sample sizes and methodological problems resulted in a complete lack of useful conclusions being drawn from the analysis. In particular, there was no difference in recurrence rates between abdominal and perineal approaches.[15]

Perineal approaches

The principal perineal approaches are the Delorme and Altemeier procedures. Delorme's procedure involves resection of the sleeve of redundant rectal mucosa and plication of the prolapsed muscle wall without resection.[18,19] Altemeier's procedure (perineal rectosigmoidectomy) involves dissection into the peritoneal cavity via the prolapsed peritoneal lining of the pouch of Douglas, followed by excision of the rectosigmoid and a coloanal anastomosis (**Figs 12.1 and 12.2**). The latter is usually done by hand but is occasionally described with a circular stapler.[20] Pelvic floor repair or levatorplasty may be used in conjunction with perineal procedures to treat symptoms of incontinence.[21]

Delorme's procedure for full-thickness rectal prolapse has remained in favour as it is well tolerated in the elderly population, has low morbidity and mortality,[22–24] and minimal impact on continence and bowel function.[23–25] However, recurrence rates after Delorme's procedure are high, varying between 5% and 26.5%,[19,22–24,26] although the procedure may be repeated.

Altemeier's procedure[27] carries the potential complication of pelvic sepsis from anastomotic dehiscence, but nevertheless appears well tolerated, even in the elderly.[28] The largest published series report complication rates of 12–14% with very low mortality rates and improved continence in around half of patients, but rates of recurrent prolapse are still high at 10–16%.[29,30]

A small randomised trial with a total of 20 participants compared Altemeier's procedure with abdominal resection rectopexy, both procedures being combined with pelvic floor repair.[31] One patient in the Altemeier's arm had recurrent full-thickness prolapse, although two patients in each arm also developed mucosal prolapse. Both groups experienced significant postoperative morbidity, but symptoms of incontinence were significantly improved only in the abdominal resection rectopexy group.[31]

Abdominal approaches

Abdominal surgery may be performed either open or laparoscopically. Abdominal rectopexy entails rectal mobilisation and fixation to the sacrum with either non-absorbable sutures or mesh. Rectopexy may be performed either posteriorly with Ivalon sponge (Wells's procedure), fascia lata

Table 12.1 • Randomised controlled trials in rectal prolapse surgery

Authors (reference)	Year	n	Length of follow-up	Trial procedures	Outcomes
Speakman et al.[37]	1991	26	Median 12 months	Open polypropylene mesh rectopexy with division vs. preservation of lateral ligaments	Lateral ligament preservation was associated with less postoperative constipation but an increased rate of recurrent prolapse
Luukkonen et al.[46]	1992	30	6 months	Open resection suture rectopexy vs. open polyglycolic acid mesh rectopexy	Resection rectopexy resulted in less postoperative constipation
McKee et al.[47]	1992	18	Mean 20 months	Open resection rectopexy vs. open suture rectopexy (with division of the lateral ligaments)	Resection rectopexy resulted in less postoperative constipation but less improvement in faecal incontinence
Selvaggi et al.[38]	1993	20	Mean 14 (range 6–24) months	Open Marlex®/Mersilene® rectopexy with division vs. preservation of lateral ligaments	Lateral ligament preservation was associated with less postoperative constipation
Winde et al.[43]	1993	49	Mean 50.5 months	Open abdominal rectopexy (with anterior mesh sling) comparing polyglycolic acid vs. polyglactin mesh	No significant differences in postoperative complications or recurrence rates
Novell et al.[42]	1994	63	Median 47 (range 44–50) months	Open abdominal Ivalon® sponge rectopexy vs. suture rectopexy	No significant difference in recurrence rates but a significantly higher incidence of postoperative constipation in the Ivalon® sponge group
Deen et al.[31]	1994	20	Median 17 (8–22) months	Altemeier's procedure with pelvic floor repair vs. abdominal resection rectopexy with pelvic floor repair	Similar recurrent full thickness and mucosal prolapse rates. Significant postoperative morbidity in both groups. Incontinence significantly improved in resection rectopexy group only
Galili et al.[44]	1997	37	Mean 3.7 years	Open abdominal mesh rectopexy (with anterolateral rectal mesh fixation) comparing polyglycolic acid vs. polypropylene mesh	No significant differences in postoperative complications or recurrence rates
Boccasanta et al.[50]	1998	21	Mean 29.5 (range 8–45) months	Laparoscopic vs. open Marlex®/Mersilene® mesh rectopexy versus open suture mesh (with anterolateral rectal mesh fixation)	No significant difference in recurrence rates

195

Reference	Year	Number	Follow-up	Comparison	Outcome
Mollen et al.[39]	2000	18	Mean 3.5 years	Posterior mesh rectopexy with division vs. preservation of lateral ligaments	No statistical difference in functional outcome
Solomon et al.[49]	2002	40	Mean 24.2 (range 2–52) months	Laparoscopic vs. open abdominal mesh rectopexy	No significant difference in recurrence rates but the laparoscopic approach was associated with significantly less morbidity, shorter hospital stays and longer operating times
Boccasanta et al.[20]	2006	40	Mean 28 months	Altemeier's procedure with levatorplasty comparing monopolar electrocautery dissection and handsewn anastomosis vs. harmonic scalpel dissection and circular stapled anastomosis	No significant difference in functional outcomes or recurrence rates but operating time, blood loss and hospital stay were significantly reduced in the stapled group
PROSPER (Prolapse Surgery: Perineal or Rectopexy) trial, www.prosper.bham.ac.uk		292	90% of patients recruited by January 2007	First randomisation or surgeon preference to select abdominal vs. perineal approach. Second randomisation in abdominal approach of suture vs. resection rectopexy and in perineal approach of Delorme's vs. Altemeier's operations (see Fig. 12.1)	48 patients randomised to approach, 78 to abdominal methods and 212 to perineal methods. Primary end-point of recurrent prolapse abandoned in favour of secondary end-points of bowel function and quality of life when recruitment one-third of anticipated

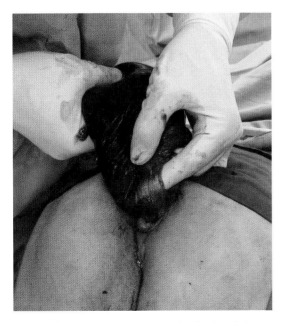

Figure 12.1 • Division of peritoneal reflection during Altemeier's procedure. Photograph printed with permission of Dr Tracy Hull, Cleveland Clinic, Cleveland, Ohio.

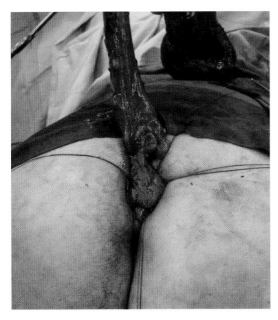

Figure 12.2 • Resection of rectosigmoid prior to coloanal anastomosis during Altemeier's procedure. Photograph printed with permission of Dr Tracy Hull, Cleveland Clinic, Cleveland, Ohio.

(Orr–Loygue operation) or non-absorbable mesh, or anteriorly with an anterior mesh sling around the rectum to the sacrum (Ripstein's procedure) or ventral mesh rectopexy. Resection during an abdominal rectopexy (Frykman–Goldberg procedure) usually involves resection of the sigmoid colon with a handsewn or stapled anastomosis at the sacral promontory.[32]

A multicentre pooled analysis of 643 patients who underwent abdominal procedures for rectal prolapse over a 22-year period found age, gender, surgical technique, means of approach (open or laparoscopic) and method of rectopexy had no impact on recurrence rates.[33] Nevertheless this study was retrospective and probably not powered to show significant differences between the different surgical techniques of rectal mobilisation only, mobilisation with resection and rectopexy, or mobilisation and rectopexy.[33] Another retrospective meta-analysis using data from six studies on abdominal approaches to rectal prolapse repair again found no difference in recurrence rates with age, sex or surgical technique.[34]

Defecatory disorders are common after abdominal rectopexy and may present either as novel or worsening constipation, evacuatory difficulties or faecal incontinence. Although many studies include analysis of these problems, the actual extent of the problem is difficult to quantify. A small series of 23 patients undergoing abdominal rectopexy were evaluated prospectively for bowel function: symptoms of incontinence improved in 82%, 36% of patients with preoperative constipation improved with surgery, and 42% developed new-onset constipation.[35] Faecal incontinence is reportedly improved in most series of abdominal rectopexy.[36]

Three trials have compared the effects of conservation versus division (with potential rectal denervation) of the lateral ligaments during posterior mesh rectopexy,[37–39] although all studies only involved small numbers of participants. Two of these trials found that preservation of the lateral ligaments was associated with less postoperative constipation,[37,38] although one also found an increased rate of recurrent prolapse with this technique.[37] A more recent, but still small, prospective randomised study found that division of the lateral ligaments during posterior Teflon® mesh rectopexy had no impact on postoperative constipation.[39]

A number of studies have looked at different methods of rectal fixation during rectopexy. The principal concern with mesh is infection and extrusion. Although the incidence of infection is low,[40,41] when it occurs the consequences are serious. Complete peritoneal closure over non-absorbable meshes may also reduce the incidence of postoperative small bowel obstruction.

A randomised trial in 63 patients comparing Ivalon® sponge to suture rectopexy found no difference in recurrence rates, although there was a significantly higher incidence of postoperative constipation in the Ivalon® sponge arm.[42] The authors concluded that there was no need to use prosthetic materials to perform successful rectopexy.

Two trials looking at the relative benefits of different types of mesh in rectopexy surgery found no significant differences in either postoperative complications or recurrence rates with either absorbable or non-absorbable meshes.[43,44]

Resection is usually performed in combination with suture rectopexy in view of the excess risk of infection if non-absorbable mesh is used for the rectopexy.[41] However, a small series of 35 cases of resection rectopexy with non-absorbable mesh in young patients reported good functional outcomes and no instances of mesh infection or anastomotic leakage.[45]

Two trials with a combined total of 48 patients have examined the impact of concomitant sigmoid resection during open abdominal rectopexy.[46,47] One trial randomised patients between resection rectopexy and polyglycolic acid mesh rectopexy[46] and the other compared resection rectopexy with suture rectopexy.[47] If the results of these two small studies are combined, there is a statistically significant difference in rates of postoperative constipation with a lower incidence in the resection arms of each trial.[15] However, one of the trials involved division of the lateral ligaments,[47] which may in itself have contributed to the high incidence of postoperative constipation. This trial also demonstrated that there was no improvement in incontinence symptoms in the resection group.[47]

Laparoscopic approaches

No prospective randomised trial has been conducted with a treatment arm including either laparoscopic suture rectopexy or laparoscopic resection rectopexy. A meta-analysis conducted to compare open and laparoscopic rectopexy in 195 patients[48] included six studies, only one of which was prospective and randomised.[49] The rectopexy techniques included resection, suture and mesh. The meta-analysis concluded that laparoscopic rectopexy was safe and had a similar recurrent prolapse rate to open surgery.[48]

Two randomised trials have compared open and laparoscopic approaches to mesh rectopexy.[49,50] The first small trial (21 patients) involved anterolateral rectal fixation of non-absorbable mesh (either Marlex® or Mersilene®) to the sacral promontory and found no difference in recurrence rates between the different approaches at just over 2 years.[50] The second trial (40 patients) described full rectal mobilisation with posterior mesh rectopexy to the sacral promontory with a single spiked chromium staple and lateral fixation with hernia staples.[49] It too confirmed no difference in recurrence rates at 2 years (with one recurrence in the open group) but did show that the laparoscopic approach was associated with significantly less morbidity, a shorter hospital stay but a longer operating time.[49]

The surgical management of combined rectal and urogenital prolapse is probably best carried out from an abdominal approach and laparoscopic repairs are particularly amenable to repairing abnormalities of the rectum, vagina, bladder and pelvic floor.[51,52] The advantages of laparoscopic approaches in these patients include nerve-sparing surgery and minimally invasive techniques. A combined approach may also serve to lessen the impact of prolapse repair in one compartment on symptoms in another.

Working on the premise that rectal prolapse is always initiated by anterior rectal wall intussusception, ventral rectosacropexy with no other rectal mobilisation was introduced. The operation can be performed open or laparoscopically. Laparoscopic ventral rectopexy involves peritoneal mobilisation over the pouch of Douglas to gain access via the rectovaginal septum to the pelvic floor, mesh fixation to the septum distally and with either sutures or a ProTack™ stapling device proximally to the sacrum, and extraperitonealisation of the mesh by full peritoneal closure.[52] A simultaneous colporrhaphy to treat an enterocele or vaginal prolapse may be performed by anchoring the posterior vagina to the mesh with sutures. A prospective series of 109 cases treated using this technique reported low morbidity (minor complications in 7%) and low recurrent prolapse rates (4%).[52] Another series of 80 patients reported complications in 21% but no recurrence at a median follow-up of 54 months; there was also marked improvement in symptoms of either faecal incontinence or obstructed defecation.[51] There was no instance of mesh infection or erosion in either series.

The PROSPER trial

Uncertainty as to the best surgical procedure for rectal prolapse led to the PROSPER (Prolapse Surgery: Perineal or Rectopexy) trial being initiated in the UK in 2001.

The PROSPER trial had an unusual pragmatic design in that randomisation occurred at either one or two steps within the treatment pathway (**Fig. 12.3**). The first potential randomisation was based on the surgeon's uncertainty as to whether an abdominal or perineal approach was the more appropriate. If the surgeon had a preference, then this randomisation was avoided. The second potential point for randomisation occurred in the decision between suture or resection rectopexy if the abdominal approach was elected or allocated at randomisation, or between Delorme's and Altemeier's operations if the perineal approach was selected.

The primary outcome measure for the first randomisation between abdominal and perineal approaches in the PROSPER trial was recurrent rectal prolapse, but this was later relegated to a secondary outcome measure in favour of bowel function and quality-of-life scores when recruitment to the trial failed to meet anticipated levels. The primary outcome measures for the second randomisation between procedures were bowel function and quality of life. The trial saw substantially more patients randomised in the perineal than the abdominal arm. The original target number of participants was set at 1000 and the trial was completed in 2007 after a revised target of 300. The final results on the 292 patients recruited are awaited; 48 were randomised to the approach, 78 to abdominal method (resection/suture rectopexy) and 212 to the perineal method (Delorme's/Altemeier's).

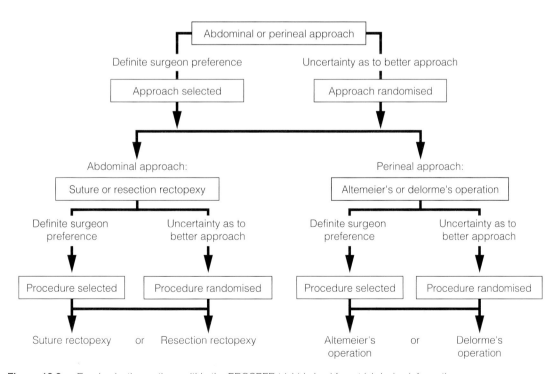

Figure 12.3 • Randomisation options within the PROSPER trial (derived from trial design information, www.prosper.bham.ac.uk).

An interim report on the first 153 patients in the PROSPER trial reported five (3.7%) serious adverse events including three (2%) deaths. There were 23 (15%) episodes of recurrent (11 mucosal and 12 full-thickness) prolapse. Thirty-two patients (20.9%) experienced postoperative complications (www.prosper.bham.ac.uk/poster.pdf). Initial assessment of defecatory function using Kamm scores showed a dramatic improvement in continence and evacuation.

Recurrent rectal prolapse

Recurrence rates following rectal prolapse surgery vary widely. As all of the approaches carry a risk of recurrent rectal prolapse, a number of patients will come to a second procedure. There is, however, little in the reported literature on management of recurrent rectal prolapse. Abdominal approaches are used more commonly than perineal approaches for recurrent full-thickness prolapse by some groups,[53] while others point out that perineal procedures can be safely repeated.[54] Recurrent prolapse in more than one compartment may be best treated via an abdominal approach.[55] Irrespective of approach, surgery for recurrent prolapse carries a significant risk of postoperative bowel dysfunction, either with obstructive or incontinent symptoms.[53,54]

Obstructive defecation and rectocele

The cardinal symptoms of obstructive defecation are straining at stool, a sense of incomplete evacuation, and the need for rectal, vaginal or perineal digitation in order to achieve evacuation. Paradoxical contraction of the puborectalis muscle during straining at stool is more aptly called pelvic floor dyssynergia. The latter is more commonly associated with urogynaecological, gastrointestinal and psychological problems than with slow-transit constipation. Many 'constipated' patients will have improvement in their symptoms with treatment of obstructive defecation. The treatment is predominantly medical with dietary manipulation, use of laxatives and biofeedback training.[56]

An anterior rectocele and/or rectal intussusception (internal rectal prolapse) are often found in association with obstructive defecation symptoms. Nevertheless the syndrome is very complex and the symptomatology variable. Symptoms of obstructive defecation may mask a number of occult disorders including anxiety and depression, gynaecological prolapse, anismus, rectal hyposensitivity and slow-transit constipation. This has led the syndrome of obstructive defecation to be called an 'iceberg' disorder, as many of the associated problems may not be immediately apparent.[57] Recognition and anticipation of occult pathology allows treatment to be tailored to the individual patient.

Objective assessment of the symptoms of obstructive defecation is particularly important when trying to assess the impact of new surgical interventions for the condition. The Cleveland Clinic Constipation Scoring System is already widely used but is not specific for obstructive defecation.[58] A new scoring system using a structured questionnaire and giving a possible maximum score of 31 points has recently been suggested.[59] This system gives weight to time spent at defecation, the number of attempts at defecation each day, use of digitation, use of laxatives and enemas, the presence of incomplete evacuation, straining at stool, and stool consistency.[59]

Rectocele

A rectocele is a hernia of the anterior rectal wall through the rectovaginal septum. It arises from muscular and nerve damage sustained during vaginal delivery, as a result of hormonal changes following the menopause, or due to paradoxical contraction of puborectalis. Rectoceles occur due to a pressure gradient between the rectum and vagina during coughing and straining due to weakness in the puborectalis and bulbocavernosus muscles.[60] Suspensory surgery on the anterior vaginal wall, e.g. anterior colporrhaphy or Burch colposuspension, may predispose to the development of a rectocele.[61] Posterior rectoceles are only rarely found, and usually result from traumatic injury or surgical interventions breaching the anococcygeal ligament.

An anterior rectocele is a common finding in patients with obstructive defecation syndrome, but may also occur in asymptomatic patients. It is a common finding on defecography[62] and magnetic resonance proctography.[63] Symptoms associated with rectoceles include difficulty in evacuation, constipation, the need for perineal or vaginal digitation during defecation and rectal discomfort. Anal digitation is not usually a symptom caused by a rectocele. Rectoceles vary in size, both in the extent of protrusion into the vagina as well as in the length of involvement of the rectovaginal septum, but size does not necessarily correlate with severity of symptoms.

The mainstay of treatment of symptomatic rectoceles is dietary manipulation and biofeedback.[64,65] Surgical repair by either gynaecologists or colorectal surgeons gives highly variable results and can be performed via transvaginal, perineal, transanal or transabdominal routes. A variety of techniques employ suture plication, mesh reinforcement of the rectovaginal septum, resection of redundant tissue, fixation of the rectum, vagina or perineal body, or reinforcement of the pelvic floor musculature. There has been a recent vogue for excision of rectoceles using linear[66,67] and circular staplers (see section on stapled transanal rectal resection).

The Block procedure involves full-thickness suture plication of the rectocele with absorbable sutures via a transanal approach.[68] The Sarles procedure consists of an elliptical transanal mucocutaneous flap, plication of the anterior rectal muscle with non-absorbable sutures, resection of redundant mucosa and reapplication of the flap to the anal verge with absorbable sutures[69] (much like an anterior Delorme operation). Transanal approaches may compromise the integrity of the sphincter complex with consequent faecal incontinence,[70,71] although other studies have shown no effect on continence or sexual function.[72]

Abdominal repair may be performed by open or laparoscopic approaches and involve dissection of the rectovaginal septum via the pouch of Douglas; repair of the rectocele can then be carried out with or without concomitant rectopexy or sacrocolpopexy.

Although a number of authors report series of varying numbers, there have been very few prospective randomised controlled trials (Table 12.2).

A retrospective multicentre study examined the results of rectocele repair in 317 patients by transanal approaches (*n* = 141), perineal levatorplasty (*n* = 126) or combined transanal repair and perineal levatorplasty (*n* = 50).[73] None of the procedures was functionally superior, but bleeding complications were more common in transanal procedures, and dyspareunia and delayed perineal wound healing were more frequent after perineal levatorplasty. About half of the patients studied who had preoperative faecal incontinence and who underwent perineal levatorplasty had improved continence scores postoperatively.[73]

A small Finnish prospective randomised trial in 30 patients compared transanal rectocele repair with posterior colporrhaphy.[74] Both resulted in improved defecatory function, with a greater proportion of patients in the vaginal approach group achieving successful outcomes (see Table 12.2). Although the latter difference was not significant, this may be due to a type II error as the numbers enrolled in the trial were small. The transanal group also had a significantly higher rate of symptomatic recurrent posterior vaginal wall prolapse.[74]

Stapled transanal rectal resection (STARR)

STARR was first used in obstructive defecation syndrome following the introduction of the procedure for prolapse and haemorrhoids (PPH) technique. The latter uses a circular stapling device called Proximate PPH-01™ made by Ethicon Endo-Surgery®. The STARR technique was described by Altomare et al. in 2002,[75] who combined dissection of the rectovaginal septum via a perineal incision with a single transanal firing of the PPH-01™ stapling gun. The PPH technique was modified for STARR by using a purse string suture which was full thickness anteriorly and only mucosal posteriorly. The initial study described the results in eight female patients, all of whom had symptoms of obstructive defecation in association with an anterior rectocele.[75]

Early concern about introduction of the STARR procedure arose from a report of 29 patients of whom half had severe postoperative complications or recurrent symptoms.[76] Complications included severe intraoperative or early postoperative bleeding requiring re-operation or rectal tamponade, pelvic and retroperitoneal sepsis, persistent severe perianal pain, and new onset of faecal incontinence. Seven patients had recurrent symptoms of obstructive defecation, and one patient underwent resection of recurrent rectal internal mucosal prolapse.[76] The authors discussed potential errors in technique, including the possibility of stapling too close to the dentate line, undetected co-pathology including pelvic floor dyssynergia, or poor patient selection. The study suggested that parity, pelvic floor dyssynergia and anxiety states were risk factors predisposing to failure of STARR.[76]

Table 12.2 • Randomised controlled trials in rectocele surgery

Authors	Year	n	Length of follow-up	Procedures	Outcomes
Sand et al.[102]	2001	160	12 months	Anterior and posterior colporrhaphy without vs. with Vicryl™ mesh (Ethicon)	• No difference in rates of recurrent rectocele at 1 year 10% vs. 8.2% ($P = 0.7$) • Cystocele recurrence greater in group without mesh (43%) than with mesh (25%) ($P = 0.02$)
Boccasanta et al.[78]	2004	50	23.4 ± 5.1 months vs. 22.3 ± 4.8 months	Stapled transanal prolapsectomy with perineal levatorplasty vs. STARR procedure	• STARR group had less postoperative pain ($P < 0.0001$) and greater decrease in rectal sensitivity threshold volume ($P = 0.012$) • No differences in functional outcomes or early and late complication rates • Significantly higher incidence of dyspareunia in prolapsectomy with levatorplasty group (20%) over STARR group (none) ($P = 0.018$)
Nieminen et al.[74]	2004	30	12 months	Posterior colporrhaphy (15) vs. Transanal repair (15)	• Improved defecatory function 93% vs. 73% ($P = 0.08$) • Recurrent symptomatic rectocele/enterocele 7% vs. 40% ($P = 0.04$)
Paraiso et al.[103]	2006	106	17.5 ± 7 months	Posterior colporrhaphy (37) vs. site-specific rectocele repair (37) vs. site-specific rectocele repair with graft augmentation (32)	• No difference in symptom improvement among groups (15% functional failure rate overall) • Anatomical failure rate 46% in graft augmentation group compared to 14% and 22% in other groups ($P = 0.02$) • No differences in improvement in sexual function or dyspareunia rates • Bowel symptoms at 12 months were improved significantly in all groups[104]

A prospective non-randomised multicentre study of 90 patients was undertaken in Italy in order to assess the STARR procedure.[77] The majority of patients experienced a short hospital stay and minimal postoperative pain. Symptoms of constipation in association with obstructive defecation improved significantly without any concomitant deterioration in incontinence. There was, however, a significant functional complication rate with 17.8% of patients subsequently experiencing urgency, 8.9% flatus incontinence, 5.5% urinary retention, 4.4% postoperative bleeding and 3.3% anastomotic stenosis. Patient satisfaction at 12 months was excellent in 53.3%, good in 36.7%, fairly good in 5.6% and poor in 4.4%.[77]

The same group from Milan reported on a randomised controlled trial between single stapled transanal prolapsectomy with perineal levatorplasty and the STARR procedure.[78] The STARR group had consistently lower postoperative pain scores but there were otherwise no differences in operative time, hospital stay or return to work. The stapled prolapsectomy group had improvement in constipation symptoms in 76% as compared to 88% in the STARR group. Both groups experienced similar complication rates, with a significant incidence of delayed perineal wound healing in the prolapsectomy group. Late complications were again similar, with urgency of defecation, incontinence to flatus and anal stenosis occurring in both groups. Dyspareunia affected 20% of the prolapsectomy group but did not occur within the STARR group.[78]

STARR became widely used without good published evidence for its efficacy and safety, raising concerns in the surgical press about the need for evidence-based practice with this procedure.[79] It became apparent that there was no good procedure against which STARR could be compared and that patient selection was of paramount importance in ensuring the success of the procedure. It was recommended that prospective audit and adequate training of appropriately experienced coloproctologists should be implemented in order to ensure the safe introduction of a novel procedure.[79]

These words of caution were particularly poignant in view of reports about complications of the STARR procedure, including rectovaginal fistula,[80,81] proctalgia due to retained staples,[82] postoperative bleeding and new-onset incontinence.[76] In addition

to the earlier report of retroperitoneal sepsis,[78] there has been a further report of necrotising pelvic fasciitis requiring emergency laparotomy with Hartmann's procedure and hysterectomy and subsequent early death from multiorgan failure.[81] Patient selection continues to be a problem, and cost-effectiveness has yet to be proven.[83]

More recent series have been reported from a number of European centres;[81,84–87] the results are summarised in Table 12.3. The indication for STARR in all these studies was obstructive defecation unresponsive to conservative measures and/or biofeedback. The largest series[81] reported a significant number of complications both in the authors' own patients and in a tertiary referral practice. Univariate analysis suggested that poor outcomes were associated with preoperative digital manipulation of defecation, pelvic floor dyssynergia, enterocele, a large rectocele, low frequency of bowel action and a sense of incomplete evacuation.[81] Bleeding was again the most common complication in this series, and one-fifth of patients required further surgery, most often for recurrent disease. The reasons for tertiary referral after STARR were perineal pain (53%), persistent symptoms with recurrent rectocele and/or rectal intussusception (50%), new onset of faecal incontinence (28%) and rectovaginal fistula.[81]

Another large series in the literature[85] looked at 71 patients with obstructive defecation. The complication rate in this series was much lower, with perineal bruising in 23.5%, acute urinary retention in 4.4% and postoperative bleeding in 2.9%. This series reported an excellent or good functional outcome at 6-month follow-up in 77.3%.[85]

The European STARR registry recently reported 6-month follow-up analysis on a total of 1682 patients;[88] 1404 patients had complete records and were suitable for analysis. The mean age for undergoing a STARR procedure was 53.5 years and 73% of the patients were female. Just over half of the patients had a rectocele and about half had internal prolapse. A significant reduction in obstructive defecation symptoms was seen at 6 months and an improvement in quality-of-life scores was also observed; 31.7% of this series of patients experienced complications, with bleeding in 4.3%, urgency of defecation in 14.3%, postoperative perineal pain in 8.1%, new onset of faecal incontinence in 1.3% and sepsis in 1.1%.[88]

Table 12.3 • Reported series of stapled transanal rectal resection (STARR)

Authors	Year	n	Length of follow-up	Complication rates	Outcomes
Altomare et al.[75]*	2002	8	Median 12 months	Vaginal injury 12.5% Urgency 12.5%	Reduction in median Cleveland Clinic Constipation Scores from 14.3 to 5.0 ($P < 0.04$)
Dodi et al.[76]	2003	14	Median 12 months	Intraoperative bleeding 7.1% Postoperative bleeding 14.3% Retroperitoneal sepsis 7.1% Persistent severe anal pain 50% Faecal incontinence 21.4% Stenosis 7.1%	Recurrent rectal mucosal prolapse occurred in 42.9% Recurrent symptoms of ODS occurred in 50%
Boccasanta et al.[77]	2004	90	Mean 16.3 ± 4.8 months	Total 40% Urinary retention 5.6% Bleeding 4.4% Urgency 10% (3 months) and 1.1% (12 months) Flatus incontinence 6.7% (3 months) and 1.1% (12 months) Stenosis 3.3%	Reduct on in mean Constipation Score from 13.02 to 4.52 ($P < 0.001$) Patient satisfaction good or excellent in 86.6% at 3 months and 90% at 12 months
Boccasanta et al.[78]	2004	25	Mean 22.3 ± 2.9 months	Total 40% Urinary retention 8% Bleeding 4% Urgency 16% Flatus incontinence 8% Stenosis 4%	Reduction in mean Constipation Score from 18.01 to 5.65 ($P < 0.001$) Reduction in mean rectal sensitivity threshold from 154.7 to 135.0 ($P = 0.0117$)
Ommer et al.[84]	2006	14	Mean 19 ± 9 months	Bleeding 14.3% Urinary retention 28.6% Severe postoperative pain 7.1% resolved Urgency 21.4% resolved at 3 months Faecal incontinence 7.1%	Reduction in defecation score[†] from 13.0 to 4 at 1 month ($P < 0.05$)

(Continued)

Table 12.3 • (cont.) Reported series of stapled transanal rectal resection (STARR)

Authors	Year	n	Length of follow-up	Complication rates	Outcomes
Renzi et al.[85]	2006	68	6 months	Perineal haematoma 23.5% Urinary retention 4.4% Bleeding 2.9% Urgency 4.4% resolved at 6 months Flatus incontinence 2.9% resolved at 6 months Dyspareunia 1.4% resolved at 6 months Stenosis 1.4% requiring reoperation	Reduction in ODS score[†] from 15.1 to 5.1 ($P < 0.0001$) Reduction in mean Cleveland Clinic Constipation Score from 17.0 to 7.9 ($P < 0.001$) Patient satisfaction good or excellent in 79.3% at 6 months
Pechlivanides et al.[87]	2007	16	9 months	Bleeding 6.3%	Reduction in defecation score[†] from 9.5 to 3 at 9 months ($P < 0.001$) 43.8% had persistent mild symptoms of obstructive defecation Reduction in mean maximum anal resting pressure ($P = 0.002$), rectal compliance ($P < 0.001$) and maximum tolerated rectal volume ($P < 0.001$)
Arroyo et al.[86]	2007	37	Mean 24 months	Urgency 24.3% at 3 months resolved by 6 months Flatus incontinence 18.9% at 4 weeks resolved by 3 months Recurrence 5.4 Stenosis 2.7%	51.4% of patients required intraoperative haemostatic sutures on staple line Reduction in mean Symptom Score from 12.77 to 4.12 at 12 months ($P < 0.01$) No significant change in mean anal resting pressure, squeeze, rectal sensitivity or compliance
Jayne et al.[88]	2007	1404	6 months	Total 31.7% Bleeding 4.3% Urgency 14.3% Pain 8.1% Incontinence 1.3% Sepsis 1.1%	Reduction in ODS from 15.18 to 4.13 ($P < 0.001$) Reduction in SSS from 24.26 to 12.93 ($P < 0.001$) Improvement in QoL scores ($P < 0.001$)

ODS, obstructive defecation symptoms; QoL, quality of life; SSS, symptom severity scores.
* STARR included perineal repair in addition to stapled resection.
† Unvalidated symptom scoring system.

Technique

STARR is normally carried out in the Lloyd–Davies position, although some surgeons prefer the prone jack-knife or Kraske position. The anal retractor provided with the PPH gun is inserted into the anal canal with some surgeons also using a flat spatula behind the anal retractor to protect the posterior wall while operating on the anterior wall. Purse-string sutures are placed in the anterior wall first with three or four sutures at 1-cm intervals starting at 4 cm above the dentate line and well above the haemorrhoidal plexus. The circular stapling gun is inserted into the anus fully opened above the purse strings, which are then tied together. The stapler is closed completely with a finger in the vagina to ensure that the rectovaginal septum is protected as the stapler closes. The anterior rectal wall is then stapled and excised. The posterior surface is plicated with two or three hemicircumferential purse strings. Surgeons may choose to use either mucosal or full-thickness sutures posteriorly. The end result should be a circumferential row of staples. Any bleeding points are oversewn manually with an absorbable suture.

PPH-01™ was originally designed for stapled haemorrhoidectomy. The PPH-03™ (Ethicon Endo-Surgery®) stapling device has been modified to reduce the risk of haemorrhagic complication during STARR.[86] Some groups have started using a circumferential technique involving four or five firings of a curved linear stapler (Contour Transtar™, Ethicon Endo-Surgery®), which allows more accurate placement of the purse strings and each firing of the stapler to be done under direct observation. No major series has yet been published using this technique.

One of the major concerns about the STARR technique is the potential threat to structures lying anterior to the rectal wall in the pouch of Douglas. As an enterocele is a fairly common finding in patients with pelvic floor disorders, it is important to exclude the presence of an enterocele with defecography or magnetic resonance imaging prior to performing a STARR procedure. A German group has recently advocated the use of laparoscopic surveillance during the STARR procedure in patients known to have an enterocele preoperatively.[89]

The external pelvic rectal suspension (EXPRESS) procedure

The EXPRESS procedure was developed as an alternative surgical repair for patients with symptoms of obstructive defecation in conjunction with rectal intussusception with or without a rectocele. The aim of developing the procedure was to develop a less invasive procedure than abdominal rectopexy which did not carry the potential complications of worsening constipation afterwards. The procedure was first described using Gore-Tex® mesh[90] and then Permacol® (Tissue Science Laboratories).[91]

There is one reported series of 17 patients treated with the EXPRESS procedure for obstructive defecation. Intraoperative complications included small vaginal perforations in two patients and anterior rectal wall perforations in three patients; all injuries were recognised at the time of surgery and repaired. One patient developed sepsis in the rectovaginal plane and required subsequent surgical drainage and a diverting stoma. Two other patients also developed postoperative sepsis, one requiring surgical drainage. Three patients complained of neuralgic pain, either in the perineal wound or over the anterior aspect of the thigh, but all resolved with time. There was significant improvement in symptom and quality-of-life scores, and no reported changes in sexual function. The authors concluded that the postoperative morbidity was lower than in the STARR procedure, with similar functional results.[90–92] The EXPRESS procedure requires longer-term follow-up and replication in other centres before it can be more widely adopted.

Technique

The EXPRESS procedure is carried out in the Lloyd–Davies position. A crescentic incision is made over the perineal body following the curvature of the external anal sphincter. The plane through the rectovaginal septum into the pouch of Douglas is developed to a level above the rectocele with mobilisation of the lateral rectal wall. Two small incisions are made in the suprapubic region on either side of the symphysis pubis to allow blunt dissection via each incision into the retropubic space anterior to the bladder. Anchoring sutures are placed in the tendinous insertions of the recti muscles. A curved tunnelling device with a blunt tip is passed upwards from the perineal wound via a channel created with blunt finger dissection lateral to the rectum and vagina and into the retropubic space to join the suprapubic wounds. Vaginal integrity is checked after passage of the tunnelling device. The bladder is protected superiorly with a finger in the suprapubic wound.

Two T-shaped strips of Permacol® are pre-soaked in gentamicin solution. Each strip is marked on the T crossbar with the right and left sides to avoid twisting during passage in the extrarectal plane. A suture is attached to the central part of the T piece and secured to a special olive; the olive is then clipped on to the tip of the tunnelling device. Each strip of Permacol® can then be withdrawn from the suprapubic wound back into the perineal wound. The T bar is secured to the anterolateral wall of the rectal serosa with absorbable sutures on the other side of the rectum. The long central piece of Permacol® is shortened via the suprapubic wound on each side and anchored to the rectus muscle tendon insertion with the suture placed earlier.

Any associated rectocele is repaired via the perineal wound by dissecting into the ischiorectal fossa on either side to expose the ischial tuberosity. A winged piece of Permacol® is inserted into the rectovaginal space, each wing passed underneath the puborectalis muscle and sutured to the ischial tuberosity on either side. The main part of the Permacol® mesh is anchored to the rectum with sutures.

Rectal intussusception

Rectal intussusception refers to the invagination of the rectal wall during the act of defecation. The bowel wall will descend to varying degrees which are classified to the leading edge of the intussusception. The intussusception may remain entirely within the rectum, reach the dentate line, protrude into the anorectum or (in the case of full-thickness prolapse) protrude through the anus. There is, however, little correlation between the degree of prolapse seen on evacuation defecography and the symptoms experienced by the patient. Rectal intussusception is also seen in asymptomatic individuals.

Rectal intussusception may be associated with symptoms of obstructive defecation. It may be diagnosed at rigid sigmoidoscopy by an experienced practitioner on asking the patient to strain during withdrawal of the sigmoidoscope. It is more commonly seen during contrast or magnetic resonance defecography. Internal rectal intussusception is initially treated with conservative measures. Surgical procedures in the event of failure of conservative management have included abdominal rectopexy,[93,94] an internal Delorme procedure[95] and more recently the STARR procedure.[84,87]

Solitary rectal ulcer syndrome (SRUS)

SRUS may be caused by paradoxical contraction of the anal sphincter muscle during defecation, is frequently associated with anal digitation, and results in anterior mucosal trauma and ulceration. It is characterised by classical symptoms, endoscopic findings and histopathological changes.[96] Treatment involves dietary changes, bulking agents and biofeedback to reverse the underlying defecatory disorder.[97] Surgical intervention is only rarely indicated and should only be used for patients with concomitant demonstrable prolapse or intractable symptoms refractory to conservative management. A number of surgical options have been described in SRUS management, including transanal excision of the ulcer, stapled mucosal resection, modified anterior Delorme's procedure, abdominal rectopexy and colostomy formation.[98] Simple resection without biofeedback does not resolve the symptoms.[99] Rectopexy has high associated failure rates of up to 50%,[98,100] although early results of the STARR procedure in refractory SRUS appear encouraging.[101]

Key points

- Patients being considered for surgical management of functional disorders of defecation are best managed within the setting of a multidisciplinary clinic or team.
- The management of full-thickness prolapse is almost exclusively surgical.
- There is no current evidence to support the superiority of abdominal or perineal approaches to rectal prolapse repair, although the results of the PROSPER trial are awaited.
- Mesh and suture techniques give equivalent results in abdominal rectopexy.
- Preservation of the lateral ligaments during rectal mobilisation is associated with fewer postoperative defecatory symptoms.
- Laparoscopic approaches to abdominal rectopexy are as effective as open approaches, and may have benefits in terms of recovery times and lower morbidity.

- Laparoscopic surgery may have particular benefits for management of combined genital and rectal prolapse.
- Rectocele repairs should only be offered to patients who remain symptomatic after conservative management of obstructed defecation with dietary manipulation, bulking agents and biofeedback, and who digitate vaginally or perineally (i.e. not anal digitators).
- The STARR procedure may offer symptomatic relief in carefully selected patients with obstructive defecation syndrome.
- The EXPRESS procedure provides an alternative surgical repair for patients with symptoms of obstructive defecation associated with rectal intussusception or rectocele but needs validation by others.

References

1. Davis K, Kumar D. Posterior pelvic floor compartment disorders. Best Pract Res Clin Obstet Gynaecol 2005; 19(6):941–58.
2. Kapoor DS, Sultan AH, Thakar R et al. Management of complex pelvic floor disorders in a multidisciplinary pelvic floor clinic. Colorectal Dis 2008; 10(2):118–23.
3. Finco C, Luongo B, Savastano S et al. Selection criteria for surgery in patients with obstructed defecation, rectocele and anorectal prolapse. Chir Ital 2007; 59(4):513–20.
4. Carley ME, Schaffer J. Urinary incontinence and pelvic organ prolapse in women with Marfan or Ehlers Danlos syndrome. Am J Obstet Gynecol 2000; 182(5):1021–3.
5. Dreznik Z, Vishne TH, Kristt D et al. Rectal prolapse: a possibly underrecognized complication of anorexia nervosa amenable to surgical correction. Int J Psychiat Med 2001; 31(3): 347–52.
6. Karasick S, Spettell CM. The role of parity and hysterectomy on the development of pelvic floor abnormalities revealed by defecography. Am J Roentgenol 1997; 169(6):1555–8.
7. Swift S, Woodman P, O'Boyle A et al. Pelvic Organ Support Study (POSST): the distribution, clinical definition, and epidemiologic condition of pelvic organ support defects. Am J Obstet Gynecol 2005; 192(3):795–806.
8. Chew SS, Marshall L, Kalish L et al. Short-term and long-term results of combined sclerotherapy and rubber band ligation of hemorrhoids and mucosal prolapse. Dis Colon Rectum 2003; 46(9):1232–7.
9. Gupta PJ. Randomized controlled study: radiofrequency coagulation and plication versus ligation and excision technique for rectal mucosal prolapse. Am J Surg 2006; 192(2):155–60.
10. Kleinubing H Jr, Pinho MS, Ferreira LC. Longitudinal multiple rubber band ligation: an alternative method to treat mucosal prolapse of the anterior rectal wall. Dis Colon Rectum 2006; 49(6):876–8.
11. Araki Y, Ishibashi N, Kishimoto Y et al. Circular stapling procedure for mucosal prolapse of the rectum associated with outlet obstruction. Kurume Med J 2001; 48(3):201–4.
12. Orrom W, Hayashi A, Rusnak C et al. Initial experience with stapled anoplasty in the operative management of prolapsing hemorrhoids and mucosal rectal prolapse. Am J Surg 2002; 183(5):519–24.
13. Johnson DB, DiSiena MR, Fanelli RD. Circumferential mucosectomy with stapled proctopexy is a safe, effective outpatient alternative for the treatment of symptomatic prolapsing hemorrhoids in the elderly. Surg Endosc 2003; 17(12):1990–5.
14. Corman ML, Carriero A, Hager T et al. Consensus conference on the stapled transanal rectal resection (STARR) for disordered defecation. Colorectal Dis 2006; 8(2):98–101.
15. Bachoo P, Brazzelli M, Grant A. Surgery for complete rectal prolapse in adults. Cochrane Database Syst Rev 2000; 2:CD001758.

Cochrane meta-analysis of randomised controlled trials in prolapse surgery identified eight trials with 264 patients. There was no difference in recurrence rates between abdominal and perineal approaches.

16. Brown AJ, Anderson JH, McKee RF et al. Strategy for selection of type of operation for rectal prolapse based on clinical criteria. Dis Colon Rectum 2004; 47(1):103–7.
17. Farouk R, Duthie GS. The evaluation and treatment of patients with rectal prolapse. Ann Chir Gynaecol 1997; 86(4):279–84.
18. Christiansen J, Kirkegaard P. Delorme's operation for complete rectal prolapse. Br J Surg 1981; 68(8):537–8.
19. Senapati A, Nicholls RJ, Thomson JP et al. Results of Delorme's procedure for rectal prolapse. Dis Colon Rectum 1994; 37(5):456–60.
20. Boccasanta P, Venturi M, Barbieri S et al. Impact of new technologies on the clinical and functional outcome of Altemeier's procedure: a randomized, controlled trial. Dis Colon Rectum 2006; 49(5):652–60.

21. Agachan F, Reissman P, Pfeifer J et al. Comparison of three perineal procedures for the treatment of rectal prolapse. South Med J 1997; 90(9):925–32.

22. Lechaux JP, Lechaux D, Perez M. Results of Delorme's procedure for rectal prolapse. Advantages of a modified technique. Dis Colon Rectum 1995; 38(3):301–7.

23. Watts AM, Thompson MR. Evaluation of Delorme's procedure as a treatment for full-thickness rectal prolapse. Br J Surg 2000; 87(2):218–22.

24. Watkins BP, Landercasper J, Belzer GE et al. Long-term follow-up of the modified Delorme procedure for rectal prolapse. Arch Surg 2003; 138(5):498–502; discussion 502–3.

25. Pascual Montero JA, Martinez Puente MC, Pascual I et al. Complete rectal prolapse clinical and functional outcome with Delorme's procedure. Rev Esp Enferm Dig 2006; 98(11):837–43.

26. Marchal F, Bresler L, Ayav A et al. Long-term results of Delorme's procedure and Orr–Loygue rectopexy to treat complete rectal prolapse. Dis Colon Rectum 2005; 48(9):1785–90.

27. Altemeier WA, Culbertson WR, Schowengerdt C et al. Nineteen years' experience with the one-stage perineal repair of rectal prolapse. Ann Surg 1971; 173(6):993–1006.

28. Kimmins MH, Evetts BK, Isler J et al. The Altemeier repair: outpatient treatment of rectal prolapse. Dis Colon Rectum 2001; 44(4):565–70.

29. Williams JG, Rothenberger DA, Madoff RD et al. Treatment of rectal prolapse in the elderly by perineal rectosigmoidectomy. Dis Colon Rectum 1992; 35(9):830–4.

30. Kim DS, Tsang CB, Wong WD et al. Complete rectal prolapse: evolution of management and results. Dis Colon Rectum 1999; 42(4):460–6; discussion 466–9.

31. Deen KI, Grant E, Billingham C et al. Abdominal resection rectopexy with pelvic floor repair versus perineal rectosigmoidectomy and pelvic floor repair for full-thickness rectal prolapse. Br J Surg 1994; 81(2):302–4.

A randomised controlled trial of Altemeier's procedure with pelvic floor repair compared to abdominal resection rectopexy with pelvic floor repair. Similar recurrent prolapse rates and significant postoperative morbidity were observed in both groups. Incontinence significantly improved in the resection rectopexy group only.

32. Madoff RD, Williams JG, Wong WD et al. Long-term functional results of colon resection and rectopexy for overt rectal prolapse. Am J Gastroenterol 1992; 87(1):101–4.

33. Raftopoulos Y, Senagore AJ, Di Giuro G et al. Recurrence rates after abdominal surgery for complete rectal prolapse: a multicenter pooled analysis of 643 individual patient data. Dis Colon Rectum 2005; 48(6):1200–6.

Analysis of outcomes from a large series of patients treated with abdominal prolapse procedures over a 22-year period found that age, gender, surgical technique, means of approach (open or laparoscopic) and method of rectopexy had no impact on recurrent rectal prolapse rates.

34. DiGiuro G, Ignjatovic D, Brogger J et al. How accurate are published recurrence rates after rectal prolapse surgery? A meta-analysis of individual patient data. Am J Surg 2006; 191(6):773–8.

35. Madden MV, Kamm MA, Nicholls RJ et al. Abdominal rectopexy for complete prolapse: prospective study evaluating changes in symptoms and anorectal function. Dis Colon Rectum 1992; 35(1):48–55.

36. Marderstein EL, Delaney CP. Surgical management of rectal prolapse. Nat Clin Pract Gastroenterol Hepatol 2007; 4(10):552–61.

37. Speakman CT, Madden MV, Nicholls RJ et al. Lateral ligament division during rectopexy causes constipation but prevents recurrence: results of a prospective randomized study. Br J Surg 1991; 78(12):1431–3.

38. Selvaggi F, Scotto di Carlo E, Silvestri L et al. Surgical treatment of rectal prolapse: a randomised study (Abstract). Br J Surg 1993; 80:89.

39. Mollen RM, Kuijpers JH, van Hoek F. Effects of rectal mobilization and lateral ligaments division on colonic and anorectal function. Dis Colon Rectum 2000; 43(9):1283–7.

40. Keighley MR, Fielding JW, Alexander-Williams J. Results of Marlex mesh abdominal rectopexy for rectal prolapse in 100 consecutive patients. Br J Surg 1983; 70(4):229–32.

41. Athanasiadis S, Weyand G, Heiligers J et al. The risk of infection of three synthetic materials used in rectopexy with or without colonic resection for rectal prolapse. Int J Colorectal Dis 1996; 11(1):42–4.

42. Novell JR, Osborne MJ, Winslet MC et al. Prospective randomized trial of Ivalon sponge versus sutured rectopexy for full-thickness rectal prolapse. Br J Surg 1994; 81(6):904–6.

A prospective randomised trial comparing Ivalon® sponge to suture rectopexy found no difference in recurrence rates, although there was a significantly higher incidence of postoperative constipation in the Ivalon® sponge arm.

43. Winde G, Reers B, Nottberg H et al. Clinical and functional results of abdominal rectopexy with absorbable mesh-graft for treatment of complete rectal prolapse. Eur J Surg 1993; 159(5):301–5.

44. Galili Y, Rabau M. Comparison of polyglycolic acid and polypropylene mesh for rectopexy in the treatment of rectal prolapse. Eur J Surg 1997; 163(6):445–8.

45. Lechaux JP, Atienza P, Goasguen N et al. Prosthetic rectopexy to the pelvic floor and sigmoidectomy for rectal prolapse. Am J Surg 2001; 182(5):465–9.

46. Luukkonen P, Mikkonen U, Jarvinen H. Abdominal rectopexy with sigmoidectomy vs. rectopexy alone for rectal prolapse: a prospective, randomized study. Int J Colorectal Dis 1992; 7(4):219–22.

47. McKee RF, Lauder JC, Poon FW et al. A prospective randomized study of abdominal rectopexy with and without sigmoidectomy in rectal prolapse. Surg Gynecol Obstet 1992; 174(2):145–8.

48. Purkayastha S, Tekkis P, Athanasiou T et al. A comparison of open vs. laparoscopic abdominal rectopexy for full-thickness rectal prolapse: a meta-analysis. Dis Colon Rectum 2005; 48(10):1930–40.

49. Solomon MJ, Young CJ, Eyers AA et al. Randomized clinical trial of laparoscopic versus open abdominal rectopexy for rectal prolapse. Br J Surg 2002; 89(1):35–9.

No significant difference was found in recurrence rates but the laparoscopic approach was associated with significantly less morbidity, shorter hospital stays and longer operating times.

50. Boccasanta P, Rosati R, Venturi M et al. Comparison of laparoscopic rectopexy with open technique in the treatment of complete rectal prolapse: clinical and functional results. Surg Laparosc Endosc 1998; 8(6):460–5.

51. Slawik S, Soulsby R, Carter H et al. Laparoscopic ventral rectopexy, posterior colporrhaphy and vaginal sacrocolpopexy for the treatment of recto-genital prolapse and mechanical outlet obstruction. Colorectal Dis 2008; 10(2):138–43.

52. D'Hoore A, Penninckx F. Laparoscopic ventral recto(colpo)pexy for rectal prolapse: surgical technique and outcome for 109 patients. Surg Endosc 2006; 20(12):1919–23.

53. Hool GR, Hull TL, Fazio VW. Surgical treatment of recurrent complete rectal prolapse: a thirty-year experience. Dis Colon Rectum 1997; 40(3):270–2.

54. Fengler SA, Pearl RK, Prasad ML et al. Management of recurrent rectal prolapse. Dis Colon Rectum 1997; 40(7):832–4.

55. Gauruder-Burmester A, Koutouzidou P, Rohne J et al. Follow-up after polypropylene mesh repair of anterior and posterior compartments in patients with recurrent prolapse. Int Urogynecol J Pelvic Floor Dysfunct 2007; 18(9):1059–64.

56. Lau CW, Heymen S, Alabaz O et al. Prognostic significance of rectocele, intussusception, and abnormal perineal descent in biofeedback treatment for constipated patients with paradoxical puborectalis contraction. Dis Colon Rectum 2000; 43(4):478–82.

57. Pescatori M, Spyrou M, Pulvirenti d'Urso A. A prospective evaluation of occult disorders in obstructed defecation using the 'iceberg diagram'. Colorectal Dis 2006; 8(9):785–9.

58. Agachan F, Chen T, Pfeifer J et al. A constipation scoring system to simplify evaluation and management of constipated patients. Dis Colon Rectum 1996; 39(6):681–5.

59. Altomare DF, Spazzafumo L, Rinaldi M et al. Set-up and statistical validation of a new scoring system for obstructed defecation syndrome. Colorectal Dis 2008; 10(1):84–8.

60. Shafik A, El-Sibai O, Shafik AA et al. On the pathogenesis of rectocele: the concept of the rectovaginal pressure gradient. Int Urogynecol J Pelvic Floor Dysfunct 2003; 14(5):310–5; discussion 315.

61. Wiskind AK, Creighton SM, Stanton SL. The incidence of genital prolapse after the Burch colposuspension. Am J Obstet Gynecol 1992; 167(2):399–404; discussion 404–5.

62. Agachan F, Pfeifer J, Wexner SD. Defecography and proctography. Results of 744 patients. Dis Colon Rectum 1996; 39(8):899–905.

63. Kaufman HS, Buller JL, Thompson JR et al. Dynamic pelvic magnetic resonance imaging and cystocolpoproctography alter surgical management of pelvic floor disorders. Dis Colon Rectum 2001; 44(11):1575–83; discussion 1583–4.

64. Mimura T, Roy AJ, Storrie JB et al. Treatment of impaired defecation associated with rectocele by behavorial retraining (biofeedback). Dis Colon Rectum 2000; 43(9):1267–72.

65. Heymen S, Scarlett Y, Jones K et al. Randomized, controlled trial shows biofeedback to be superior to alternative treatments for patients with pelvic floor dyssynergia-type constipation. Dis Colon Rectum 2007; 50(4):428–41.

66. Ayav A, Bresler L, Brunaud L et al. Long-term results of transanal repair of rectocele using linear stapler. Dis Colon Rectum 2004; 47(6):889–94.

67. D'Avolio M, Ferrara A, Chimenti C. Transanal rectocele repair using EndoGIA: short-term results of a prospective study. Tech Coloproctol 2005; 9(2):108–14.

68. Block IR. Transrectal repair of rectocele using obliterative suture. Dis Colon Rectum 1986; 29(11):707–11.

69. Sarles JC, Arnaud A, Selezneff I et al. Endo-rectal repair of rectocele. Int J Colorectal Dis 1989; 4(3):167–71.

70. Ho YH, Ang M, Nyam D et al. Transanal approach to rectocele repair may compromise anal sphincter pressures. Dis Colon Rectum 1998; 41(3):354–8.

71. Ayabaca SM, Zbar AP, Pescatori M. Anal continence after rectocele repair. Dis Colon Rectum 2002; 45(1):63–9.

72. Heriot AG, Skull A, Kumar D. Functional and physiological outcome following transanal repair of rectocele. Br J Surg 2004; 91(10):1340–4.

73. Boccasanta P, Venturi M, Calabro G et al. Which surgical approach for rectocele? A multicentric

report from Italian coloproctologists. Tech Coloproctol 2001; 5(3):149–56.

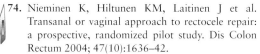

74. Nieminen K, Hiltunen KM, Laitinen J et al. Transanal or vaginal approach to rectocele repair: a prospective, randomized pilot study. Dis Colon Rectum 2004; 47(10):1636–42.

   A small prospective randomised trial comparing transanal rectocele repair with posterior colporrhaphy. Both procedures resulted in an improvement in defecatory function. The transanal group had a greater proportion of patients with successful outcomes, but also had a significantly higher rate of symptomatic recurrent posterior vaginal wall prolapse.

75. Altomare DF, Rinaldi M, Veglia A et al. Combined perineal and endorectal repair of rectocele by circular stapler: a novel surgical technique. Dis Colon Rectum 2002; 45(11):1549–52.

76. Dodi G, Pietroletti R, Milito G et al. Bleeding, incontinence, pain and constipation after STARR transanal double stapling rectotomy for obstructed defecation. Tech Coloproctol 2003; 7(3):148–53.

77. Boccasanta P, Venturi M, Stuto A et al. Stapled transanal rectal resection for outlet obstruction: a prospective, multicenter trial. Dis Colon Rectum 2004; 47(8):1285–96; discussion 1296–7.

78. Boccasanta P, Venturi M, Salamina G et al. New trends in the surgical treatment of outlet obstruction: clinical and functional results of two novel transanal stapled techniques from a randomised controlled trial. Int J Colorectal Dis 2004; 19(4):359–69.

   A randomised controlled trial between single stapled transanal prolapsectomy in association with perineal levatorplasty compared to the STARR procedure. Constipation symptoms improved in 76% of the stapled prolapsectomy group and 88% of the STARR group. Late complications included urgency, flatus incontinence and anal stenosis. Dyspareunia affected 20% of the prolapsectomy group but none of the STARR group.

79. Jayne DG, Finan PJ. Stapled transanal rectal resection for obstructed defecation and evidence-based practice. Br J Surg 2005; 92(7):793–4.

80. Pescatori M, Dodi G, Salafia C et al. Rectovaginal fistula after double-stapled transanal rectotomy (STARR) for obstructed defecation. Int J Colorectal Dis 2005; 20(1):83–5.

81. Gagliardi G, Pescatori M, Altomare DF et al. Results, outcome predictors, and complications after stapled transanal rectal resection for obstructed defecation. Dis Colon Rectum 2008; 51(2):186–95.

82. De Nardi P, Bottini C, Faticanti Scucchi L et al. Proctalgia in a patient with staples retained in the puborectalis muscle after STARR operation. Tech Coloproctol 2007; 11(4):353–6.

83. Binda GA, Pescatori M, Romano G. The dark side of double-stapled transanal rectal resection. Dis Colon Rectum 2005; 48(9):1830–1; author reply 1831–2.

84. Ommer A, Albrecht K, Wenger F et al. Stapled transanal rectal resection (STARR): a new option in the treatment of obstructive defecation syndrome. Langenbeck's Arch Surg 2006; 391(1):32–7.

85. Renzi A, Izzo D, Di Sarno G et al. Stapled transanal rectal resection to treat obstructed defecation caused by rectal intussusception and rectocele. Int J Colorectal Dis 2006; 21(7):661–7.

86. Arroyo A, Perez-Vicente F, Serrano P et al. Evaluation of the stapled transanal rectal resection technique with two staplers in the treatment of obstructive defecation syndrome. J Am Coll Surg 2007; 204(1):56–63.

87. Pechlivanides G, Tsiaoussis J, Athanasakis E et al. Stapled transanal rectal resection (STARR) to reverse the anatomic disorders of pelvic floor dyssynergia. World J Surg 2007; 31(6):1329–35.

88. Jayne D, Schwandner O, Stuto A. The European STARR Registry: 6-month follow-up analysis (abstr). Colorectal Dis 2007; 9(Suppl 3):11.

   The European STARR registry report on follow-up in 1404 patients undergoing the STARR procedure. A significant reduction in obstructive defecation symptoms and an improvement in quality-of-life scores were seen at 6 months. Complication rate was 31.7%, with bleeding 4.3%, urgency 14.3%, postoperative perineal pain 8.1%, new-onset faecal incontinence 1.3% and sepsis 1.1%.

89. Petersen S, Hellmich G, Schuster A et al. Stapled transanal rectal resection under laparoscopic surveillance for rectocele and concomitant enterocele. Dis Colon Rectum 2006; 49(5):685–9.

90. Williams NS, Giordano P, Dvorkin LS et al. External pelvic rectal suspension (the Express procedure) for full-thickness rectal prolapse: evolution of a new technique. Dis Colon Rectum 2005; 48(2):307–16.

91. Williams NS, Dvorkin LS, Giordano P et al. EXternal Pelvic REctal SuSpension (Express procedure) for rectal intussusception, with and without rectocele repair. Br J Surg 2005; 92(5):598–604.

92. Dench JE, Scott SM, Lunniss PJ et al. Multimedia article. External pelvic rectal suspension (the Express procedure) for internal rectal prolapse, with or without concomitant rectocele repair: a video demonstration. Dis Colon Rectum 2006; 49(12):1922–6.

93. Kruyt RH, Delemarre JB, Gooszen HG et al. Selection of patients with internal intussusception of the rectum for posterior rectopexy. Br J Surg 1990; 77(10):1183–4.

94. Christiansen J, Zhu BW, Rasmussen OO et al. Internal rectal intussusception: results of surgical repair. Dis Colon Rectum 1992; 35(11):1026–8; discussion 1028–9.

95. Trompetto M, Clerico G, Realis Luc A et al. Transanal Delorme procedure for treatment of rectocele associated with rectal intussusception. Tech Coloproctol 2006; 10(4):389.

96. Vaizey CJ, van den Bogaerde JB, Emmanuel AV et al. Solitary rectal ulcer syndrome. Br J Surg 1998; 85(12):1617–23.

97. Malouf AJ, Vaizey CJ, Kamm MA. Results of behavioral treatment (biofeedback) for solitary rectal ulcer syndrome. Dis Colon Rectum 2001; 44(1):72–6.

98. Sitzler PJ, Kamm MA, Nicholls RJ et al. Long-term clinical outcome of surgery for solitary rectal ulcer syndrome. Br J Surg 1998; 85(9):1246–50.

99. Marchal F, Bresler L, Brunaud L et al. Solitary rectal ulcer syndrome: a series of 13 patients operated with a mean follow-up of 4.5 years. Int J Colorectal Dis 2001; 16(4):228–33.

100. Tweedie DJ, Varma JS. Long-term outcome of laparoscopic mesh rectopexy for solitary rectal ulcer syndrome. Colorectal Dis 2005; 7(2):151–5.

101. Boccasanta P, Venturi M, Calabro G et al. Stapled transanal rectal resection in solitary rectal ulcer associated with prolapse of the rectum: a prospective study. Dis Colon Rectum 2008; 51(3):348–54.

102. Sand PK, Koduri S, Lobel RW et al. Prospective randomized trial of polyglactin 910 mesh to prevent recurrence of cystoceles and rectoceles. Am J Obstet Gynecol 2001; 184(7):1357–62; discussion 1362–4.

103. Paraiso MF, Barber MD, Muir TW et al. Rectocele repair: a randomized trial of three surgical techniques including graft augmentation. Am J Obstet Gynecol 2006; 195(6):1762–71.

104. Gustilo-Ashby AM, Paraiso MF, Jelovsek JE et al. Bowel symptoms 1 year after surgery for prolapse: further analysis of a randomized trial of rectocele repair. Am J Obstet Gynecol 2007; 197(1):76e1–5.

13

Functional problems and their medical management

Anton V. Emmanuel

Introduction

Symptoms related to functional gastrointestinal disorders (FGIDs) are highly prevalent. In community-based studies, up to 22% of 'normal' UK subjects can be diagnosed as having irritable bowel syndrome (IBS) and up to 28% have functional constipation.[1] These disorders are constellations of symptoms – they are not diseases. As such, the emphasis of management of these patients is based on simple principles: the exclusion of organic disease, making a confident diagnosis, explaining why symptoms occur, alteration of lifestyle where appropriate and avoidance of surgery. Education about healthy lifestyle behaviours, reassurance that the symptoms are not due to a life-threatening disease such as cancer and establishment of a therapeutic relationship are essential, and patients have a greater expectation of benefit from lifestyle modification than drugs. This chapter will deal primarily with IBS and functional constipation, leaving the treatment of faecal incontinence to Chapter 11. Similarly, rectal prolapse, which is a frequent comorbidity of chronic constipation, is dealt with in Chapter 12.

The prevalence of functional disorders depends on the exact diagnostic criteria used; the current standards are the Rome III criteria.[2] The core diagnostic requirement for IBS is abdominal pain related to bowel function in association with altered stool form or frequency. The definition of functional constipation requires the presence of at least two

of the following: less than three bowel actions a week, need to strain or manually assist evacuation on >25% of occasions, passage of hard stools on >25% of occasions or a sensation of abnormal evacuation on >25% of occasions. These symptoms need to be chronic, and organic disease needs to have been excluded. Although these criteria can be criticised for being over-inclusive, what is clear is that FGIDs represent a major burden on secondary and tertiary outpatient clinics and IBS is the commonest diagnosis in gastrointestinal clinics.[3] An important confounding factor to be borne in mind when reviewing the literature on FGIDs is that the overwhelming majority of studies originate from tertiary centres. Patients attending such institutions are known to have disproportionately high scores on scales of depression, health-related anxiety and somatisation,[4] representing a potentially biased, self-selected group. One further compounding variable in assessing studies of FGIDs is that there is a notoriously high placebo response, ranging from 30% to 80%.[5]

Irritable bowel syndrome

The key to successful management of IBS is empathic reassurance. This will need to be individually directed according to the patient's symptoms, beliefs and anxieties.[6] Early and positive diagnosis is essential. Helpful factors in establishing a diagnosis are: (i) presence of symptoms for more than 6 months; (ii) frequent consultations for non-gastrointestinal symptoms; (iii) self-report that stress aggravates symptoms.

A key component of the reassurance is provision of a simple explanation of the benign nature and prognosis of the condition. Patients should be advised that no more than 2% of patients need their diagnosis of IBS to be revised at 30 years of follow-up.[1] Equally, it is important to remember that 88% of patients had recurring episodes of gastrointestinal symptoms, and so reassurance should be allied to advice about the need for long-term symptom control.[1]

Investigation

The presence of alarm features such as symptom onset after age 50, rectal bleeding, significant weight loss or abdominal mass mandates serological and luminal investigation to exclude organic disease. Investigations in these frequently young patients (the majority of patients at presentation are aged less than 35[1]) should otherwise be avoided since they may both exacerbate patients' anxieties and undermine their confidence in the clinician.

 An important diagnosis to consider, especially in the presence of low-grade anaemia, is coeliac disease.

Approximately 5% of patients fulfilling IBS diagnostic criteria will have histological evidence of coeliac disease compared to 0.5% of controls without IBS symptoms.[7]

Treatment

Lifestyle modification

No strong, reproducible clinical trial evidence exists in favour of any particular dietary intervention in IBS.

 Behavioural training to encourage patients to alter patterns of phobic avoidance of public toilets is a central component of biofeedback, and is of undoubted value in some patients.[8]

True food allergies are much rarer than lay perception would predict,[9] and food fads and avoidances should be discouraged. One helpful dietary intervention worth considering in diarrhoea-predominant IBS patients (d-IBS) is reduction of excess caffeine and sorbitol (found in chewing gum and sweeteners).[10]

Studies have been carried out on the effect of dietary fibre augmentation in some constipation-predominant IBS (c-IBS) patients.[11,12] Early placebo-controlled crossover studies showed some acceleration of transit but no significant effect on symptoms.[11] Later studies have corroborated the absence of beneficial effect on symptoms and suggested that there is an increase in abdominal bloating, discomfort and flatulence during dietary fibre supplementation.[12] In summary, the effect of dietary fibre in IBS is not significantly beneficial, and the diet is frequently difficult to adhere to in the long term.[13]

Pharmacological treatments

Most patients with FGIDs do not need drug therapy. The strongest evidence for a single agent in IBS patients is in d-IBS, where loperamide is a well-tolerated and effective treatment of diarrhoea and urgency.[14]

The popular aetiological theory that IBS symptoms relate to gut spasm has led to a huge number of uniformly low-quality studies of antispasmodics in IBS patients. These have been subject to meta-analysis.[15] In essence, what can be concluded is that, even allowing for publication bias in favour of positive studies, there is no evidence that anticholinergic (such as discycloverine, hyoscine) or antispasmodic drugs (mebeverine, peppermint) have any advantage over placebo in treating the symptoms of IBS.

 In contrast, the data for the efficacy of tricyclic antidepressants show unequivocal benefit in favour of low-dose usage of these agents.[16] Doses of amitryptilline or nortryptilline of 10–50 mg act at both the central (anxiety and depression) and peripheral (neuromodulatory) mechanisms of IBS.

One putative mechanism of action of tricyclic agents is through an effect on gut serotonin receptors.

Many drugs that agonise or antagonise these receptors have been developed, although the effect of all these drugs seems at best to be modest, amounting to no more than a 10–20% advantage over placebo.[17]

None of these agents are licensed for use in the UK at the time of writing, with some having been withdrawn due to safety concerns. In contrast to studies of low-dose tricyclics, standard doses of newer antidepressants (selective serotonin reuptake inhibitors) lead to a less impressive improvement in IBS, and at greater cost.[18] Finally, preliminary evidence suggests the possibility that some probiotic strains of bacteria may have a beneficial influence in patients with IBS, though this is very much emerging information.[19]

Psychological treatments

A landmark study by Creed et al. showed that cognitive behavioural therapy directed towards bowel symptoms is effective in treating women with IBS, with a 'number needed to treat' of 3.[20]

The essence of such treatment is that it is gut focussed, since general cognitive behavioural and relaxation therapies are no more effective than standard care. The Creed study also showed that such treatment is cost-effective and beneficial in the long-term.[20]

A number of studies in the literature show the benefit of hypnotherapy in IBS including, in the long-term setting, at up to 6 years following the cessation of therapy.[17]

In brief, three-quarters of patients report symptom alleviation after hypnotherapy, and over 80% of these responders remain well at a median follow-up of 5 years.[21]

Surgery

Patients with IBS are disproportionately more likely to undergo abdominal and pelvic surgery than age- and sex-matched controls.[22,23] IBS patients have a prevalence of cholecystectomy of 4.6% compared with 2.4% in controls, and a prevalence of hysterectomy of 18% versus 12% in controls. There is also evidence that IBS patients are more likely to undergo appendicectomy (35% prevalence compared to 8% in control patients with ulcerative colitis).[23] [Editor's comment: although patients with ulcerative colitis may have a lower than normal prevalence of appendicectomy.] Furthermore, these examinations are more likely to yield normal findings macroscopically and histologically in IBS patients.[24]

Abdominal or pelvic surgery may predispose to the development of functional symptoms through mechanical, neural or hormonal impairments. Heaton et al. reported that 44% of subjects develop new symptoms of urgency after cholecystectomy and 27% report constipation symptoms beginning after hysterectomy.[25] In contrast, women undergoing gynecological surgery for non-pain indications did not develop IBS more often than non-operated controls.[26] What these studies do highlight is the key importance of trying to minimise surgery in patients with FGIDs. In those patients who do undergo an operation it is implicit that there is complete explanation of the possibility of developing new symptoms postoperatively. The corollary of this is that patients in whom there is a high suspicion of FGID (based on symptoms and normal investigations) should be dissuaded from undergoing diagnostic laparoscopy which is not usually revealing and which may result in new complaints.

Functional constipation

Estimates from the USA suggest that 1.2% of the population consult a physician every year with the complaint of constipation.[27] Since 85% of these consultations result in the prescription of a laxative, it should come as no surprise that the estimated annual expenditure on prescription laxatives in the UK is £48 million,[28] more than is spent on treating hypertension. This figure does not include the cost of over-the-counter laxatives nor the costs of specialist investigation and work absenteeism. What these figures reflect is the importance of the role of the hospital specialist in identifying appropriate patients to put through further investigation and specific treatments.

In terms of pathophysiology, functional constipation is considered to be due to either slow whole-gut transit ('colonic inertia'), rectal evacuatory dysfunction or a combination of both of these abnormalities.

The commonest cause of slow transit in general practice is as a side-effect of drug therapy for other reasons. The commonest culprit drugs are opiates, anticholinergics, antihypertensives, iron supplements, antacids and non-steroidal anti-inflammatory drugs.[28]

Investigation

As with the case of patients with IBS, luminal investigation is reserved for patients with a short history or alarm symptoms, in whom there is the need to exclude colorectal cancer. In addition to the drug causes listed above, which can be identified from careful history-taking, the other common associations are with neurological disease (multiple sclerosis, Parkinson's disease and diabetic autonomic neuropathy). Causes of constipation that can be identified from simple serological testing include hypothyroidism, hypercalcaemia and hypokalaemia.

Whereas the diagnosis of IBS is one of exclusion, there are investigations available both to define the pathophysiological abnormality and confirm the presence of constipation. Colonic transit can be simply measured by use of radio-opaque markers followed by a plain abdominal X-ray. One well-described assessment comprises ingestion of three sets of radiologically distinct markers that are ingested at 24-hour intervals and an abdominal X-ray taken 120 hours after the first ingestion; retention of more than the normal range for any one of the three sets of markers reflects slow transit.[29] The test is cheap, sensitive and reproducible, and provides clinically helpful information in the management of patients with constipation.[28]

Defecating proctography (using barium or magnetic resonance contrast gel) and the balloon expulsion test are means of quantifying the anatomical and physiological disturbances of rectal evacuation in patients with functional constipation. Abnormalities such as paradoxical anal sphincter contraction, impaired pelvic floor relaxation, anal intussusception and rectal prolapse can be demonstrated by these techniques.[30] No firm evidence exists as to the value of these abnormalities in the management of patients with constipation.[30] The place of anorectal manometry in patients with chronic constipation is primarily in the exclusion of Hirschsprung's disease.[30]

Treatment

Dietary fibre supplementation

This is the traditional first line of therapy for chronic constipation, and by the time of specialist referral most patients would have already undertaken trials of such therapy. Fibre supplementation increases gut transit and stool bulk by a fraction of the starting value, and as such is only effective in patients with mild constipation.[31] In those small number of patients seen in hospital who have not tried fibre supplementation, advice needs to be offered about a gradual stepwise increase in fibre intake. Patients need to be counselled that the effect is not apparent until therapy has been established for several weeks.

 Patients need to continue with the diet in the long term,[32] and there is evidence that this can be difficult for a significant proportion. Increasing liquid intake and attempting to maintain regular meal-time patterns seem also to have a place in improving symptoms, although the evidence is strongest in the elderly.[31]

Laxatives, suppositories, enemas and novel prokinetics

There are widely held misconceptions of the danger of 'self-poisoning' without a daily bowel action. Given the limited evidence base for the use of laxatives, the first step in the management of constipation is to discourage laxative overuse.[28,33] The effect of laxatives in chronic constipation is modest at best. Only a very small number of trials have compared a laxative regimen with placebo, and meta-analysis would not be statistically or clinically meaningful.[33] Compared to the dearth of placebo-controlled studies, there are a number of open and blinded comparisons between different laxatives. These have been systematically reviewed recently[33] and as might be predicted the opinion of the reviewers is that methodological flaws and inconsistencies prevent meaningful conclusions being drawn. The conclusions that can be drawn are listed below. Overall there is an increase in stool frequency with bulking agents of 1.4 bowel movements per week, and with other laxative classes of 1.5 bowel movements per week.

Bulk laxatives have a limited role in chronic constipation. They should be reserved for patients who are unable to consume adequate dietary fibre.

They have no role in either patients with severe constipation or those who need rapid relief of symptoms.

 Osmotic agents comprise either poorly absorbed ionic salts or non-absorbed sugars and alcohols. Dose titration is possible with osmotic laxatives, which have a particular place in the management of megacolon and megarectum once the patient has been disimpacted.

 Stimulant laxatives (anthranoid compounds such as senna, or polyphenolic compounds such as bisacodyl) usually have an effect on stool output within 24 hours of ingestion, and are most suitable for occasional, rather than regular, use.

The effect of these drugs is unpredictable and dose escalation is often required. Nevertheless, they appear to be harmless and are frequently used in chronic severe constipation. What is clear is that the previous fears that chronic use of anthranoid laxatives may result in enteric nerve damage is highly unlikely.[34] **Stool softeners** and **compound mixtures** of the above classes of laxative are also commonly used, although their efficacy has not been rigorously demonstrated.

Some **suppositories** induce a chemically induced reflex rectal contraction. **Enemas** act either by inducing rectal contraction or by softening hard stool.

 Suppositories and enemas can be effective in alleviating the symptoms of evacuation difficulty if dietary modification and behavioural therapy have been unsuccessful. Used on an as-required basis, enemas have a particular place in managing rectal impaction.

Cisapride was the first **prokinetic** to be studied in chronic functional constipation, showing limited short-lived effect. Prucalopride and tegaserod are agonists at the serotonin-4 receptor and seem to accelerate both upper and lower gut transit.[35] Both drugs rapidly improve symptoms, although the optimal duration of treatment remains uncertain.

Behavioural therapy (biofeedback)

Gut-directed behavioural therapy, biofeedback, is now an established therapy for functional constipation, and in a number of specialist centres is first-line therapy for new referrals.[36,37] Biofeedback is a learning strategy based on operant conditioning. The main focus is on abdominal and pelvic coordination and it is undoubtedly beneficial in patients with dyssynergic evacuation,[36] but it also seems benificial in patients with slow transit.[37]

 Short- and long-term benefit is evident in over 60% of unselected patients in specialist centres.[8,37,38]

The effect of treatment is seen not only in symptoms (improved bowel frequency, reduced need to strain), but also in terms of reduced laxative use and improved quality-of-life scores.[8]

Biofeedback seems to have its effect through alteration of a variety of pathophysiological disturbances. There is evidence that successful outcome with biofeedback is associated with specifically improved autonomic innervation to the colon, and improved transit time for patients with slow and normal transit.[8]

 Additionally, treatment may improve pelvic floor coordination,[37] thereby allowing antegrade peristalsis and preventing retrograde movement of colonic content. What is important is that biofeedback is successful not just in patients with mild symptoms, but also in those with intractable symptoms who are being considered for surgery.[38]

Surgical treatment for constipation

In those patients with proven slow transit who have failed to respond to dietary modification, biofeedback, long-term trials of laxatives and prokinetics, the traditional algorithm dictates consideration of a surgical approach. The standard surgical procedure has been total colectomy (performed to the level of the sacral promontory) and ileorectal anastomosis.[39] Ileorectostomy is reported as being more successful than ileosigmoidostomy in terms of successful relief of constipation and, providing greater than 7–10 cm of rectum is left intact, then bowel frequency and urgency are not unacceptably frequent.[39]

Almost every major colorectal institution and a huge number of other centres have published on their experience of subtotal colectomy for slow transit constipation. Results vary widely with satisfaction rates varying from 39% to 100%.[40] Whilst median scores of bowel frequency tend to show statistically significant improvements, what these composite figures mask are the facts that, firstly, approximately one in three patients do not improve at all and, secondly, that some patients develop diarrhoea.

 The strongest argument against colectomy for slow transit constipation is that the disorder is a pan-enteric one, and so mere removal of the colon is unlikely to yield sustained benefit.[40,41]

There are two unequivocal conclusions that come out of the welter of small studies in the literature. Firstly, adverse effects occur in over half of all patients. Most common is episodic subacute small bowel obstruction (occurring in up to two-thirds of some series), need for further abdominal surgery (in up to one-third of patients), persisting constipation (in up to one-quarter), diarrhoea (in up to one-quarter) and faecal incontinence (in up to 10%).

 The second conclusion, related to the incidence of adverse events, is the importance of careful patient selection.

Thus, of the many patients complaining of constipation in the community, only a tiny proportion (approximately 1%) are referred to tertiary care, of whom only a small fraction (less than 5%) would benefit from surgical treatment.[42] Patient selection must initially be on clinical grounds (including careful consideration of potential psychiatric disorders) and the physiological demonstration of slow transit. Some authors have recommended extensive anorectal sensory and motor physiological testing, defecating proctography and upper gut motility studies to aid identification of subgroups in whom surgery may be more successful.[43] In contrast, Rantis et al.[44] identified only 23% of patients in whom such extensive testing altered clinical management; additionally the cost of this testing was great (US $140 000 in 1997).

In view of the controversy about subtotal colectomy, a vogue for alternative surgical therapies arose. Two particular surgical approaches have received sustained study: stoma formation and segmental colonic resection. However, the data on efficacy and morbidity of these techniques are little different and no less controversial than those for subtotal colectomy.[45] There is unequivocally no place for division of puborectalis in an attempt to treat rectal evacuatory dysfunction.[46]

A less invasive surgical approach to functional constipation has been the antegrade continence enema (the Malone procedure). Initially used in patients with constipation secondary to neurological disease, the technique has been widely reported in functional constipation.[47] Patients intubate their stoma (appendix or plastic conduit) and irrigate with either water, a stimulant or osmotic laxative. Although there are stomal complications in over 50% of patients (stenosis, mucus leak, pain), three-quarters of patients report 'high' or 'very high' satisfaction with the procedure.[47]

Current trials of medical therapy for FGIDs require quality-of-life data to complement conventional efficacy data. The surgical literature to date shows that although stool frequency may improve, gut-specific quality of life does not.[48]

Putative treatments for constipation

 Recent surgical developments have looked at modifications of subtotal colectomy. Small, short-term studies have shown that ileosigmoid or antiperistaltic caecorectal anastomoses may improve bowel frequency and quality of life.[49,50]

However, the major recent development with regard to surgical therapy for constipation has been sacral nerve stimulation.[51] In the single publication to date, two patients were studied in a double-blind crossover fashion with their sacral nerve stimulator either turned on or off.

 There was a clear improvement in both symptoms and quality of life with the stimulator turned on, potentially extending the role of sacral nerve stimulation from its existing licence for the treatment of faecal incontinence.

Idiopathic megarectum and megacolon

Megarectum and megacolon are uncommon clinical conditions of unknown aetiology that present typically, but not exclusively, with intractable constipation in the first two decades of life.[52] Other conditions presenting with constipation in the context of gut dilatation (e.g. Hirschsprung's disease, chronic intestinal pseudo-obstruction) are not included since the aetiology of these disorders is known. Patients with idiopathic megarectum tend to present with faecal incontinence in the context of recurrent faecal impaction frequently requiring surgical disimpaction. In contrast, patients with idiopathic megacolon more frequently present with abdominal pain and distension in the context of chronic constipation.[52]

The majority of patients with idiopathic megarectum and megacolon can be successfully managed by disimpaction followed by the use of osmotic laxatives. The osmotic agent needs titration in order that the patient obtains a semiformed ('porridgey') stool which is passed three times a day. Occasionally, rectal evacuation techniques (such as suppository use or biofeedback therapy) are required actually to empty the rectum of the semiformed stool.[53]

When medical therapy fails (due to compliance failure or lack of success in avoiding recurrent impaction), surgical therapy is warranted. A number of surgical procedures have been performed, with variable reports of success. As with reports of surgery for idiopathic constipation, the longer the duration of follow-up, the worse the documented outcome. Anorectal physiology, whole-gut transit studies and evacuation proctography do not help identify patients who may benefit or help with choice of surgical procedure.[54] Anorectal physiology testing does have a role in identifying the presence of a rectoanal inhibitory reflex, which excludes the differential diagnosis of Hirschsprung's disease.

With regard to resectional surgery, colectomy offers good results in the majority of patients (80%), with ileorectal anastomosis yielding the greatest levels of patient satisfaction.[54]

Outcomes with the Duhamel procedure, anal myomectomy and restorative proctocolectomy are also favourable in the majority of cases, approaching 70% in the majority of series. Restorative proctocolectomy is suitable in patients with dilatation of both the colon and rectum, whilst the recent procedure of vertical reduction rectoplasty has been proposed for those with dilatation confined to the rectum.[54]

In situations where initial surgery has failed, formation of a stoma (colostomy or ileostomy) is associated with excellent results.[55]

Stoma formation as a primary procedure is also successful in the vast majority of cases.[55] The ultimate choice of surgical procedure will depend on available expertise, patient physical and psychological factors, and the patient's choice.

Key points

- Dietary manipulation is rarely helpful in managing symptoms in hospital-referred patients with functional disorders.
- Drug therapy is rarely needed in treating patients with IBS.
- Loperamide is unequivocally beneficial in patients with loose stools and urgency.
- Low-dose tricyclic antidepressants are effective in relieving functional abdominal pain.
- A comprehensive approach to therapy of functional disorders requires close liaison with psychological services.
- The effect of laxatives in chronic constipation is minimally superior to placebo.
- Biofeedback is effective in almost two-thirds of patients with constipation, whether due to slow transit or evacuatory dysfunction.
- Subtotal colectomy and ileorectal anastomosis is beneficial in a small number of highly selected patients, although surgical morbidity is frequently high.
- The majority of patients with idiopathic megarectum and megacolon can be managed by disimpaction and initiation of osmotic laxatives.

References

1. Jones R, Lydiard S. Irritable bowel syndrome in the general population. BMJ 1991; 304:87–90.

2. Longstreth GF, Thompson WG, Chey WD et al. Functional bowel disorders. Gastroenterology 2006; 130:1480–91.

3. Drossman DA, Sandler RS, McKee DC et al. Bowel patterns among subjects not seeking health care: use of a questionnaire to identify a population with bowel dysfunction. Gastroenterology 1982; 83:529–34.

4. Emmanuel AV, Mason HJ, Kamm MA. Relationship between psychological state and level of activity of extrinsic gut innervation in patients with a functional gastrointestinal disorder. Gut 2001; 49:214–19.

5. Patel SM, Stason WB, Legezda A et al. The placebo effect in irritable bowel syndrome trials: a meta-analysis. Neurogastroenterol Motil 2005; 17:332–40.

6. Thompson WG. Review article: the treatment of the irritable bowel syndrome. Aliment Pharm Ther 2002; 16:1395–406.

7. Sanders DS, Carter MJ, Hurlstone DP et al. Association of adult coeliac disease with irritable bowel syndrome: a case control study in patients fulfilling the Rome II criteria referred to secondary care. Lancet 2001; 358:1504–8.

8. Emmanuel AV, Mason HJ, Kamm MA. Response to a behavioural treatment, biofeedback, in constipated patients is associated with improved gut transit and autonomic innervation. Gut 2001; 49:209–13.

9. Pearson DJ. Pseudo food allergy. BMJ 1986; 292:221–2.

10. Hyams JS. Sorbitol intolerance: an unappreciated cause of functional gastrointestinal complaints. Gastroenterology 1983; 84:30–3.

11. Lucey MR, Clark ML, Lowndes J et al. Is bran efficacious in irritable bowel syndrome? A double blind placebo-controlled crossover study. Gut 1987; 28:221–5.

12. Snook J, Shepherd HA. Bran supplementation in the treatment of irritable bowel syndrome. Aliment Pharm Ther 1994; 8:511–14.

   Whilst some patients can expect improvement in stool output with bran, the majority of patients experience an increase in abdominal distension and discomfort.

13. Hillman LC, Stace NH, Pomare EW. Irritable bowel patients and their long-term response to a high fibre diet. Am J Gastroenterol 1984; 79:1–7.

14. Cann PA, Read NW, Holdsworth CD et al. Role of loperamide and placebo in management of irritable bowel syndrome. Dig Dis Sci 1984; 29:239–47.

   Loperamide is effective in slowing gut transit, reducing stool frequency and urgency in patients with IBS.

15. Poynard T, Regimgeau C, Benhamou Y. Meta-analysis of smooth muscle relaxants in the treatment of irritable bowel syndrome. Aliment Pharm Ther 2001; 15:355–61.

16. Jackson AL, O'Malley PG, Tomkins G et al. Treatment of functional gastrointestinal disorders with antidepressant medications. Am J Med 2000; 108:65–72.

   Meta-analysis of studies using a variety of tricyclic antidepressants in varying doses in patients with FGIDs showing clear benefit for low-dose tricyclics over placebo.

17. Spiller R, Aziz Q, Creed F, Emmanuel A et al. Guidelines on the irritable bowel syndrome: mechanisms and practical management. Gut 2007; 56:1770–98.

   Practical and up-to-date review of management options available for IBS, encompassing minimum investigation, pharmacological, dietary and lifestyle treatment.

18. Tack J, Broekaert D, Fischler B et al. A controlled crossover study of the selective serotonin reuptake inhibitor citalopram in irritable bowel syndrome. Gut 2006; 55:1095–103.

19. Whorwell PJ, Altringer L, Morel J et al. Efficacy of an encapsulated probiotic Bifidobacterium infantis 35624 in women with irritable bowel syndrome. Am J Gastroenterol 2006; 101:1581–90.

20. Creed F, Fernandes L, Guthrie E et al. The cost-effectiveness of psychotherapy and paroxetine for severe irritable bowel syndrome. Gastroenterology 2003; 124:303–17.

21. Gonsalkorale WM, Miller V, Afzal A et al. Long term benefits of hypnotherapy for irritable bowel syndrome. Gut 2003; 52:1623–9.

22. Kennedy TM, Jones RH. Epidemiology of cholecystectomy and irritable bowel syndrome in a UK population. Br J Surg 2000; 87:1658–63.

23. Kennedy TM, Jones RH. The epidemiology of hysterectomy and irritable bowel syndrome in a UK population. Int J Clin Pract 2000; 54:647–50.

24. Lu CL, Liu CC, Fuh JL et al. Irritable bowel syndrome and negative appendectomy: a prospective multivariable investigation. Gut 2007; 56:655–60.

25. Heaton KW, Parker D, Cripps H. Bowel function and irritable bowel symptoms after hysterectomy and cholecystectomy – a population based study. Gut 1993; 34:1108–11.

26. Sperber AD, Morris CB, Greemberg L et al. Development of abdominal pain and IBS following gynecological surgery: a prospective, controlled study. Gastroenterology 2008; 134:75–84.

27. Sonnenberg A, Koch TR. Physician visits in the United States for constipation: 1958–1986. Dig Dis Sci 1989; 34:606–11.

28. Emmanuel AV. The use and abuse of laxatives in the elderly. In: Potter J, Norton C, Cottenden AM (eds) Bowel care in frail older people. London: Royal College of Physicians, 2002; Chapter 6.

29. Evans RC, Kamm MA, Hinton JM et al. The normal range and a simple diagram for recording whole gut transit. Int J Colorectal Dis 1992; 7:15–17.

30. Diamant NE, Kamm MA, Wald A et al. AGA technical review on anorectal testing techniques. Gastroenterology 1999; 116:735–54.

31. Harari D, Gurwitz JH, Minaker KL. Constipation in the elderly. J Am Geriatr Soc 1993; 41:1130–40.

32. Jones MP, Talley NJ, Nuyts G et al. Lack of objective evidence of efficacy of laxatives in chronic constipation. Dig Dis Sci 2002; 47:2222–30.

33. Tramonte SM, Brand MB, Mulrow CD et al. The treatment of chronic constipation in adults. J Gen Intern Med 1997; 12:15–24.

    Systematic review of the placebo-controlled laxative studies and those comparing different laxative classes. The limited benefit of these drugs over placebo is highlighted.

34. Kieman JA, Heinicke EA. Sennosides do not kill myenteric neurons in the colon of the rat or mouse. Neuroscience 1989; 30:837–42.

35. Emmanuel AV, Roy AJ, Nicholls TJ. Prucalopride, a systemic enterokinetic, for the treatment of constipation. Aliment Pharm Ther 2002; 16:1347–56.

    Large, single-centre study of the effect of a serotonin agonist on gut physiology and symptoms in patients with functional constipation.

36. Heymen S, Scarlett Y, Jones K et al. Randomized, controlled trial shows biofeedback to be superior to alternative treatments for patients with pelvic floor dyssynergia-type constipation. Dis Colon Rectum 2007; 50:428–41.

37. Chiotakakou-Faliakou E, Kamm MA, Roy AJ et al. Biofeedback provides long term benefit for patients with intractable slow and normal transit constipation. Gut 1998; 42:517–21.

    Demonstration of long-term efficacy of biofeedback in patients who have an initially good response to treatment.

38. Brown SR, Donati D, Seow-Chen F et al. Biofeedback avoids surgery in patients with slow transit constipation: report of four cases. Dis Colon Rectum 2001; 44:737–9.

39. Vasilevsky CA, Nemer FD, Balcos EG et al. Is subtotal colectomy a viable option in the management of chronic constipation? Dis Colon Rectum 1988; 31:679–81.

40. Knowles CH, Scott M, Lunniss PJ. Outcome of colectomy for slow transit constipation. Ann Surg 1999; 230:627–38.

    Systematic review of most of the small reports of subtotal colectomy showing that efficacy is inversely related to duration of follow-up. A rationale for patient selection is presented.

41. Altomare DF, Portincasa P, Rinaldi M et al. Slow transit constipation: solitary symptom of a systemic gastrointestinal disease. Dis Colon Rectum 1999; 42:231–40.

42. Rex DK, Lappas JC, Goulet RC et al. Selection of constipated patients as subtotal colectomy candidates. J Clin Gastroenterol 1992; 15:212–17.

43. Redmond JM, Smith GW, Barofsky I et al. Physiologic tests to predict long-term outcome of total abdominal colectomy for intractable constipation. Am J Gastroenterol 1995; 90:748–53.

44. Rantis PC, Vernava AM, Daniel GL et al. Chronic constipation – is the work-up worth the cost? Dis Colon Rectum 1997; 40:280–6.

45. Lundin E, Karlbom U, Pahlman L et al. Outcome of segmental colonic resection for slow-transit constipation. Br J Surg 2002; 89:1270–4.

46. Kamm MA, Hawley PR, Lennard-Jones JE. Lateral division of puborectalis in the management of severe constipation. Br J Surg 1988; 75:661–3.

47. Marshall J, Hutson JM, Anticich N et al. Antegrade continence enemas in the treatment of slow-transit constipation. J Pediatr Surg 2001; 36:1227–30.

48. FitzHarris GP, Garcia-Aguilar J, Parker SC et al. Quality of life after subtotal colectomy for slow-transit constipation: both quality and quantity count. Dis Colon Rectum 2003; 46:433–40.

49. Feng Y, Jianjiang L. Functional outcomes of two types of subtotal colectomy for slow-transit constipation: ileosigmoidal anastomosis and cecorectal anastomosis. Am J Surg 2008; 195:73–7.

50. Marchesi F, Sarli L, Percalli L et al. Subtotal colectomy with antiperistaltic cecorectal anastomosis in the treatment of slow-transit constipation: long-term impact on quality of life. World J Surg 2007; 31:1658–64.

51. Kenefick NJ, Vaizey CJ, Cohen CR et al. Double-blind placebo-controlled crossover study of sacral nerve stimulation for idiopathic constipation. Br J Surg 2002; 89:1570–1.

52. Gattuso JM, Kamm MA. Clinical features of idiopathic megarectum and idiopathic megacolon. Gut 1997; 41:93–9.

    The only true prospective comparison of symptoms, pathophysiology and management between patients with idiopathic megarectum and megacolon.

53. Mimura T, Nicholls T, Storrie JB et al. Treatment of constipation in adults associated with idiopathic megarectum by behavioural retraining including biofeedback. Colorectal Dis 2002; 4:477–82.

54. Gladman MA, Scott SM, Lunniss PJ et al. Systematic review of surgical options for idiopathic megarectum and megacolon. Ann Surg 2005; 241:562–74.

    A definitive systematic review of the published data on surgical procedures for idiopathic megacolon and megarectum in adults.

55. Stabile G, Kamm MA, Hawley PR et al. Results of stoma formation for idiopathic megarectum and megacolon. Int J Colorectal Dis 1992; 7:82–4.

14

Anal fistula: evaluation and management

Peter J. Lunniss
Robin K.S. Phillips

Introduction

Anorectal sepsis is common, presenting as either an acute abscess or a chronic anal fistula. The majority of cases can be dealt with avoiding complication, but a small minority can present a major challenge to both sufferer and surgeon.

Although fistula in ano may be found in association with a variety of specific conditions, the majority seen in the UK today are classified as non-specific, idiopathic or cryptoglandular, their exact aetiology having not been fully proven, although the diseased anal gland in the intersphincteric space is considered central. Fistulas may be seen in association with Crohn's disease, tuberculosis, pilonidal disease, hidradenitis suppurativa, lymphogranu-loma venereum, presacral dermoids, rectal duplication, actinomycosis, trauma and foreign bodies.[1] An important association is malignancy, which may manifest itself as a discharging opening on the perineum from a pelvic source, but which may also arise in long-standing fistulas, either cryptoglandu-lar, as part of perianal Crohn's disease, or even in hidradenitis suppurativa.

The exact incidence of idiopathic anal fistula in the general population is not known, as most data come from hospital analysis in tertiary referral centres, which attract only the more difficult cases. Perhaps the most accurate information comes from Scandinavia, where incidences of between 8.6 and 10 per 10 000 have been reported.

All reported series have demonstrated a male pre-dominance, most reporting a male to female ratio of between 2:1 and 4:1, for reasons that are unclear. McColl[2] found no sex differences in histology or distribution of anal glands in 50 normal human anal canals, and we have found no differences in circulating sex hormone concentrations between sufferers of either sex and healthy controls. Furthermore, the sex difference is not limited to humans. The German Shepherd dog is a breed particularly prone to the development of anal fistula compared with other breeds, and this is not due to any differences in anal crypt or gland anatomy. There is a 3:1 male to female ratio of the incidence of canine fistulas, compared to a 1:1 ratio for the whole dog population, and the incidence of fistula is much lower in neutered dogs and bitches compared with those that are sexually intact.

Anal fistulas most commonly afflict people in their third, fourth or fifth decades.[3–5] There is little information on racial differences in incidence, although the peak incidence has been reported at a lower age in Nigerians and in African-Americans. Sedentary occupations cannot be implicated.[4] Whether bowel habit may be influential is unclear. Some authors take the view that diarrhoea may allow easier access of bacteria to the anal glands, especially in infants; others feel that hard stools are implicated by their abrasive passage through the anal canal.

The overall morbidity from fistula is difficult to assess in either individual or economic terms.

For the majority of patients with simple fistulas, the time spent off work with the parent abscess and subsequent fistula management may be relatively short. However, it is not that uncommon for a patient with a complex fistula to have had multiple hospital admissions for attempted cure over several years, only to end up incontinent, or with a permanent stoma, and permanently incapacitated. For these patients in particular, tertiary referral centres that have gained the necessary expertise are essential, expertise lying in the hands not only of the surgeons, but also the nurses, radiologists, physiologists and psychologists who all play an important part in management.

Aetiology

Anal glands and their link with anal fistulas have been recorded since the end of the 19th century. The function of the anal glands is uncertain. They have been shown to secrete mucin, but this has a different composition from that secreted by rectal mucosa. From comparative anatomical studies, McColl[2] showed that the anal glands are not vestigial remnants of sexual scent glands, and the suggestion that they are not true glands at all but rather vestigial epithelial remnants left after proctodeal invagination into the hindgut has not been substantiated.

Current thinking lays the blame at those anal glands situated in the intersphincteric space; these may constitute one-third to two-thirds of the total number of anal glands found in an anal canal.[4]

Eisenhammer[6] considered all non-specific abscesses and fistulas to be the result of extension of sepsis from an intramuscular anal gland, the sepsis being unable to drain spontaneously into the anal lumen because of infective obstruction of its connecting duct across the internal sphincter.

Parks[7] proposed that, should the initial abscess in relation to the intersphincteric anal gland subside, the diseased gland might become the seat of chronic infection with subsequent fistula formation. The fistula is thus a granulation tissue-lined track kept open by the infective source, which is the abscess around a diseased anal gland deep to the internal sphincter. Parks[7] studied 30 consecutive cases of anal fistula and found cystic dilatation of anal glands in eight,

which he attributed to acquired duct dilatation or more probably a congenital abnormality, a precursor to infection within a mucin-filled cavity.

There have been few studies which have examined the cryptoglandular hypothesis. Goligher et al.[8] found intersphincteric space sepsis in only 8 of 28 cases of acute anorectal sepsis; of 32 cases of anal fistula, only 14 had evidence of either intersphincteric sepsis or the track travelling within (rather than simply across) the intersphincteric space. However, Goligher et al. failed to acknowledge that a proportion of cases of acute sepsis have nothing to do with fistula and that some common fistulas (e.g. superficial fistulas and those arising from a chronic anal fissure) have an aetiology separate from that postulated by Parks.

Another question arises from studies of the microbiology of fistula tissue. Although infection and its effective drainage are the primary problems in the acute stage, and although failure to treat secondary extensions and abscesses adequately will inevitably lead to recurrence, the possibility that the anal gland becomes the seat of chronic infection in the established fistula has found little support in the only two studies directed at this aspect of the hypothesis.[9,10] A more attractive theory as to why idiopathic fistulas persist is that they become (at least partly) epithelialised, a factor responsible for failure of healing of fistulas at other sites in the body. A histological study of the intersphincteric component of 18 consecutive idiopathic anal fistulas showed that although an association between anal gland and fistula may be demonstrated (as had been suggested by Gordon-Watson and Dodd[11] in 1935) in a minority of cases, epithelialisation from either or both ends of the fistula track is a more common finding.[12] Indeed, the presence of epithelium and local production of antimicrobial peptides may explain the relative paucity of organisms found in chronic fistulas.[13]

Spread of sepsis from an acutely infected anal gland may occur in any of the three planes, vertical, horizontal or circumferential. Caudal spread is the simplest and most usual way by which infection is thought to disseminate to present acutely as a perianal abscess (labelled **a** in **Fig. 14.1**). Cephalad extension in the same space will result in a high intermuscular abscess (**b** in Fig. 14.1) or a supralevator pararectal (syn. pelvirectal) abscess (**c** in Fig. 14.1), depending on the relation of the sepsis to the longitudinal muscle layer. Lateral spread across

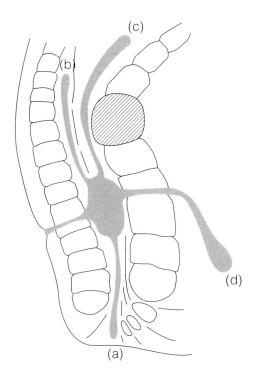

Figure 14.1 • The possible courses of spread of sepsis from the diseased anal gland in the intersphincteric space. See text for explanation. Reproduced from Parks AG. The pathogenesis and treatment of fistula-in-ano. Br Med J 1961; i:463–9. With permission from BMJ Publishing Group Ltd.

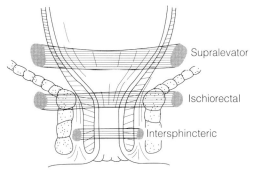

Types of horseshoe extension

Figure 14.2 • The three planes in which sepsis may spread circumferentially. Reproduced from Parks AG, Gordon PH, Hardcastle JD. A classification of fistula-in-ano. Br J Surg 1976; 63:1–12. © British Journal of Surgery Society Ltd. Permission is granted by John Wiley & Sons Ltd on behalf on the BJSS Ltd.

Management of acute sepsis

The majority of chronic anal fistulas are preceded by an episode of acute anorectal sepsis, although acute sepsis does not inevitably lead to fistula formation. The reported rates of recurrent abscess or fistula development following simple incision and drainage range from 17% to 87%. The optimal management of acute sepsis should reside in an understanding of aetiology. Pilonidal infection, hidradenitis and perianal Crohn's disease are usually fairly easy to recognise by history and examination. Pus in the perianal space may result from caudal spread of intersphincteric (cryptoglandular) infection or from simple skin appendage infection. Similarly, pus in the ischiorectal space may or may not be related to presumed anal gland disease.

Patients with acute anorectal sepsis usually present via the accident and emergency department rather than the outpatient clinic. Those with perianal sepsis tend to present early, 2 or 3 days after onset of symptoms, with pain and a palpable tender lump close to the anal margin, and usually with no constitutional symptoms. Patients with ischiorectal abscesses tend to present later with more vague discomfort, but because much more pus may accumulate in the large relatively avascular loose areolar tissue of the ischiorectal fossa, they often have fever and constitutional upset. Examination may reveal tender induration over the abscess rather than an exquisitely tender, well-defined lump as found when

the external sphincter will reach the ischiorectal fossa (**d** in Fig. 14.1), where further caudal spread will result in the abscess pointing at the skin as an ischiorectal abscess; upward spread may penetrate the levators to reach the supralevator pararectal space. Circumferential spread (**Fig. 14.2**) may occur in any of the three planes, intermuscular (synonymous with intramuscular and equivalent to intersphincteric but with no restriction to a level beneath the anorectal ring), ischiorectal or supralevator. All those conditions which Eisenhammer[14] considered not to be of cryptoglandular origin he placed into the miscellaneous group of acute anorectal non-cryptoglandular non-fistulous abscesses (**Fig. 14.3**). These included the submucous abscess (arising from an infected haemorrhoid, sclerotherapy or trauma), the mucocutaneous or marginal abscess (infected haematoma), the perianal abscess (follicular skin infection), some ischiorectal abscesses (primary infection or foreign body) and the pelvirectal supralevator abscess originating in pelvic disease.

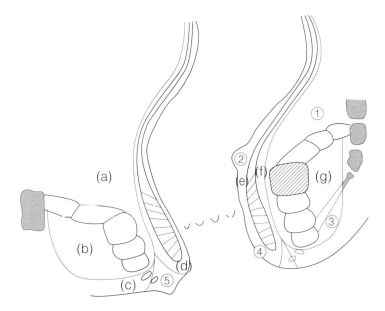

Figure 14.3 • The acute anorectal non-cryptoglandular non-fistulous abscesses of Eisenhammer: **(a)** pelvirectal supralevator space; **(b)** ischiorectal space; **(c)** perianal or superficial ischiorectal space; **(d)** marginal or mucocutaneous space; **(e)** submucous space; **(f)** intermuscular (syn. intersphincteric) space; **(g)** deep postanal space. 1, Pelvirectal supralevator abscess; 2, submucous abscess; 3, ischiorectal abscess; 4, mucocutaneous or marginal abscess; 5, perianal or subcutaneous abscess. Reproduced from Eisenhammer S. The final evaluation and classification of the surgical treatment of the primary anorectal cryptoglandular intermuscular (intersphincteric) fistulous abscess and fistula. Dis Colon Rectum 1978; 21:237–54. With permission from Lippincolf, williams and wilkins.

the sepsis is perianal. Sepsis higher up in the sphincter complex may present with rectal pain, and possibly disturbance of micturition, and there may be no external signs of pathology. The rare submucosal abscess is revealed on digital examination of the anal canal as a distinct tender bulge, and the patient may have reported the passage of pus from the anal canal with relief of symptoms.

 Clues as to the aetiology of perineal sepsis may be gleaned from microbiology of the drained pus:[15,16] if skin organisms alone are cultured and the acute abscess adequately drained, the patient may be told with confidence that recurrence should not occur and that a fistula will not result. If gut organisms are cultured, however, it is probable but not inevitable that there is an underlying fistula. The results of microbiology are therefore sensitive (100%) but not totally specific (60–80%), and of course are not available at the time of initial surgery.

Determination of the presence or absence of sepsis in the intersphincteric space (irrespective of the site of the main abscess or whether an internal opening is demonstrable) has been shown to be the most accurate way of determining the presence of an underlying fistula,[17] although it has been argued that such exploration is beyond the expertise of a general surgical trainee untrained in proctology for whom simple incision and drainage represents the safest option in the acute stage.

Those who advocate a more aggressive approach to acute sepsis do so on the basis that incision and drainage can only be effective if the abscess is not cryptoglandular,[14] that definitive treatment in the initial stage obviates further surgery, and that such a policy reduces the incidence of complex fistulas arising through incompletely drained sepsis. Certainly, the reported recurrence/fistula rate following primary fistulotomy (0–7%) would support this. There are drawbacks, however: internal openings are evident in only about one-third of cases; the acute situation lends itself to the creation of false tracks and internal openings; and the unknown proportion of patients with cryptoglandular sepsis who might be cured by incision and drainage alone would not be well served by a procedure associated with a greater risk of flatus incontinence and soiling.

A prospective randomised trial involving 200 patients presenting with anal sepsis compared simple drainage to drainage plus primary fistulotomy, when the fistula was deemed low (subcutaneous, intersphincteric or low trans-sphincteric). This yielded recurrence rates of 36.7% in the drainage-alone group and 5% in those in whom the underlying fistula was laid open.[18] There was no reported incontinence following simple drainage, compared with 2.8% in the fistulotomy group. This was the largest of five randomised trials subjected to meta-analysis[19] which concluded that fistulotomy resulted in 83% reduction in risk of recurrence at final follow-up (RR 0.17, 95% CI 0.09–0.32, $P < 0.001$), but was associated with a tendency to a higher risk of flatus incontinence and soiling (RR 2.46, 95% CI 0.75–8.06, $P = 0.140$).

A policy (in experienced hands) of simple incision when a fistula is not evident, and primary fistulotomy when a fistula is evident and low (or a draining loose seton placed if there is any doubt about the level, or concern about continence) is sensible, as long as the patient has been adequately counselled.

Patients with an established fistula usually give a history of intermittent pain and purulent discharge from an opening on the perineum, the pain building up until relief is felt when the pus escapes. Patients in whom the internal opening is rectal, and those with large internal openings irrespective of site, may pass flatus and stool through the external opening(s).

Classification of anal fistula

Successful surgical management of anal fistula depends upon accurate knowledge of anal sphincter anatomy and the fistula's course through it. Failure to understand either may result in fistula recurrence or incontinence. To this end, classification of pathology is extremely important.

The most comprehensive and practical classification, and the one most widely used presently, is that devised by Sir Alan Parks at St Mark's, based on a study of 400 fistulas treated there.[20]

The cryptoglandular hypothesis is central to this classification, which holds firstly that the majority of fistulas arise from an abscess in the inter-sphincteric plane and secondly that the relation of the primary track to the external sphincter is paramount in surgical management. Four main groups exist: intersphincteric, trans-sphincteric, supra-sphincteric and extrasphincteric. These groups can be further subdivided according to the presence and course of any extensions or secondary tracks.

Intersphincteric fistulas (**Fig. 14.4**), constituting 45% of cases in the original St Mark's series, are usually simple; however, others have a high blind track, or a high opening into the rectum or no perineal opening, or even have pelvic extension, or arise from pelvic disease. Trans-sphincteric fistulas (**Fig. 14.5**) (29%) have a primary track that passes through the external sphincter at varying levels into the ischiorectal fossa. Such fistulas may be uncomplicated, consisting only of the primary track, or can have a high blind track that may terminate below or above the levator ani muscles. Suprasphincteric fistulas (**Fig. 14.6**) (20% in the 1976 series[20]) run up to a level above puborectalis and then curl down through the levators and ischiorectal fossa to reach the skin. Extrasphincteric fistulas (**Fig. 14.7**) (5%) run without relation to the sphincters and are classified according to their pathogenesis. In addition to horizontal and vertical spread, sepsis may spread circumferentially in any of the three spaces: intersphincteric, ischiorectal or pararectal.

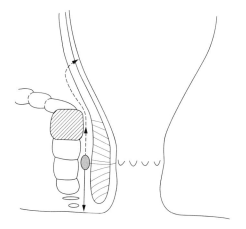

Figure 14.4 • The possible courses of an intersphincteric fistula. Reproduced from Marks CG, Ritchie JR. Anal fistulas at St Mark's Hospital. Br J Surg 1977; 64:84–91. © British Journal of Surgery Society Ltd. Permission is granted by John Wiley & Sons Ltd on behalf on the BJSS Ltd.

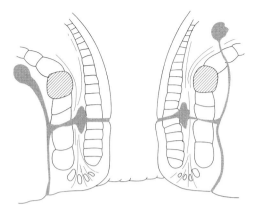

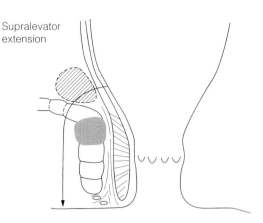

Supralevator
extension

Figure 14.5 • A trans-sphincteric fistula with blind infralevator ischiorectal extension (left) and supralevator pararectal extension (right). Reproduced from Parks AG, Gordon PH, Hardcastle JD. A classification of fistula-in-ano. Br J Surg 1976; 63:1–12. © British Journal of Surgery Society Ltd. Permission is granted by John Wiley & Sons Ltd on behalf on the BJSS Ltd.

Figure 14.7 • Extrasphincteric fistula running without relation to the sphincter complex. Reproduced from Marks CG, Ritchie JK. Anal fistulas at St Mark's Hospital. Br J Surg 1977; 64:84–91. © British Journal of Surgery Society Ltd. Permission is granted by John Wiley & Sons Ltd on behalf on the BJSS Ltd.

The St Mark's classification does have a few drawbacks,[21] but these are of little clinical significance. Superficial fistulas and those associated with bridged fissures are not acknowledged by a classification whose emphasis is the intersphincteric

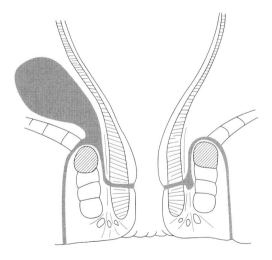

Figure 14.6 • Simple suprasphincteric fistula (right) and more complex form with associated secondary pelvic abscess (left). Reproduced from Parks AG, Gordon PH, Hardcastle JD. A classification of fistula-in-ano. Br J Surg 1976; 63:1–12. © British Journal of Surgery Society Ltd. Permission is granted by John Wiley & Sons Ltd on behalf on the BJSS Ltd.

space. There can be clinical difficulty in differentiating between a simple intersphincteric fistula and a very low trans-sphincteric fistula that crosses the lowermost fibres of the subcutaneous portion of the external sphincter. And some argue whether suprasphincteric tracks can be part of a classification based on cryptoglandular pathology (arguing indeed that many are iatrogenic). The extreme rarity of suprasphincteric fistulas and the difficulty of distinguishing them from high trans-sphincteric tracks even raise doubts about their very existence. However, clinical differentiation from high trans-sphincteric fistulas is in most cases immaterial since the same methods of treatment would be employed.

Assessment

Clinical

A full history and examination including proctosigmoidoscopy are essential in all cases to exclude any associated conditions. Clinical assessment involves five essential points, enumerated by Goodsall and Miles at the end of the 19th century:

1. location of the internal opening;
2. location of the external opening;
3. course of the primary track;
4. presence of secondary extensions;
5. presence of other diseases complicating the fistula.

The relative positions of the external and internal openings will indicate the likely course of the primary track, and the presence of any palpable induration, especially supralevator, should alert the surgeon to a secondary track. The distance of the external opening from the anal verge may assist in differentiating an intersphincteric from a trans-sphincteric fistula; the greater the distance, the greater the likelihood of a complex cephalad extension.[4] Goodsall's rule generally applies in that the likely site of the internal opening can be predicted by the position around the anal circumference of the external opening. Exceptions to this rule include anteriorly located openings more than 3 cm from the anal verge (which may be anterior extensions of posterior horseshoe fistulas) and fistulas associated with other diseases, especially Crohn's and malignancy.

Thus, the first step in examining the anus is to identify the position of the external opening (or openings). Next, the perianal area should be carefully palpated with a well-lubricated finger to feel for the presence and direction of induration, which will indicate the course of the primary track (**Fig. 14.8**). If the track is not palpable, it is probable that the fistula is not intersphincteric or low trans-sphincteric. Digital examination within the anorectal lumen is then performed with the specific intention of feeling for any indentation/induration as the sign marking the site of the internal opening. Asking the patient to contract the anal sphincters allows an assessment of the position of the primary track in relation to the puborectalis sling (if posterior) or upper border of the external anal sphincter (if anterior), although it must be remembered that in trans-sphincteric fistulas the level of the internal opening may not be the same as that at which the primary track crosses the external sphincter (which may be higher, especially if the internal opening is above the dentate line). The finger is then advanced into the rectum and any supralevator induration is sought (it feels like bone and is easier to notice when it is unilateral as there will be asymmetry) (**Fig. 14.9**). Digital assessment of the primary track by an experienced coloproctologist has been shown to be 85% accurate.[22]

Examination under anaesthesia complements examination in the awake patient. The internal opening may be easily seen at proctoscopy, aided if necessary by gentle downward retraction of the dentate line, which may expose openings concealed by prominent valves or papillae. Lateral traction of an opened Eisenhammer proctoscope may reveal dimpling at the internal opening through its underlying fibrous inelasticity. Sometimes, the site of the responsible crypt may be seen only as scar tissue if the internal opening is not patent. Digital massage of the track may reveal the site of the internal opening as a bead of pus. If the track is simple, a

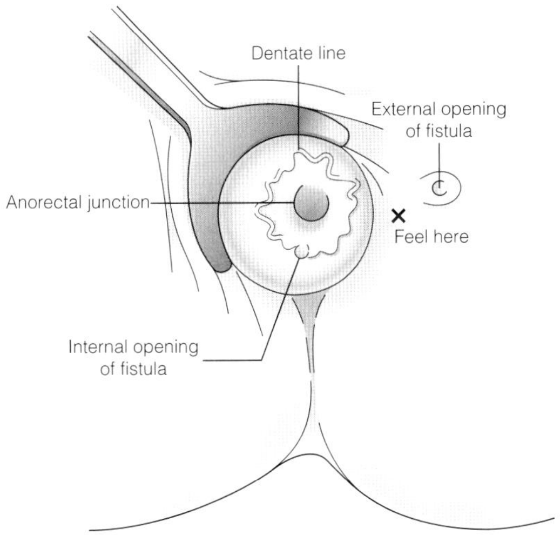

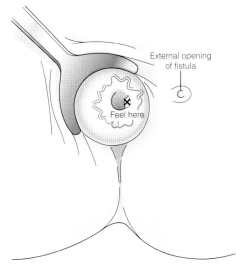

Figure 14.8 • Palpating for the direction and depth of the primary tract. Reproduced from Phillips RKS. Operative management of low cryptoglandular fistula-in-ano. Operat Tech Gen Surg 2001; 3(3):134–41. With permission from Elsevier.

Figure 14.9 • Palpating for the presence of induration, indicating either a high primary tract or secondary extension in the roof of the ischiorectal fossa or supralevator space. Reproduced from Phillips RKS. Operative management of low cryptoglandular fistula-in-ano. Operat Tech Gen Surg 2001; 3(3):134–41. With permission from Elsevier.

probe may traverse its entire length, but if the probe comes to lie above or remote from the dentate line, a direct association between the track and the adjacent anoderm cannot be assumed.[23] The instillation of various agents along the track via the external opening has also been advocated, including saline, hydrogen peroxide and dyes such as methylene blue and indigo carmine. In practical terms, instillation of dilute hydrogen peroxide is the easiest way of locating the internal opening, as staining is avoided.[23,24]

Careful probing can delineate primary and secondary tracks. If the internal and external openings are easily detected but the probe cannot easily traverse the path of the track, it is possible that there is a high extension, and a probe passed via each opening may then delineate the primary track. Failure to negotiate probes around a horseshoe posterior trans-sphincteric fistula suggests at least one acute bend in the track, within the intersphincteric space and crossing the external sphincter, or in the roof of the ischiorectal fossa, in which case anatomy will only be defined once surgery is under way (**Fig. 14.10**). Persistence of granulation tissue after curettage during the operation is an indication of a secondary extension.[24]

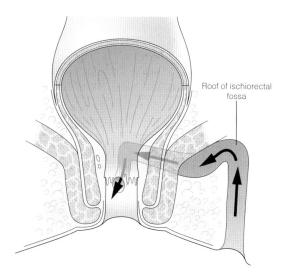

Roof of ischiorectal fossa

Figure 14.10 • Trans-sphincteric horseshoe fistulas may have several sharp bends along their course, preventing exact delineation unless the ischiorectal fossa is opened widely (to reach the acute bend in the roof of the ischiorectal fossa), and often necessitating dislocation of the posterior sphincter from its ligamentous attachments (to ascertain the site at which the tract crosses the external sphincter). Reproduced from Phillips RKS. Operative management of low cryptoglandular fistula-in-ano. Operat Tech Gen Surg 2001; 3(3):134–41. With permission from Elsevier.

Imaging

Careful examination of a fistula under anaesthesia has been considered the most important part of any assessment.[23] However, previous surgery leads to scarring and deformity, as well as the creation of unusual primary tracks, which can make clinical assessment extremely difficult. Until recently, techniques aimed at helping in fistula assessment have proved disappointing. The advent of endoanal ultrasound and magnetic resonance imaging (MRI), however, has resulted in a plethora of reports assessing and comparing imaging modalities, which has been recently comprehensively reviewed.[25]

In summary, the introduction of more accurate methods has rendered fistulography almost obsolete, but the technique should be considered if an extrasphincteric track is a possibility. Computed tomography suffers other disadvantages, and similarly is indicated only when there is suspicion that the fistula arises from an intra-abdominal or pelvic source.

Anal endosonography (AES) is relatively cheap and easy to perform, but is operator dependent and has limited focal range, which makes evaluation of pathology beyond the sphincters (either lateral to or above) difficult to assess, areas from which difficulty in clinical assessment often arises. Also, sepsis and scarring can confuse fistula assessment in those who have undergone previous surgery. Given the superiority of MRI, perhaps the main role of AES in patients with anal fistula is in the determination of internal and external sphincter integrity, although AES is superior to clinical evaluation.[26] Good agreement has been found between the newer imaging modalities of hydrogen peroxide-enhanced three-dimensional AES and endoanal MRI, but findings have not been compared to the best standard, i.e. healing after surgery, and neither technique is widely available.

The potential advantages of MRI include the lack of ionising radiation, the ability to image in any plane and the high soft-tissue resolution.

 Short tau inversion recovery (STIR) sequencing (a fat-suppression technique) to highlight the presence of pus and granulation tissue without the need for any contrast media[27] was used in a prospective study involving 35 patients at St Mark's Hospital that favourably compared MRI interpretations with the independently documented operative findings.[28]

Further prospective studies have confirmed that the technique certainly challenges operative assessment by an experienced coloproctologist as the 'gold standard'. A recent prospective study has demonstrated a therapeutic impact of MRI in the management of 10% of patients treated for primary anal fistulas,[29] although the therapeutic impact is much greater when used to assess recurrent fistulas.[30]

Perhaps a logical approach is that patients with (suspected) primary anal fistulas undergo AES, and those in whom there is clinical or sonographic suspicion of complexity go on to MRI. There is strong evidence that all recurrent fistulas should be examined using MRI preoperatively, and that the surgeon uses the scans to aid surgery. The accuracy of MRI also means that we are now able to refute or confirm the presence of sepsis in those patients with symptoms but in whom clinical examination is unrevealing, and in the prospective assessment of newer methods of attempted fistula eradication.

Physiological

The correlation between subjective assessment of an individual's continence and physiological static measurements recorded in a laboratory may be debatable, but the argument for physiological assessment (anal canal length, pressures along it, anorectal sensitivity, sphincter integrity and pudendal nerve conduction studies) in the clinical context of a patient with a complex fistula (or one deemed to have, or be at risk of, compromise in function) is nowadays strong. Continence may be regarded as a balance between rectal pressure and the power of the sphincters to overcome this, orchestrated by anorectal sensation.

 Milligan and Morgan[31] stressed the importance of the anorectal ring in fistula surgery: 'If this ring be cut, loss of control surely results, yet as long as the narrowest complete ring of muscle remains, control is preserved. All the anal sphincter muscles below this ring may be divided in any manner without harmful loss of control.'

Certainly, complete division of the puborectalis sling in suprasphincteric and extrasphincteric fistulas results in total incontinence to all rectal contents, but division of muscles below the ring may

result in equally devastating consequences. It is reasonable to suppose that the higher the level at which the primary track crosses the sphincter complex, the greater the possibility of impaired function after fistulotomy; and the weaker the sphincters before surgical intervention, the greater the likelihood of such morbidity.

Traditionally, more importance has been apportioned to the external than to the internal anal sphincter in the context of muscle preservation in anal fistula surgery. Indeed, the importance of eradication of the presumed aetiological source, the diseased anal gland in the intersphincteric space, led Parks[7] to advocate internal sphincterectomy (excision of that segment of internal sphincter overlying the diseased gland) as an essential part of surgical management. Nowadays, most surgeons divide rather than excise the circular muscle, but the concept of getting rid of the intersphincteric source remains widely held.

To determine the physiological and functional effects of fistula surgery, we conducted a prospective study[32] of 37 patients successfully treated for either intersphincteric (15 patients) or trans-sphincteric fistulas. All patients underwent division of the internal anal sphincter and anoderm below the level of the primary track; 15 of the 22 patients with trans-sphincteric fistulas also underwent division of the external sphincter, at least to the level of the dentate line, whereas the remaining seven patients with trans-sphincteric fistulas were successfully treated without recourse to external sphincter division. As might be predicted, distal anal canal and maximum resting pressures were reduced in all patients after surgery, external sphincter division resulting in no greater reduction of maximum resting pressure than occurred after internal sphincter division alone. Squeeze pressures were unaffected in those in whom the external sphincter had been preserved, but division in the 15 patients who underwent fistulotomy of trans-sphincteric tracks resulted in significant reductions in distal anal canal squeeze pressures and maximum squeeze pressure.

However, functional outcome was not related to division of the external sphincter, with an equal incidence of minor disturbances of continence reported by those in whom it had been preserved (53% vs. 50% respectively). Furthermore, the severity of postoperative symptoms was no different between the two groups, being related to reduced postoperative resting pressures, reduced maximum resting pressure and higher thresholds of anal electro-sensitivity in the sector of surgery, rather than to postoperative squeeze pressures.

It appears that total sphincter conservation would be optimal in terms of functional outcome, but the drawback is that no sphincter-preserving method heals the underlying fistula as surely as lay-open. This is important, because although this study revealed a relatively high incidence of functional disturbance, the vast majority of patients were satisfied with their management and tolerated a reduction in function as a reasonable price to pay in order to be rid of chronic anal sepsis. Nevertheless, there is a functional price to pay, even for curing the more minor forms of fistula, and this justifies continued attempts at methods that preserve sphincter integrity and function when appropriate. Perhaps preoperative physiology highlights those at most risk of functional disturbance after fistulotomy, but normal results do not render the patient immune from risk.

Principles of fistula surgery

Acute sepsis is an indication for early surgical intervention and drainage. However, in cases where a more complex procedure than lay-open is contemplated, acute sepsis should have been eradicated long before, leaving well-established chronic tracks. A loose seton may be required to achieve adequate drainage of the primary track. Secondary tracks should be either laid open, curetted or drained, according to their position in relation to the levators. Some authors advise bowel preparation before fistula surgery, although laid-open wounds in the perineum heal remarkably well despite the continual bacterial load. Most authors recommend parenteral antibiotics peroperatively and postoperatively for any of the more complex procedures.

In the UK, fistula surgery is usually performed under general anaesthesia, but in North America local or regional anaesthesia is more widely employed. Similarly, in the UK most anal fistula surgery is performed with the patient in the lithotomy position, although the prone jack-knife position is gaining in popularity, at least among some surgeons. Prophylaxis against development of venous thrombosis is advised, and in the UK is usually achieved with a combination of low-dose subcutaneous heparin and elasticated stockings. Finally, the oper-

ative findings and treatment should be recorded. The St Mark's Hospital fistula operation sheet (**Fig. 14.11**) based on Parks' classification provides an excellent standardised format for documentation both by description and by illustration.

Surgical treatment

Lay-open remains the surest way of eliminating an anal fistula. The multiplicity of techniques designed to preserve sphincter function and at the same time eradicate fistula pathology reflects their relative lack of success. A degree of caution and scepticism may be appropriately apportioned when assessing reported results of the various approaches towards complex fistula, since:

1. patient populations may be markedly different;
2. fistula classification may be variable;
3. reports of successes may not be tempered by honest reporting of failures;
4. reports of success in terms of fistula cure have historically not always been accompanied by reports of changes in continence;
5. despite the increasing drive for evidence-based medicine, the use of adequately powered prospective randomised trials is perhaps unachievable, because of individual fistula (and sphincter) variability and individual surgeon preference and skill;
6. follow-up may be inadequate.

Fistulotomy

Fistulotomy means laying open and allowing to heal by secondary intention. Its application should, in the first instance, be restricted to situations where a significant degree of incontinence would not result. In principle, high trans-sphincteric (especially anterior tracks in women) and suprasphincteric tracks should not be treated by one-stage fistulotomy. Intersphincteric and low trans-sphincteric tracks are probably best treated by this method, but the decision whether to lay open rests on the skill and experience of the surgeon after informed advice to the patient.

Abcarian[33] recommends the following technique: after initial assessment of the track, a crypt hook is placed into the internal opening which is laid open by diathermy cautery, the latter maintaining a dry operative field and thus allowing easy identification of granulation tissue. If examination with the

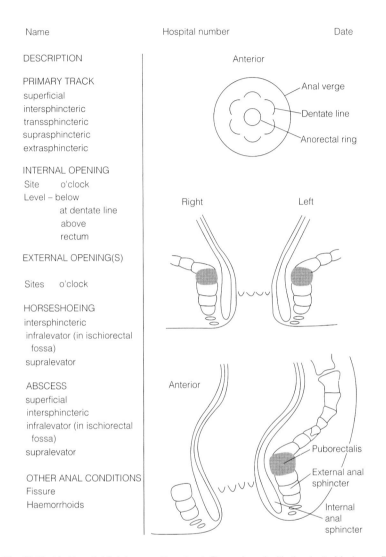

ST. MARK'S HOSPITAL
FISTULA OPERATION NOTES

Name   Hospital number   Date

DESCRIPTION   Anterior

PRIMARY TRACK
superficial
intersphincteric
transsphincteric
suprasphincteric
extrasphincteric

Anal verge
Dentate line
Anorectal ring

INTERNAL OPENING
Site   o'clock
Level – below
          at dentate line
          above
          rectum

Right   Left

EXTERNAL OPENING(S)

Sites   o'clock

HORSESHOEING
intersphincteric
infralevator (in ischiorectal
   fossa)
supralevator

ABSCESS   Anterior
superficial
intersphincteric
infralevator (in ischiorectal
   fossa)
supralevator

Puborectalis
External anal
sphincter

OTHER ANAL CONDITIONS
Fissure
Haemorrhoids

Internal
anal
sphincter

Figure 14.11 • The St Mark's Hospital fistula operation sheet. Reproduced with thanks to Mr James P.S. Thomson Emeritus Consultant Surgeon, St Mark's.

crypt hook reveals the primary track to be intersphincteric or to involve only the lowermost fibres of the external anal sphincter, the tissue overlying the probe is divided along its length. If, however, the probe enters the depths outside the external sphincter, it is left in place and a second probe gently passed via the external opening, and the two probes manipulated until they can be felt or heard to touch. That portion of the track outside the external sphincter is laid open, and the internal sphincter divided over the crypt hook. An assessment is then made as to how much voluntary muscle lies below the track and the decision is made either to lay the track open or to resort to a sphincter-saving procedure.

 Marsupialisation, i.e. suturing the divided wound edge to the edges of the curetted fibrous track, results in a smaller wound and faster healing.[34,35]

Secondary extensions from the primary track can be dealt with in two ways. The traditional method in the UK is to lay these open widely to allow maximal drainage, which is followed by healing by secondary intention. As long as the external sphincter is intact, the residual scarring after healing is remarkably little. In the USA, the use of incisions, counter-incisions and the placement of encircling drains is sometimes preferred; these drains are left in for 2–4 weeks, with more rapid healing and less deformity claimed.

Fistulotomy and immediate reconstitution

Parkash et al.[36] reported a series of 120 patients treated by fistulotomy and immediate reconstruction of the divided musculature, and with primary wound closure. The reported results were impressive: 88% of wounds had healed by 2 weeks, there was a 4% recurrence rate and all patients were satisfied with the functional outcome. However, 118 of the 120 fistulas were classified as low intersphincteric or simple trans-sphincteric, and the authors admitted that similar success would not be expected with more complex fistulas. The technique has been applied to a small cohort of patients with recurrent complex fistulas, not amenable to fistulotomy, with impressive results in terms of healing rates, manometric and functional outcomes, and with no report of dehiscence of the reconstituted sphincter.[37]

 A randomised trial of 55 patients with non-recurrent complex fistulas comparing fistulotomy combined with immediate sphincter reconstitution and advancement flap repair yielded equivalent results in respect to healing and functional outcomes.[38]

Fistulectomy

 The technique of fistulectomy, which excises rather than incises the fistula track, has been criticised on the basis that the greater tissue loss leads to delayed healing.[39]

However, Lewis[40] advocates fistulectomy, but by a core-out technique rather than excision of the track, because he claims that:

1. the precise course of the track is more accurately determined by core-out under direct vision, and does not involve the passage of probes along the track and thus creation of false tracks – a probe is used only to open the external opening and assist in inserting a stay suture around it;
2. coring out the primary track reduces the risk of missing secondary tracks, which are seen as transected granulation tissue and which may be followed by the same technique;
3. the relation of the primary track to the external anal sphincter may be correctly ascertained before any sphincter muscle is divided;
4. a complete specimen is available for histology.

Once the track has been cored out, from the external towards the internal opening using either scissors or cautery dissection, the decision as to whether the tunnel left after the core-out can be safely laid open is made. For a non-recurrent single trans-sphincteric track, Lewis recommends simple anatomical closure of the cored-out tunnel, with mucosal closure and closure of the holes in the muscles. The wound outside the sphincters is lightly packed.

Of 67 low fistulas treated by Lewis[41] between 1985 and 1992 by coring out and laying open the resultant tunnel, there was one recurrence. Of 32 patients with high trans-sphincteric or supra-sphincteric fistulas treated between 1972 and 1992 by core-out and simple anatomical closure, a temporary colostomy was raised in four and there were three recurrences. In the case of recurrent or more complex fistulas, Lewis recommends the adoption of other sphincter-conserving methods, since excessive scarring and the larger defect created by coring out this tissue makes simple anatomical closure inappropriate.

Setons

The loose seton

Setons may be classified as loose, tight or chemical according to their different properties and modes of action. A thread, loosely tied, is often used as a marker of a fistula track when its exact position and level in relation to the external sphincter is unclear at surgery, perhaps because of scarring from previous surgery or because of the depth of sphincter muscle relaxation under anaesthesia. In such circumstances, the proportions of muscle above and below the fistula may be more accurately determined when the patient is awake and with the track palpably delineated by the thread. Similarly, a loosely tied thread can be used as a drain of acute sepsis, to allow subsidence of acute inflammatory changes and safer definitive fistula surgery.

More specifically in the field of sphincter and continence preservation, the loose seton can be used in three ways: to preserve the entire external sphincter; to preserve part of the voluntary muscle; or as part of a staged fistulotomy in order to reduce the consequences of division of large amounts of muscle in one procedure.

The key points of a staged fistulotomy are the amount of muscle divided at each stage and the time allowed for fibrosis to develop between the divided muscle edges before a further length of sphincter is divided. Ramanujan et al.[42] reported a series of 45 patients with suprasphincteric fistulas in whom the first stage involved laying open the upper sphincter while preserving the distal sphincter within a seton; the seton-enclosed muscle was divided about 2 months later. There was just one recurrence and in only one patient did any disturbance of continence (intermittent leakage of flatus) result. Others have preserved the upper sphincter within a seton while laying open the lower portion. Kuypers[43] described this technique in 10 patients with trans-sphincteric fistulas with supralevator extensions opening into the rectum. The seton-enclosed muscle was divided 3 months after the first stage. There were no recurrences, one patient was incontinent and six reported minor soiling.

Parks and Stitz[44] reported a series of 80 patients from St Mark's Hospital with trans-sphincteric and suprasphincteric fistulas in whom, at the first stage, the lower one-third to one-half of the sphincter was divided and at the second stage a few months later either the seton removed (if all had healed) or the seton-enclosed muscle divided (if there were high tracks or cavities that had failed to close in). About 38% of patients required division of the upper sphincter to achieve healing; unfortunately, the functional outcome in the two groups of patients was not clearly described.

Later at St Mark's the loose seton was used with the aim of entire external sphincter preservation. Tracks and extensions outside the sphincters were widely laid open, and in the past the internal sphincter was then divided to the level of the internal opening (or higher if there was a cephalad intersphincteric extension). Subsequently, attempts at internal sphincter conservation were made. In the case of the high posterior trans-sphincteric track, the passage of the primary track across the sphincter complex may sometimes be accurately judged only after division of the anococcygeal ligaments, thereby dislocating the posterior sphincter attachments but allowing access to the deep postanal space.[45] The seton, passed along the primary track across the external sphincter, is then tied loosely to encircle the denuded voluntary muscle. Postoperatively, the wounds are managed by daily digitation and irrigation rather than by tight packing, with a possible repeat examination under anaesthesia at 7–10 days to ensure that all tracks have been dealt with and that healing is progressing correctly. At outpatient review, if there is evidence of good healing both of the wounds and around the seton, the latter is removed at 2–3 months. Any suspicion of ongoing sepsis requires repeat examination under anaesthesia.

A series of 34 consecutive patients with complex idiopathic trans-sphincteric fistulas treated at St Mark's Hospital between 1977 and 1984 showed that cure of the fistula without recourse to external sphincter division occurred in 44%.[46] Of those in whom the method had been successful, 83% reported full continence compared with only 32% of those in whom the external sphincter had subsequently been divided. Of the 16 patients in whom the technique failed, nine reported some degree of incontinence to formed stool; none of the patients in whom the external sphincter had been preserved reported any such disturbance of sphincter function.

A success rate of 67% was achieved in the 24 patients with similar fistulas treated in the same way between 1990 and 1991.[45] Kennedy and Zegarra[47] used a loose silk seton to treat 32 patients with high trans-sphincteric and suprasphincteric anal fistulas, and reported a success rate of 78%; the method was more successful with anterior (88%) than posterior (66%) fistulas. However, of the 25 patients successfully treated, nine had some alteration of continence. The importance of adequate follow-up to determine long-term outcomes following a particular technique has been exemplified by Buchanan et al.,[48] who reviewed 20 patients treated by this method a minimum of 10 years following surgery. Although in the short term 13 of the 20 healed, by 10 years only four had remained so.

If the technique fails and it is certain that this is not due to any missed secondary extensions (detectable by MRI), untoward aetiology, etc., there are several options available: (i) the patient may be happy living with a 'controlled' fistula with a long-term draining seton [Editor's note: my own personal preference is for a permanent loose seton made of No. 1 Ethibond with just one knot to avoid bulkiness and to give comfort (nylon setons tend to be sharp, silastic setons to have bulky knots)]; (ii) the tight seton method may be employed; (iii) a fistulotomy may be performed and the functional results assessed postoperatively; or (iv) fistulotomy may be combined with the raising of a defunctioning colostomy, time allowed for full healing, before sphincter repair and then restoration of intestinal continuity at a final stage. The decision made must be between the individual patient and the surgeon.

The tight seton

The rationale of the tight or cutting seton is similar to that of the staged fistulotomy technique, in that the divided muscle is not allowed to spring apart but there is supposed to be gradual severance through the sphincter followed by fibrosis. Goldberg and Garcia-Aquilar[49] recommend the use of a tight seton whenever the fistula encircles more than 30% of the sphincter complex and when local sepsis or fibrosis precludes the raising of an advancement flap. The portion of the track outside the sphincters is laid open, although others in the USA have recommended Penrose drainage of horseshoe limbs. The anoderm and perianal skin overlying that portion of the sphincter encircled by the seton are incised and the intersphincteric space drained by internal sphincterotomy, extended cephalad if necessary to drain any high intersphincteric (intermuscular) extension. Tightening of the seton (Goldberg uses a rubber band) does not commence until any suppuration has resolved, usually at 3 weeks postoperatively. Tightening is repeated every 2 weeks using a silk tie or Barron band until the seton has cut through.

Goldberg described the use of the cutting seton in 13 patients with trans-sphincteric fistulas between 1988 and 1992, and found that the average time for the seton to cut through was 16 weeks (range 8–36 weeks) with no recurrences at a median follow-up of 24 months (range 4–60 months). As might be expected, this cure rate was tempered by a relatively high incidence of functional morbidity: one patient suffered major incontinence, and a further seven patients (54%) complained of minor persistent loss of control to flatus or episodic loss of liquid stool.

The critical aspects of management by the cutting seton must be firstly the elimination of acute sepsis and secondary extensions before sphincter division, and secondly the speed with which the seton cuts through the sphincter. In a series of 24 patients with high trans-sphincteric fistulas, Christensen et al.[50] tightened the seton every second day; 62% of patients reported some degree of incontinence postoperatively, including 29% who wore a pad constantly. The 'snug' silastic (elastic) seton method, in which the muscle is cut through much more slowly but without the need for tightening, in the treatment of inter- and transphincteric fistulas, was associated with healing in all cases but with a 25% incidence of continence disturbance in the 16 patients followed up at a median 42 months after the seton had cut through.[51]

The chemical seton

This method, enjoying a resurgence in India where it is known as *Kshara sutra*, involves the weekly reinsertion of a specially prepared thread along the fistula track. The thread is prepared in a multistage process involving multiple layers of agents derived from plants. Apart from its antibacterial and anti-inflammatory properties, the alkalinity of the thread (about pH 9.5) would appear to be the means by which the thread slowly cuts through the tissues. Indeed, the chemical nature might be the reason behind the rather slow rate of cutting, about 1 cm of track every 6 days.

 In a prospective randomised trial involving 502 patients,[52] apart from a longer healing time (8 weeks vs. 4 weeks), the results of this outpatient treatment were comparable with fistulotomy (incontinence rate 5% vs. 9%; recurrence rate at 1 year 4% vs. 11%).

Recurrences usually occur for the same reasons as after conventional surgery, such as a missed secondary track or another internal opening, but the economic advantages of such a method in a less privileged country are obvious.

 For low fistulas, however, a more recent prospective randomised study from Singapore concluded that the method has no advantage over conventional fistulotomy.[53]

Advancement flaps

The use of an advancement flap was first proposed in 1902 for the repair of rectovaginal fistulas. Elting[54] described its use in managing anal fistula in 1912, supported by two principles: separation of the track from the communication with the bowel; and adequate closure of that communication with eradication of all diseased tissue in the anorectal wall. To Elting's principles, modern surgeons have added adequate flap vascularity and anastomosis of the flap to a site well distal to the site of the (previously excised) internal opening as important tenets. Modifications have included the use of full-thickness rectal flaps, partial-thickness flaps, curved incisions and rhomboid flaps, with or without closure of the defect in and outside the external sphincter,[55] and distally based (anocutaneous flaps transposed upwards) flaps. Most authors agree that the flap should include part if not all of the underlying internal sphincter in order to maintain vascularity. Apart from the presence of acute sepsis, large internal openings (>2.5 cm) would be considered a contraindication as the risks of anastomotic breakdown are high,[56] and a heavily scarred, indurated, wooden perineum precludes adequate exposure and flap mobilisation.

Although the technique has not enjoyed much popularity because of a low success rate at St Mark's Hospital, there are several studies that have reported excellent results, with cure rates of 90–100% for idiopathic anal fistulas and little in the way of functional morbidity. A review of the technique and its results has been published.[57] The report by Athanasiadis et al.[58] is interesting for several reasons. In the larger series of patients (*n* = 224), internal sphincterotomy was performed

aiming to eradicate the presumed aetiological source, but this led, as might be expected, to a much higher incidence of significant postoperative continence disorders than when internal sphincterotomy had not been performed. The persistence/recurrent fistula rate was 18% for transsphincteric fistulas and 40% for suprasphincteric fistulas. Preservation of the internal sphincter in a subsequent group of 55 patients resulted in a much lower incidence of functional morbidity, but unfortunately fistula persistence/recurrence was not reported. Physiological assessment has revealed that the technique may[55] or may not[59] be associated with preservation of resting and squeeze pressures, and success rates in terms of fistula healing decrease with time.[60]

Biological agents

Fibrin glue

There are several studies that have reported the successful use of fibrin glue in sealing off fistula tracks.[61,62] Autologous glues have been largely replaced by commercially available virus-inactivated fibrinogen solution from donor plasma. The glue aims to plug the tube from internal opening to external opening and promote healing through fibroblast migration and activation, and the formation of a collagen meshwork. The importance of thorough curettage to remove all granulation tissue and debris (some have used laser to destroy the chronic inflammatory lining) is stressed; the authors suspect that this, and complete plugging of the tracks, may be very difficult when dealing with serpiginous secondary tracks. Use of antibiotics is variable, but some go as far as to try to 'sterilise' the fistula track preoperatively according to the results of microbiological culture. Again, the technique is contraindicated when there is acute sepsis, this being dealt with first (and in some series always the first stage) with a loose draining seton. The internal opening itself is plugged with sealant, closed simply, or an advancement flap raised.

 Poorer outcomes were observed following advancement flap repair of the internal opening and fibrin obliteration of the track than following advancement flap alone.[63]

Notwithstanding the various modifications employed, it is difficult to explain the highly variable reported success rates (0–100%). Paradoxically, treatment of short tracks appears less successful than that of longer tracks, which might relate to extrusion of the fibrin plug from the track. Some reports are victims of short follow-up (most failures occur early but some occur in the long term; postoperative MRI, despite apparent healing at that time, has shown much lower true healing rates, of the order of 10–20%[64]), and efficacy in fistulas with tortuous primary tracks or secondary extensions is unknown (strengthening the case for preoperative MRI, which would make evaluation of the technique much more comprehensive).

 A randomised controlled trial has recently demonstrated no benefit in terms of healing over fistulotomy in treating low fistulas, but for those fistulas deemed unsafe to lay open, a cumulative (a second application offered in the event of initial failure) 69% success rate at 3 months[65] appears at least as good as other techniques aimed at avoiding any sphincter division.

The attractions of such a relatively simple technique are self-evident. It may be that further developments will produce glues that are more effective, although claims for success will need to be backed up by MRI validation of deep healing.

Bioprosthetic plugs

More recently, reports of the use of bioabsorbable xenografts in plugging fistula tracks have somewhat replaced those of fibrin glue in the literature, following a prospective non-randomised study which suggested that outcomes in the short term using lyophilised porcine intestinal submucosa were superior to those using fibrin glue,[66] and that success was sustained at a median of 6 months in 38 of 46 (83%) patients,[67] with failure often attributed to plug extrusion. As we have learnt from the story of fibrin glue, where the initial enthusiasm waned markedly with time and more rigorous measures of healing, so we now need MRI

validation that fistulas really can be healed with these new plugs.

Management of the recurrent fistula

Failure of sphincter-preserving methods and persistent symptoms may make lay-open the most sensible option (although some patients may prefer to live with a long-term loose seton). After fistulotomy some patients are able to lead normal lives with the narrowest of (often fibrotic) anorectal rings, as Milligan and Morgan had stated in 1934.[31] However, some may request sphincter repair. MRI is a useful way of making sure that there is no covert pathology before embarking on repair. Over a 3-year period at St Mark's Hospital 20 patients underwent sphincteroplasty for incontinence after previous surgery for idiopathic fistulas. A good outcome (Parks' grade 1 or 2 continence score) was obtained in 13 (65%).[68]

It is important to consider the possibility of an extrasphincteric fistula when a high 'blind' track is encountered, arising from pelvic or abdominal disease or from a presacral dermoid cyst. Failure to perform imaging (fistulography, barium studies or MRI) is a major reason for delayed diagnosis of extrasphincteric fistulas. If a track is truly high and blind, this might be because the internal opening has closed, or because surgery has dealt with the primary track and recurrence is because of an overlooked secondary extension.[69] In such cases, the component of the track outside the sphincters should be laid open and curetted. As the resulting wound may be large, it is often wise to make a circular rather than a radial incision to avoid sphincter damage. Following granulation tissue with curette and probe must be done extremely carefully if false tracks and iatrogenic openings are to be avoided. If the track peters out before reaching the intersphincteric space, it is safest to stop and come back another day. If the track enters the intersphincteric space but no internal opening can be identified, it is reasonable to assume that the opening has healed or is extremely small; internal sphincterectomy of that quadrant is then justified to try to prevent recurrence.

Key points

- A fistula has a primary track and may have secondary extensions.
- Complete eradication of both will lead to cure.
- All lay-open procedures divide some of the internal sphincter, so patients should be warned of a 1 in 4 chance of flatus incontinence and mild mucus leakage.
- Lay-open is the most certain treatment where it is possible and when the risks have been properly explained and accepted.
- Advancement flaps are intuitively attractive but practically uncertain.
- Glue is only rarely effective – bioprosthetic plugs are more attractive but long-term results of healing validated by MRI are awaited.
- In the balance between minor soiling with almost certain cure vs. potential recurrence with a less than certain technique, many patients allowed the choice will choose the former.
- Anterior fistulas in women are dangerous and should only rarely be laid open.
- STIR sequence MRI is the gold standard for imaging.
- A permanent, comfortable, loose seton will preserve continence and prevent much (but not all) future abscess formation, but continual discharge means all patients need continuing outpatient support and reassurance, and a minority find it unacceptable in the long term.

References

1. Phillips RKS, Lunniss PJ. Anorectal sepsis. In: Nicholls RJ, Dozois RR (eds) Surgery of the colon and rectum. New York: Churchill Livingstone, 1997; pp. 255–84.

2. McColl I. The comparative anatomy and pathology of anal glands. Ann R Coll Surg Engl 1967; 40:36–67.

3. Marks CG, Ritchie JK. Anal fistulas at St Mark's Hospital. Br J Surg 1977; 64:1003–7.

4. Lilius HG. Fistula-in-ano: a clinical study of 150 patients. Acta Chir Scand 1968; 383(Suppl):3–88.

5. Sainio P. A manometric study of anorectal function after surgery for anal fistula, with special reference to incontinence. Acta Chir Scand 1985; 151:695–700.

6. Eisenhammer S. The internal anal sphincter and the anorectal abscess. Surg Gynecol Obstet 1956; 103:501–6.

7. Parks AG. The pathogenesis and treatment of fistula-in-ano. Br Med J; i:463–9.

8. Goligher JC, Ellis M, Pissides AG. A critique of anal glandular infection in the aetiology and treatment of idiopathic anorectal abscesses and fistulae. Br J Surg 1967; 54:977–83.

9. Seow-Choen F, Hay AJ, Heard S et al. Bacteriology of anal fistulae. Br J Surg 1992; 79:27–8.

10. Lunniss PJ, Faris B, Rees H et al. Histological and microbiological assessment of the role of microorganisms in chronic anal fistulae. Br J Surg 1993; 80:1072.

11. Gordon-Watson C, Dodd H. Observations on fistula in ano in relation to perianal intermuscular glands. Br J Surg 1935; 22:703–9.

12. Lunniss PJ, Sheffield JP, Talbot IC et al. Persistence of anal fistula may be related to epithelialization. Br J Surg 1995; 82:32–3.

13. Kiehne K, Fincke A, Brunke G et al. Antimicrobial peptides in chronic anal fistula epithelium. Scand J Gastroenterol 2007; 42:1063–9.

14. Eisenhammer S. The final evaluation and classification of the surgical treatment of the primary anorectal, cryptoglandular intermuscular (intersphincteric) fistulous abscess and fistula. Dis Colon Rectum 1978; 21:237–54.

15. Grace RH, Harper IA, Thompson RG. Anorectal sepsis: microbiology in relation to fistula-in-ano. Br J Surg 1982; 69:401–3.

16. Toyonaga T, Matsushima M, Tanaka Y et al. Microbiological analysis and endoanal ultrasonography for diagnosis of anal fistula in acute anorectal sepsis. Int J Colorect Dis 2007; 22:209–13.

17. Lunniss PJ, Phillips RKS. Surgical assessment of acute anorectal sepsis is a better predictor of fistula than microbiological analysis. Br J Surg 1994; 81:368–9.

18. Oliver I, Lacueva FJ, Perez Vicente F et al. Randomized clinical trial comparing simple drainage of anorectal abscess with and without fistula track treatment. Int J Colorect Dis 2003; 18:107–10.
   Largest randomised trial of its kind.

19. Quah HM, Tang CL, Eu KW et al. Meta-analysis of randomized clinical trials comparing drainage alone vs primary sphincter-cutting procedures for anorectal abscess-fistula. Int J Colorectal Dis 2006; 21:602–9.

Primary fistulotomy in experienced hands is safe and effective.

20. Parks AG, Gordon PH, Hardcastle JD. A classification of fistula-in-ano. Br J Surg 1976; 63:1–12.

21. Marks CG. Classification. In: Phillips RKS, Lunniss PJ (eds) Anal fistula. Surgical evaluation and management. London: Chapman & Hall, 1996; pp. 33–46.

22. Choen S, Burnett S, Bartram CI et al. Comparison between anal endosonography and digital examination in the evaluation of anal fistulae. Br J Surg 1991; 78:445–7.

23. Fazio V. Complex anal fistulae. Gastroenterol Clin North Am 1987; 16:93–114.

24. Seow-Choen F, Phillips RKS. Insights gained from the management of problematical anal fistulas at St. Mark's Hospital, 1984–88. Br J Surg 1991; 78:539–41.

25. Halligan S, Stoker J. Imaging of fistula in ano. Radiology 2006; 239:18–33.

26. Buchanan GN, Halligan S, Bartram CI et al. Clinical evaluation, endosonography and MR imaging in preoperative assessment of fistula-in-ano: comparison with outcome derived gold standard. Radiology 2004; 233:674–81.

27. Lunniss PJ, Armstrong P, Barker PG et al. Magnetic resonance imaging of anal fistulae. Lancet 1992; 340:394–6.

28. Lunniss PJ, Barker PG, Sultan AH et al. Magnetic resonance imaging of fistula-in-ano. Dis Colon Rectum 1994; 37:708–18.

29. Buchanan GN, Halligan S, Williams AB et al. Magnetic resonance imaging for primary fistula *in ano*. Br J Surg 2003; 90:877–81.

30. Buchanan G, Halligan S, Williams A et al. Effect of MRI on clinical outcome of recurrent fistula-in-ano. Lancet 2003; 360:1661–2.

31. Milligan ETC, Morgan CN. Surgical anatomy of the anal canal with special reference to anorectal fistulae. Lancet 1934; ii:1150–6, 1213–17.

32. Lunniss PJ, Kamm MA, Phillips RKS. Factors affecting continence after surgery for anal fistula. Br J Surg 1994; 81:1382–5.

33. Abcarian H. The 'lay open' technique. In: Phillips RKS, Lunniss PJ (eds) Anal fistula. Surgical evaluation and management. London: Chapman & Hall, 1996; pp. 73–80.

34. Ho YH, Tan M, Leong FPK et al. Marsupialisation of fistulotomy wounds improves healing: a randomized controlled trial. Br J Surg 1998; 85:105–7.

35. Pescatori M, Ayabaca SM, Cafaro D et al. Marsupialization of fistulotomy and fistulectomy wounds improves healing and decreases bleeding: a randomized controlled trial. Colorectal Dis 2006; 8:11–14.

Marsupialisation does have some advantages.

36. Parkash S, Lakshmiratan V, Gajendran V. Fistula-in-ano: treatment by fistulectomy, primary closure and reconstitution. Aust NZ J Surg 1985; 55:23–7.

37. Perez F, Arroyo A, Serrano P et al. Prospective clinical and manometric study of fistulotomy with primary sphincter reconstruction in the management of recurrent complex fistula-in-ano. Int J Colorectal Dis 2006; 21:522–6.

38. Perez F, Arroyo A, Serrano P et al. Randomized clinical and manometric study of advancement flap versus fistulotomy with sphincter reconstruction in the management of complex fistula-in-ano. Am J Surg 2006; 192:34–40.

39. Kronborg O. To lay open or excise a fistula-in-ano. A randomised trial. Br J Surg 1985; 72:970.

40. Lewis A. Excision of fistula in ano. Int J Colorectal Dis 1986; 1:265–7.

41. Lewis A. Core out. In: Phillips RKS, Lunniss PJ (eds) Anal fistula. Surgical evaluation and management. London: Chapman & Hall, 1996; pp. 81–6.

42. Ramanujan PS, Prasad ML, Abcarian H. The role of seton in fistulotomy of the anus. Surg Gynecol Obstet 1983; 157:419–22.

43. Kuypers HC. Use of the seton in the treatment of extrasphincteric anal fistula. Dis Colon Rectum 1984; 27:109–10.

44. Parks AG, Stitz RW. The treatment of high fistula-in-ano. Dis Colon Rectum 1976; 19:487–99.

45. Lunniss PJ, Thomson JPS. The loose seton. In: Phillips RKS, Lunniss PJ (eds) Anal fistula. Surgical evaluation and management. London: Chapman & Hall, 1996; pp. 87–94.

46. Thomson JPS, Ross AHMcL. Can the external sphincter be preserved in the treatment of trans-sphincteric fistula-in-ano? Int J Colorectal Dis 1989; 4:247–50.

47. Kennedy HL, Zegarra JP. Fistulotomy without external sphincter division for high anal fistula. Br J Surg 1990; 77:898–901.

48. Buchanan GN, Owen HA, Torkington J et al. Long-term outcome following loose-seton technique for external sphincter preservation in complex anal fistula. Br J Surg 2004; 91:476–80.

49. Goldberg SM, Garcia-Aquilar J. The cutting seton. In: Phillips RKS, Lunniss PJ (eds) Anal fistula. Surgical evaluation and management. London: Chapman & Hall, 1996; pp. 95–102.

50. Christensen A, Nilas L, Christiansen J. Treatment of trans-sphincteric anal fistulas by the seton technique. Dis Colon Rectum 1986; 29:454–5.

51. Hammond TH, Knowles CH, Porrett T et al. The snug seton: short and medium term results of slow fistulotomy for idiopathic anal fistulae. Colorectal Dis 2006; 8:328–37.

52. Shukla NK, Narang R, Nair NG et al. Multicentric randomized controlled clinical trial of Kshaarasootra (Ayurvedic medicated thread) in the management of fistula-in-ano. Ind J Med Res 1991; 94:177–85.

53. Ho KS, Tsang C, Seoew-Choen F et al. Prospective randomized trial comparing ayurvedic cutting seton and fistulotomy for low fistula-in-ano. Tech Coloproctol 2001; 5:137–41.

54. Elting AW. The treatment of fistula in ano. Ann Surg 1912; 56:744–52.

55. Finan PJ. Management by advancement flap technique. In: Phillips RKS, Lunniss PJ (eds) Anal fistula. Surgical evaluation and management. London: Chapman & Hall, 1996; pp. 107–14.

56. Kodner IJ, Mazor A, Shemesh EL et al. Endorectal advancement flap repair of rectovaginal and other complicated anorectal fistulas. Surgery 1993; 114:682–90.

57. Lunniss PJ. The role of the advancement flap technique. Semin Colon Rectal Surg 1998; 9:192–7.

58. Athanasiadis S, Kohler A, Nafe M. Treatment of high anal fistulae by primary occlusion of the internal ostium, drainage of the intersphincteric space, and mucosal advancement flap. Int J Colorectal Dis 1994; 9:153–7.

59. Uribe N, Millan M, Minguez M et al. Clinical and manometric results of endorectal advancement flaps for complex anal fistula. Int J Colorectal Dis 2007; 22:259–64.

60. van der Hagen SJ, Baeten CG, Soeters PB et al. Long-term outcome following mucosal advancement flap for high perianal fistulas and fistulotomy for low perianal fistulas. Int J Colorectal Dis 2006; 21:784–90.

61. Hammond TH, Grahn MF, Lunniss PJ. Fibrin glue in the management of anal fistulae. Colorectal Dis 2004; 6:308–19.

62. Swinscoe MT, Ventakasubramaniam AK, Jayne DG. Fibrin glue for fistula-in-ano: the evidence reviewed. Tech Coloproctol 2005; 9:89–94.

63. Ellis CN, Clark S. Fibrin glue as an adjunct to flap repair of anal fistulas: a randomized controlled study. Dis Colon Rectum 2006; 49:1736–40.

64. Buchanan GN, Bartram CI, Phillips RKS et al. Efficacy of fibrin sealant in the management of complex anal fistula. Dis Colon Rectum 2003; 46:1167–74.

65. Lindsey I, Smilgin-Humphreys MM, Cunningham C et al. A randomized, controlled trial of fibrin glue vs. conventional treatment for anal fistula. Dis Colon Rectum 2002; 45:1608–15.

66. Johnson EK, Gaw, JU, Armstrong DN. Efficacy of anal fistula plug vs. fibrin glue in closure of anorectal fistulas. Dis Colon Rectum 2006; 49:371–6.

67. Champagne BJ, O'Connor LM, Ferguson M et al. Efficacy of anal fistula plug in closure of cryptoglandular fistulas: long-term follow-up. Dis Colon Rectum 2006; 49:1817–21.

68. Engel AF, Lunniss PJ, Kamm MA et al. Sphincteroplasty for incontinence after surgery for idiopathic fistula-in-ano. Int J Colorectal Dis 1997; 12:323–5.

69. Phillips RKS, Lunniss PJ. Approach to the difficult fistula. In: Phillips RKS, Lunniss PJ (eds) Anal fistula. Surgical evaluation and management. London: Chapman & Hall, 1996; pp. 177–82.

15

Minor anorectal conditions

Francis Seow-Choen
Chung Ming Chen

Haemorrhoids

It is now widely accepted that haemorrhoids are derived from anal cushions. Anal cushions are normal structures found in the anal canal, consisting of mucosa, submucosal fibroelastic connective tissues and smooth muscles in an arteriovenous channel system. Anal cushions complement anal sphincter function by providing fine control over the continence of liquids and gases.

Pathogenesis and aetiology

The anal cushions function normally when they are fixed in their proper sites within the anal canal by submucosal smooth muscle and elastic fibres (Treitz's muscle). These fibres may be fragmented by prolonged downward stress related to straining during defecation of hard stools.

When the supporting submucosal fibres fragment, the anal cushions are no longer restrained from engorging excessively with blood and this results in bleeding and prolapse. Veins that traverse the anal sphincter are blocked whereas arterial inflow continues, leading to increasing haemorrhoidal congestion. Defecation in the squatting position may also aggravate the tendency to prolapse as is easily attested by anyone with prolapsible piles.

Constipation certainly aggravates the symptoms of haemorrhoids. Interestingly, diarrhoea is also a potential risk factor and the tenesmus from diarrhoea causes straining that aggravates haemorrhoids. Other factors have been implicated, such as heredity, erect posture, absence of valves within the haemorrhoidal plexus and draining veins, as well as impedence of venous return from raised intra-abdominal pressure. Portal hypertension may lead to engorgement of the haemorrhoidal plexus. Pregnancy is associated with a higher risk of haemorrhoids and undoubtedly aggravates pre-existing disease.

Anatomy and nomenclature

External haemorrhoids comprise dilated vascular plexuses located below the dentate line, covered by squamous epithelium. They may swell and cause some discomfort. Bleeding is not usually the predominant complaint but quite severe pain can arise as a result of acute thrombosis. If left untreated, the thrombosed external haemorrhoids will become external skin tags.

Internal haemorrhoids are symptomatic arteriovenous channels sited above the dentate line and covered by transitional and columnar epithelium. They are divided into subcategories in order of severity, from first-degree to fourth-degree haemorrhoids. The definitions of each, as well as their management, are outlined in Box 15.1.

Management

Firstly, it must be recognised that haemorrhoids may coexist with other conditions such as rectal cancer or inflammatory bowel disease. Patients who have symptoms including blood or mucus mixed in the stools, change in bowel habit, abdominal symptoms and family history of colorectal cancer should have further evaluation of the colon and rectum.

Secondly, the anal cushions are normal functional anatomical structures contributing to anal continence. Treatment is thus reserved for 'haemorrhoidal diseases' that are abnormal and cause symptoms. Therapeutic strategies then depend upon symptoms and the amount of haemorrhoidal tissue prolapsing beyond the anal verge.

Non-prolapsing or mildly prolapsing haemorrhoids

If the piles are not permanently prolapsed, non-operative methods should be attempted first. The primary problems of constipation and straining at stool need to be addressed. In some patients, improving bowel action with laxatives may help to control the symptoms.

Other forms of treatment that can/may give more immediate symptomatic relief include rubber band ligation, injection sclerotherapy, medications such as Daflon 500 (currently not available in the UK), as well

as toilet re-education. Topical applications are popular with many patients who testify to relief from bleeding and pain. There are, however, no clinical trials to demonstrate any benefit from such applications.

Rubber band ligation

In this technique, rubber bands are applied at the apex of the haemorrhoidal tissue. The strangulated tissue then becomes necrotic and sloughs off in a few days, after which the wound fibroses, resulting in fixation of the mucosa. The pile tissue is thus prevented from engorging and prolapsing. Up to three haemorrhoids can be banded on the same occasion but we prefer to only do one at a time. This process is relatively painless if the bands are placed above the dentate line, but some patients may experience severe tenesmus and a feeling of engorgement that is only partially relieved by analgesia. Banding is usually 60–80% effective, depending on proper selection of cases. There is a 2–5% risk of secondary haemorrhage.

Rubber band ligation is the treatment of choice for grade 2 haemorrhoids when compared with excisional haemorrhoidectomy. It achieved similar results but without the effects of surgery. Surgery should be reserved for grade 3 haemorrhoids or recurrent haemorrhoids after rubber band ligation.[1]

Injection sclerotherapy

Sclerosant agents used include phenol (5%) in almond oil or sodium tetradecyl sulphate. These are injected into the submucosa around the pedicle of the pile, at the level of the anorectal ring. The sclerosant is likely to cause inflammation, leading to reduced blood flow into the haemorrhoid. This technique is about 70% effective. The sclerosant also causes fibrosis, which draws minor prolapse back into the anal canal.

The correct plane is shown by elevation of the mucosa without blanching during injection. Inappropriately deep injections can cause perirectal fibrosis, infection and urethral irritation. Prostatic injection is intensely painful and the patient may develop an erection, a strong desire to void, haematuria or haemospermia. Severe sepsis is not uncommon and such patients should be admitted for antibiotics and observation until completely well.

Box 15.1 • Management of internal haemorrhoids

First-degree haemorrhoids (bleeding but no prolapse)
- Stool softeners
- Local creams or Daflon (not available in the UK)

Second-degree haemorrhoids (prolapse but spontaneously reducible)
- Rubber band ligation
- Sclerotherapy
- Electrocoagulation
- (Haemorrhoidectomy)

Third-degree haemorrhoids (prolapse requiring manual reduction)
- Rubber band ligation
- Sclerotherapy
- Electrocoagulation
- (Haemorrhoidectomy)

Fourth-degree haemorrhoids (irreducible prolapse)
- Haemorrhoidectomy

Other methods

There are several available phlebotonics but Daflon 500 is by far the best evaluated in the medical literature, and is widely used in Europe and the Far East as first-line treatment for piles.[2] Daflon 500, not currently available in the UK, is micronised diosmin and hesperidin, which belong to the hydroxyethylrutoside group of drugs.[3] Its pharmacological properties include noradrenaline-mediated venous contraction,[4] reduction in blood extravasation from capillaries[5] and inhibition of prostaglandin (PGE_2, PGF_2) inflammatory response.[6]

 These properties have a proven therapeutic action in the symptomatic relief of haemorrhoidal symptoms.[7] Adverse effects have been minimal.[8,9]

Various other methods are also available. These include infrared photocoagulation, which requires additional equipment, and cryotherapy, which results in unpleasant discharge. For such reasons, these methods have not been popular. Topical preparations that may contain local anaesthetics or steroids are also available, often without prescription. To date, there is no evidence that such agents are any more effective than spontaneous remissions. Moreover, patient self-treatment may delay the diagnosis of serious diseases such as cancer and can therefore be potentially harmful.

Irreducible prolapsed piles

The majority of patients are well treated by non-surgical methods. However, when anal cushions have prolapsed or thrombosed (**Fig. 15.1**), they no longer function effectively to maintain continence and surgery may then be needed. In fact, sensory function may be impaired and this may partially account for the complaints of minor incontinence by some patients.

Traditionally, prolapsed piles are removed by excisional haemorrhoidectomy. Although there are variations to the technique,[10–13] the main problems encountered remain similar. These are mainly postoperative pain,[11,14] anal incontinence[15] and haemorrhage.

 Open haemorrhoidectomy may lead to faster and more reliable wound healing where three large prolapsed irreducible piles are excised.[10]

Some authors have described post-haemorrhoidectomy pain as like passing pieces of sharp glass

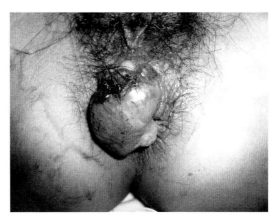

Figure 15.1 • Acute prolapsed thrombosed pile with fissure.

fragments, such that many patients would rather suffer the discomfort of large prolapsing haemorrhoids for years rather than submit to surgery.

Nonetheless, third- and fourth-degree haemorrhoids are more appropriately treated by surgery, which is conventionally performed by excision of the three primary piles. Minor variations in conventional excisional haemorrhoidectomy include whether the wounds are left to granulate or closed with sutures, whether the pedicle is ligated, or whether the piles are excised with scissors or diathermy.

Nevertheless, some patients will have more severe circumferential prolapse with massive engorgement of both external and internal haemorrhoidal plexuses. Such large haemorrhoids require extensive ablation to ensure adequate treatment in order to prevent residual or recurrent symptoms.

In the past, such haemorrhoids have been dealt with by either standard haemorrhoidectomy plus excision of the largest secondary pile with subsequent mucocutaneous reconstitution or a modification of the Whitehead or radical haemorrhoidectomy.

 In a study comparing Whitehead with four-pile haemorrhoidectomy, we concluded that four-pile haemorrhoidectomy was significantly easier to perform and although residual tags and piles were left behind, the operation was preferred to radical haemorrhoidectomy.[16,17]

Currently, however, this discussion may be immaterial as stapled haemorrhoidectomy adequately addresses most circumferential prolapses.[18]

Stapled haemorrhoidectomy

Conventional surgical haemorrhoidectomy is not based on a correction of pathophysiology but on ablation of symptoms. Hence, if prolapsed piles are bleeding, painful or otherwise symptomatic, these piles are excised.

However, prolapsed haemorrhoids are not always symptomatic. Furthermore, totally asymptomatic individuals can be made to engorge their anal cushions during proctoscopy by straining or performing the Valsalva manoeuvre. This sort of engorgement is aggravated by straining in the squatting position. Once prolapse occurs, further engorgement of these vascular cushions leads to pain and an inflammatory response. Anal spasm then prevents reduction, and pathological changes such as thrombosis, oedema and inflammation occur.

Chronicity is caused by a vicious cycle of prolapse and congestion of these vascular cushions. The vascular cushions hence prolapse easily and allow the anal sphincters to constrict, resulting in further congestion, oedema and pain.

Conventional haemorrhoidectomy deals with the symptoms alone without due regard to restoration of the normal physiology by fixation of the congested anal cushions. On the other hand, stapled haemorrhoidectomy tries to correct the primary pathology, theoretically resulting in resolution of haemorrhoidal symptoms.[19] After reduction of any prolapsed haemorrhoidal tissue, this technique then excises redundant lower rectal mucosa, fixing the prolapse back into its proper place on the wall of the anal canal. This fixation into muscle is in our opinion important to help prevent subsequent re-dislodgement and recurrence. As previously mentioned, once reduced the engorged haemorrhoidal tissue has the opportunity to decongest and shrink. We believe this theory is borne out in clinical practice. Our technique of stapled haemorrhoidectomy takes into account these pathophysiological changes and attempts to correct them all.[20] Although there are concerns of long-term pain following stapled haemorrhoidectomy, this has not been seen in larger series.[21]

 In a recent meta-analysis of 12 randomised clinical trials comparing stapled versus conventional surgery for haemorrhoids, stapled haemorrhoidectomy is associated with a higher long-term risk of recurrence and the symptoms of prolapse. It is also likely to be associated with a higher likelihood of long-term symptom recurrence and the need for additional operations compared to conventional excisional haemorrhoidal surgery.[22]

However, stapled haemorrhoidectomy on its own cannot deal adequately with the really massive haemorrhoidal prolapse. Massive haemorrhoids are prolapsed haemorrhoids more than 3–4 cm outside the anal verge. In this situation, there is not enough space within the staple housing to contain the massive redundant tissue of the prolapsed haemorrhoids.

A modified stapled haemorrhoidectomy technique has been described by us to deal with massive haemorrhoidal prolapse using one circular PPH stapler, and this has been found to be safe and effective.[23] Another more expensive alternative might be to use two staplers simultaneously. In fact, stapled haemorrhoidectomy has also been used for acute thrombosed circumferentially prolapsed piles,[24] and has been found to be feasible and perhaps even result in less pain, a more rapid resolution of symptoms and an earlier return to work when compared with conventional Milligan–Morgan haemorrhoidectomy.[25]

From our operative experience as well as from supervising junior colorectal surgeons in using the PPH stapler, we found that stapled haemorrhoidectomy is a very surgeon-dependent operation with regards to reduction of skin tags, or whether excision or leaving skin tags behind are concerned. We believe that the placement of the staple line and the selection of patients are important factors in influencing long-term results with regards to pain and recurrence.

Transanal haemorrhoidal dearterialisation

In 1995, Morinaga et al.[26] introduced a novel, less invasive and non-excisional technique for the treatment of haemorrhoids called haemorrhoidal artery ligation (HAL) or transanal haemorrhoidal dearterialisation (THD). The definition of THD was introduced by Sohn et al.[27] in 2001. This technique consists of ligating the terminal haemorrhoidal branches of the superior rectal artery using a specially designed proctoscope with a Doppler probe to locate the vessel. This results in reduction of blood flow and decongestion of the haemorrhoidal plexus. Dal Monte et al.[28] reported more than 90% resolution of symptoms with minimal complications.

Postoperative problems

Some problems that occur after haemorrhoidectomy include severe pain, urinary retention, bleeding and faecal impaction. Studies have shown that pain is significantly diminished after stapled haemorrhoidectomy and the patient is able to go home a few hours after the operation. This has led to many advocates for stapled haemorrhoidectomy in the day-surgery setting.[29–31] Nevertheless, many surgeons perform conventional haemorrhoidectomy, both open and closed, in a day-care setting with high patient satisfaction as well.

Even so, whichever technique is used, pain is still an important consideration in the postoperative period. It is multifactorial, although spasm of the internal sphincter is believed to play an important role; we believe that the actual skin wound, if present, with its exposed nerves is the most significant factor.

 Use of botulinum toxin has been shown to reduce pain towards the end of the first postoperative week.[32] The use of 0.2% glyceryl trinitrate (GTN) ointment is also associated with decreased postoperative pain, and contributes to more rapid healing of wounds after excisional haemorrhoidectomy.[33] Others have tried lateral sphincterotomy with haemorrhoidectomy with some success,[34] but we would not advocate this because of potential permanent adverse effects.

The amount of pain after stapled haemorrhoidectomy is said to depend on the height of mucosectomy above the anal verge. Removal of squamous epithelium results in greater intensity of postoperative pain and should be avoided. However, some patients with a staple line well above the dentate line have considerable pain. This situation may be caused by congestion of the haemorrhoidal plexuses, haemorrhoidal thrombosis or developing sepsis below the staple line (see later). Another less frequent problem is postoperative haemorrhage. This may be primary, presenting in the immediate postoperative period, and is usually due to technical problems, or secondary as a result of postoperative infection. Submucosal adrenaline (epinephrine) injection[35] has been shown to be effective for addressing such bleeding and avoiding a re-operation.

Post-haemorrhoidectomy anal stricture is an uncommon occurrence seen in only 3.7% of haemorrhoidectomies.[36] The stricture usually presents at 6 weeks postoperatively and up to two-thirds may be managed conservatively with stool-bulking agents and local anaesthetic gels in the outpatient setting. The remaining one-third may require an anoplasty. Although uncommon, the key to management lies in its prevention, with the maintenance of adequate skin and mucosal bridges intraopera-

tively and close follow-up postoperatively to detect stricture formation early.

 On the other hand, some believe that the use of an anal dilator in the course of stapled haemorrhoidectomy may be associated with a higher rate of anal sphincter damage. This has been shown to be true in a randomised trial.[37]

However, there were no differences in continence scores or anal pressures, the main difference being the persistence of internal anal sphincter fragmentation beyond 14 weeks postoperatively.

Sepsis after treatment of haemorrhoids

Sepsis after either conservative or operative treatment is uncommon, but when it occurs delay in treatment can be catastrophic. In one study the incidence of transient bacteraemia from blood cultures after haemorrhoidectomy was 5–11%,[38] but this did not result in any cases of clinical sepsis.

In a review by Guy and Seow-Choen,[39] injection sclerotherapy has been reported to result in life-threatening retroperitoneal sepsis and rectal perforation. Urological sepsis can result from a misplaced deep anterior injection with complications such as prostatic abscess, epididymitis, chronic cystitis, seminal vesicle abscess and urinary–perineal fistula. Even with rubber band ligation, complications such as pain and haemorrhage result in 14% of patients.

Colonisation of anal wounds occurs frequently, but the true incidence of resultant wound infection is difficult to estimate as definitions vary widely. The common colonisers include *Escherichia coli* and *Staphylococcus aureus*, followed by *Pseudomonas aeruginosa*, *Enterococcus faecalis*, *Klebsiella pneumoniae*, *Proteus vulgaris* and *Proteus mirabilis*. Culture of 'infected' haemorrhoids, on the other hand, has revealed a predominance of anaerobes like *Bacteroides fragilis* and *Peptostreptococcus*.

 In a randomised trial by Carapeti et al.,[40] metronidazole was shown to reduce pain on days 5–7 after open, largely day-case haemorrhoidectomy, resulting in a shorter time to normal activity and greater patient satisfaction. It was proposed that a reduction in bacterial colonisation was an important factor.

Secondary haemorrhage, which has often been attributed to local infection, affects approximately 5% of patients undergoing haemorrhoidectomy. The advocated treatment is antibiotics; the incidence does not seem to be increased after emergency haemorrhoidectomy.

Specifically in stapled haemorrhoidectomy, because there is a closed stapled wound with the PPH stapler, surgeons should raise their clinical suspicion of a possible underlying infective process when severe pain is the only presenting complaint. The authors have noticed a very small number of patients in whom severe pain developed in the first or second week after surgery due to an evolving and sometimes undetectable perineal abscess. Patients presenting with fever and an obvious perineal abscess are difficult to miss, but some patients in their early stages of perineal sepsis may not have fever or sufficient swelling in the anal canal to provide instant diagnosis. This is especially so in stapling large piles that may in the early postoperative period be oedematous or thrombosed, resulting in some swelling and pain during during rectal examination and hence misleading the examiner as to whether an abscess is present or not.

Conclusion

Haemorrhoidal disease is a common anorectal disease. We think its aetiology is likely to be associated with straining at defecation. As a result, the supports of the submucosal anal cushions weaken. When this happens, the anal cushions becomes susceptible to abnormal engorgement with blood, resulting in symptomatically bleeding and prolapsing haemorrhoids (**Fig. 15.2**).

When treating haemorrhoids, other possibly life-threatening diseases such as rectal cancer have first to be excluded. Non-prolapsing and reducible prolapsing piles can usually be treated with preservation of the anal cushions. However, submucosal injection and rubber band ligation may accelerate symptomatic relief. Irreducible prolapsed piles may be treated either by excisional haemorrhoidectomy or, in our view preferentially, by stapled haemorrhoidectomy. However, singular pile prolapses compared to circumferential or three/four-quadrant prolapses are still better treated by excisional procedures as pain is not severe in such cases.

Anal fissure

Anal fissures are common, representing up to 10% of new referrals to colorectal clinics. The anal pain associated with fissures classically presents during defecation and persists for a few minutes to hours afterwards. There may be associated fresh rectal bleeding and patients may have a history of an abnormal bowel habit. If there is concomitant haemorrhoidal disease, the bleeding may be more significant.

However, some patients present with chronic fissures (**Fig. 15.3**). A chronic fissure is one that has persisted for more than 6 weeks despite adequate medical therapy. If patients have signs of chronicity on examination, such as a sentinel skin tag or an intra-anal fibroepithelial polyp, then they should also be classified as having chronic fissures regardless of the duration of their symptoms, as these anatomical changes cannot have happened over a short time period.

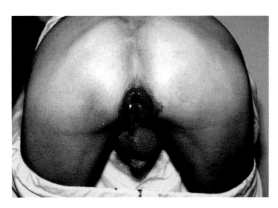

Figure 15.2 • Bleeding prolapsed piles.

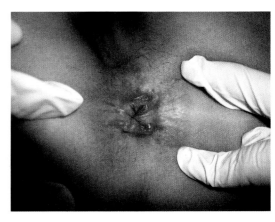

Figure 15.3 • Anterior and posterior chronic anal fissure.

Clinical findings

Pain is usually the predominant symptom in chronic fissures, but occasionally bleeding or the presence of a perianal skin tag may be more distressing to the patient. As always in history taking, symptoms like altered bowel habit and defecatory patterns must be elicited, and if there is a suspicion, a proximal colonic lesion must first be excluded.

Perianal and digital rectal examination usually demonstrates a skin tag (sentinel pile) overlying the external edge of a chronic anal fissure. Indeed, the fissure itself may be missed if the sentinel pile is not retracted to reveal the fissure. Although usually single and situated in the 6 o'clock position, some 2.5–10% may be sited in the 12 o'clock position.[41] If fissures are multiple or eccentrically located, inflammatory bowel disease, tuberculosis, syphilis or human immunodeficiency virus (HIV) infection must be considered.

When the pain is minimal, a gentle digital examination and proctoscopy may be done. This will show a fibrotic ulcer with white transverse internal sphincter fibres exposed. There may be a hypertrophic papilla at the internal edge of the fissure (**Fig. 15.4**). The presence of rectal mucosal prolapse or haemorrhoids is not unusual. It is, however, cruel to perform more than a visual examination in patients with severe pain due to an anal fissure.

Aetiology

Historically, fissures were thought to be due to the passage of a hard bolus of faeces causing a tear in the anal mucosa. A recent review by Hananel and

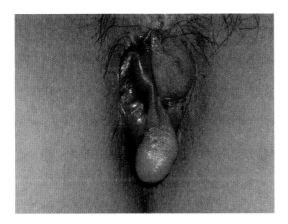

Figure 15.4 • Hypertrophic anal papilla.

Gordon showed that only 10% of patients complained of constipation and 30% needed to strain during defecation. Another 10% developed fissures after childbirth.

It has been observed that patients with chronic anal fissure commonly have a raised resting anal pressure from internal anal sphincter hypertonia.[42] Administration of pharmacological agents to relax the internal sphincter has been shown to lead to fissure healing, but the resting anal pressure returns to pretreatment levels once the fissure has healed and treatment ceased.[43] Internal sphincter hypertonia and anal spasm predate the onset of the fissure. This anal spasm does not seem to be a response to pain because application of topical local anaesthetics relieves pain but does not reduce the anal spasm.[44]

Over the past decade, local ischaemia has been gaining credence as a significant aetiological event in chronic fissures. There is a paucity of arterioles in the posterior commissure of 85% of cadaveric cases with reduced anodermal blood flow compared with controls.[45]

There are other hypotheses regarding aetiology. Brown et al.[46] suggested that an inflammatory process is responsible, with early myositis proceeding to fibrosis. Partial eversion of the anal canal during evacuation is inhibited anteriorly and posteriorly due to tethering, resulting in tearing of the tissue.[47] Finally, with decussation of the external sphincter muscle, there is weakness anteriorly and posteriorly, with tears occurring when hard stools are passed.[48]

Postpartum anal fissures are more commonly anterior, with the risk increasing in traumatic deliveries. Shearing forces from passage of the fetal head may be significant, compounded by the tethering of the anal mucosa to the skin. Although patients do not appear to have a raised internal anal sphincter resting pressure, they do complain of constipation, and this may contribute to fissure formation. The clinician should be wary of an underlying occult sphincter injury.

Medical treatment

The mainstay of treatment for chronic anal fissure used to be surgery until recently, when there was a shift towards medical therapy. Such alternatives to surgery can create an effect of temporary or reversible sphincterotomy, decreasing the anal sphincter pressure thereby allowing healing of the fissure. In a recent review of the management of chronic anal fissure, such modalities have been so popular and promising that surgery has been reserved for those who failed medical therapy.[49]

The recognition of nitric oxide as a neurotransmitter mediating the relaxation of the internal sphincter has led to many studies examining the use of isosorbide dinitrate and GTN to treat chronic fissures.

Different authors have tried oral, patch, sprayed and topical GTN, and 0.2% GTN topical ointment has become the standard as it achieves optimal healing in up to 70% of cases with minimal adverse effects (predominantly headaches).[50,51]

Comparisons of topical GTN with lateral sphincterotomy have also been made in recent trials.

The Canadian Colorectal Surgical Trials Group[52] randomised 82 patients to receive either sphincterotomy or 0.25% GTN three times a day. At 6 weeks, 34 (89.5%) in the sphincterotomy group had achieved healing compared with 13 (29.5%) in the GTN group. Of these 13 in the GTN group, five subsequently suffered a relapse.

Despite more favourable results from surgery, the enthusiasm for local creams has not diminished, mainly because of concerns of faecal incontinence, albeit usually mild after sphincterotomy.

Both diltiazem and GTN are equally effective in the treatment of chronic anal fissure, but GTN is associated with a higher rate of side-effects (headache or anal irritation). The recurrence rate of chronic anal fissure after the use of either GTN or a calcium channel blocker is equal.[53]

Both oral[54] and topical preparations have shown healing in up to 67% of patients. Patients who are already on these drugs for hypertension and ischaemic heart disease may be unsuitable for this form of treatment, although they are unlikely to have fissures.

The parasympathomimetic bethanecol has been shown to lower resting anal pressure and may be useful in conjunction with other topical medications. Indoramin, an α-adrenoceptor blocker, and salbutamol, a β-adrenoceptor agonist, are further possible alternatives.

Botulinum A toxin (Botox) reduces resting anal pressure and promotes healing of anal fissures in 70–96% of patients.[55]

In a randomised clinical trial, injection of botulinum toxin resulted in healing of 46 (92%) of 50 patients compared with 35 (70%) of 50 patients receiving topical GTN. Those treated with botulinum toxin had mild incontinence to flatus that was short-lived and resolved spontaneously, while the GTN treatment was associated with transient, moderate to severe headache.[56]

The mode of action remains unclear. The toxin binds to presynaptic cholinergic nerve terminals and inhibits the release of acetylcholine at the neuromuscular junction. This should lead to relaxation of the external sphincter but should have no corresponding effect on the internal sphincter. However, Brisinda et al.[57] have shown that maximal squeeze pressures were no different from pretreatment levels at 1–2 months after injection. The site of optimal injection is still unclear and complications include transient faecal incontinence, perianal haematoma, pain and sepsis.

In a meta-analysis of 54 randomised clinical trials, medical therapy (Botox, CCB, GTN) for chronic anal fissure is significantly better than placebo. Medications are safe and side-effects of therapy are not serious and are reversible with cessation of therapy. Surgery is then reserved for treatment failures. However, they are not as effective as surgery and late recurrence is also higher with medical therapy.[58]

For all the advantages of medical treatment, there is still no answer for sentinel piles and fibrous polyps that often accompany chronic fissures. These remain distressing to the patient as there may be associated pain and bleeding from trauma to sentinel piles or persistent tenesmus or soilage due to the presence of the fibrous polyp. Surgical excision at the time of lateral sphincterotomy offers not only good healing for the fissure but removes the sentinel pile and fibrous polyp at the same time.

Surgical treatment

We believe that uncontrolled anal stretch or dilatation should no longer be performed.[59]

An uncontrolled fracturing of the internal sphincter by this method, although shown to have good rates of healing, nevertheless results in an unacceptably high incidence of incontinence with unknown long-term consequences. Posterior midline sphincterotomy is not favoured either; its results are not superior to lateral sphincterotomy and a gutter (keyhole) defect may lead to soiling.

 Patients who have failed medical treatment or who have features of chronicity such as sentinel piles should be offered lateral sphincterotomy. This may be performed by either an open or closed method, each showing similar results.[59]

A current concern is the length of optimal internal sphincter division.[60,61] Classically, sphincterotomy was done with division of the internal sphincter up to the level of the dentate line. In a tailored sphincterotomy, the internal sphincter is divided up to the highest point of the fissure only. In practice this is gauged by eye-balling the distance between the top of the fissure and the dentate line and performing sphincterotomy accordingly. However, it is difficult to measure the exact length of division and also to study and compare the results between the two groups. There are many variations of technique but none has been shown to be superior. Most authors have described healing rates of 85–95%.

Sphincterotomy, by virtue of its division of the internal sphincter musculature, predisposes to incontinence to flatus and faecal soilage in up to 35% of patients (although the risk is usually far less than this).[60,62] Surgical removal of the fissure (fissurectomy) with subsequent use of isosorbide dinitrate cream or Botox injection has been shown to be effective, with no recurrence and no internal sphincter defects on postoperative endosonography.[63,64] This relatively new technique is as yet unverified by a randomised controlled trial, although it presents a novel approach to an age-old problem.

Recurrent or atypical fissures

If the fissure is not in the anterior or posterior midline, then Crohn's disease or immunosuppressive conditions like AIDS must be considered. These patients should not be offered surgery at the first consultation and further intestinal and anal investigation with anal manometry and anal sphincter mapping (usually by endoanal ultrasound) should be performed. Even so, in their series Fleschner et al.[65] showed that 88% of patients with Crohn's-associated fissures healed after lateral sphincterotomy compared with only 49% on medical treatment. Furthermore, no significant increase in complications was noted in the sphincterotomy group.

Authors who believe in the ischaemic nature of chronic fissures cite this as the reason behind recurrences. Internal sphincter hypertonia leads to reduced blood flow, which in turn results in tissue hypoxia and consequent failure of healing. Hyperbaric oxygen therapy ostensibly provides increased oxygenation to hypoperfused tissue and induces neovascularisation, collagen synthesis and fibroblast replication, thus enhancing the repair process. In a study by Cundall et al.,[66] five of eight patients had healed fissures at the end of 3 months, and all showed symptomatic improvement with regard to pain and bleeding.

In patients with recurrence after lateral sphincterotomy, anal manometry and anal ultrasound are essential as they separate patients with low resting anal pressures from patients with persistently raised resting pressures and will identify those who might benefit from repeat lateral sphincterotomies in the opposite lateral quadrant.

Patients with low resting sphincter pressures may be helped by anal cutaneous advancement flaps along with fissurectomy. It is reasonable to believe that these patients will not experience improved blood flow to the fissure after sphincterotomy as sphincter hypertonia was probably not a causative factor in the first place. As such, further sphincterotomy will only increase the risk of incontinence. Nyam et al.[67] and Leong and Seow-Choen[41] have shown that an island advancement flap from the perianal skin healed most fissures.

Conclusion

Anal fissures are common and aetiology is multifactorial. There are many options for chemical sphincterotomy with good results but lateral sphincterotomy remains the gold standard for chronic anal fissures. It is a simple procedure and yet achieves instant symptomatic relief.

Pruritus ani

Pruritus ani is a vexing problem to both surgeons and patients. When the cause remains elusive and cure cannot be achieved, there may be intense frustration on both sides. The actual incidence is not known as many people still view this as a minor inconvenience and do not seek medical treatment in the early stages.

Aetiology and pathogenesis

Although causes of perianal itch include many anorectal and dermatological conditions (Box 15.2), in many instances a primary cause cannot be found. Indeed, idiopathic pruritus ani is usually associated with a minor degree of faecal incontinence. The object of history taking and examination is to find the likely cause of leakage. This may be due to local pathology permitting stool to leak to the outside, such as a fissure, fistula or prolapsing haemorrhoid, or to a high-fibre diet, leading to difficulty with anal cleaning and fragments of stool becoming trapped in the anal canal, only to seep out later and set up irritation. There may be internal sphincter dysfunc-

Box 15.2 • Secondary causes of prurutis ani

Neoplasia
- Rectal adenoma
- Rectal adenocarcinoma
- Anal squamous cell carcinoma
- Malignant melanoma
- Bowen's disease
- Extramammary Paget's disease

Benign anorectal conditions
- Haemorrhoids
- Fistula in ano
- Anal fissure
- Rectal prolapse
- Anal sphincter injury or dysfunction
- Faecal incontinence
- Radiation proctitis
- Ulcerative colitis

Infections
- Condyloma acuminatum
- Herpes simplex virus
- *Candida albicans*
- Syphilis
- *Lymphogranuloma venereum*

Dermatological
- Neurogenic dermatitis
- Contact dermatitis
- Lichen simplex
- Lichen planus
- Lichen atrophicus

tion or other contributory causes such as irritative foods (spices, alcohol and caffeine). In addition, scratching, applications of inappropriate topical creams (local anaesthetics as they are sensitive to the skin; strong steroids as they lead to dependence of the skin) and excessive cleansing of the perianal skin exacerbate this condition.

Diagnosis

The diagnosis is most often revealed by good history taking and physical examination alone, especially for causes of minor anal leakage. Important facts such as duration of symptoms, dietary habits, recent travel history and change in bowel habit should be elucidated.

Physical examination should start with a general inspection of the patient for dermatological disease elsewhere on the body. Then the perineum and underclothes should be inspected for soilage. Perianal skin changes are noted, particularly excoriation and ichthyosis, as this indicates long-standing pruritus.

Specific examination of the perineum includes a digital rectal examination for anal tone and squeeze. It may help to wipe the anus with moistened gauze; a brown stain will confirm anal leakage, a frequent cause of itching. Palpation for polyps, malignancies and fistula tracks is required and patients should also be examined while straining to exclude any prolapse. Proctoscopy should be performed. Further examination using endoscopy, radiology or laboratory tests may be required in certain cases. Skin lesions should be biopsied and examined for fungal elements.

A commonly quoted cause of pruritus ani in the young is *Enterobius* or threadworm. These may be seen on sigmoidoscopy, or 'Sellotape' may reveal the diagnosis. This involves the placement of a piece of adhesive tape to the anus. This is then removed and placed onto a glass microscopy slide. The presence of ova is indicative of infection.

Treatment

Treatment is dependent on the primary pathology. Haemorrhoids can be easily treated by rubber band ligation or haemorrhoidectomy. Perianal skin tags may be excised and fissures treated as outlined in the previous section. Threadworm infections can be treated with mebendazole or piperazine.

In primary pruritus ani, the aims of treatment are the reduction of leakage, maintenance of good personal hygiene and the prevention of further injury to the perianal skin. Leakage can be reduced by avoidance of food that produces flatulence, such as fibre, which also makes stools soft and mushy. If the stool is loose, addition of an antimotility agent such as codeine or loperamide may be beneficial until the skin has healed and dietary modification has taken effect. A somewhat mushy stool frequently gets trapped in the top of the anus at the end of defecation, whereas this does not seem to happen with a harder stool. On walking, any trapped stool tends to massage out and cause irritation. Advice to patients regarding this mechanism will help them to help themselves.

Basic hygiene should be advocated. This involves daily cleansing of the anus using water, not soap, and drying the area with a soft towel or dryer. Perfumed talcum powder should be avoided. Loose underwear made of natural fibres should be worn.

If the patient feels like scratching it is usually because of fresh leakage. Further attention to hygiene may then obviate the desire to scratch, which at times can otherwise be well nigh irresistible. Short-term use of a hydrocortisone cream may help to break the cycle but this should not last for long as the skin may atrophy or become dependent upon the steroid and itch in its absence.

In a recent study by Lysy et al.,[68] topical capsaicin has been shown to be effective in treatment of idiopathic pruritus ani; 44 patients were randomised to topical capsaicin 0.006% or placebo (menthol 1%) and crossover was carried out after 4 weeks. Of these patients, 31 experienced relief with capsaicin but not with menthol. None of the patients resistant to capsaicin were relieved with menthol.

Conclusion

Pruritus ani remains a difficult problem to manage and results of treatment of primary pruritus ani remain equivocal. Treatment is aimed at reducing leakage, whether arising from a fistula, prolapsing haemorrhoid or simply increased flatulence. Good personal hygiene remains an important aspect of treatment and prevention of further irritation to the perianal skin.

Anal stenosis

Anal stenosis can be structural or functional. This section deals with structural stenosis, which is an abnormal fixed anatomical narrowing of the anal canal associated with a degree of functional obstruction at that level. This is in contrast to anal canal spasm secondary to painful lesions (commonly seen in anal fissures) or to defecatory functional abnormalities where examination shows a supple and fully compliant anus.

Aetiology

The commonest cause is postsurgical, usually after haemorrhoidectomy that has left only tenuous bridges, but other causes are given in Box 15.3. Recurrent anal fissures, perianal abscesses with repeated surgical procedures and excessive excision of perianal skin in Bowen's or Paget's disease may heal with anal canal stenosis. Chronic laxative abuse, especially those of mineral oils, over prolonged periods may anecdotally lead to anal stenosis, but frequently the patient has a functional problem with anal relaxation rather than a structural one of anal stenosis.

Clinical presentation

A history of constipation, decreasing stool calibre, difficulty in voiding with the need to strain excessively

Box 15.3 • Aetiology of anal stenosis

Congenital
- Imperforate anus
- Anal atresia

Acquired
- Irradiation
- Lacerations
- Chronic diarrhoea
- Following surgery of anal canal/low rectum

Neoplastic
- Perianal or anal cancers
- Leukaemia
- Bowen's disease
- Paget's disease

Inflammatory
- Crohn's disease
- Tuberculosis
- Amoebiasis
- *Lymphogranuloma venereum*
- Actinomycosis

Spastic
- Chronic anal fissure
- Ischaemic

and tenesmus are usually the first symptoms of anal stenosis. In severe cases, only loose stools may be passed. The clinician should be wary of some patients on laxative or enemas for their long-standing 'constipation' who may actually have a functional problem. Bleeding occurs when there is an associated anal fissure from traumatic defecation. However, a fissure in the absence of anal spasm may be seen in patients who anally digitate and thereby traumatise the anus. These patients usually have a functional problem of obstructed defecation. The diagnosis is usually obvious on perineal inspection. Often, the passage of an index finger through the narrowing is impossible. If the finger is passed (and particularly if a proctoscope can be passed), there is usually no clinically significant stenosis. Associated surgical scars may sometimes give an indication of the cause of stenosis. A biopsy is essential if a predisposing cause for the anal stenosis is suspected. The anatomical findings may not correlate well with the magnitude of the symptoms.

Treatment

The key to treatment lies firstly in its prevention. Excessive removal of the anoderm is often the cause of significant anal stenosis. Excision of the perianal skin to achieve a 'cosmetically' smooth and even skin contour does not always result in smooth anal function. Surgical judgement leaning towards adequate excision of haemorrhoidal tissue and anoderm is often more prudent. Eversion of any haemorrhoidal mass and excision may often lead to excessive removal of the anoderm. In particular, the Whitehead procedure for circumferential haemorrhoids may put the anal canal at risk of developing anal stenosis and associated mucosal ectropion as the scar contracts towards the perineum.

Anal dilatation

Treatment of anal stenosis depends on the severity and level of stenosis within the anal canal, as well as when it has arisen in relation to any precipitating anal operation. Mild or moderate stenosis (tight anal canal but permitting the passage of the index finger on pressure or forceful dilatation) may be treated with bulk laxatives, which will increase the stool calibre and provide a dilatory effect.

This may be supplemented with regular stretching, the patient using either his or her own finger or an appropriately sized anal dilator (e.g. St Mark's anal

dilator or size 18 Hagar dilator). Initial dilatation may need to be performed under anaesthesia. The patient should understand how to use the dilator before hospital discharge. This may be performed in the left lateral position or with the patient squatting and bearing down onto a well-lubricated (4% lidocaine jelly) finger or anal dilator. The patient should be guided to pass the dilator beyond the anal stricture twice daily for 2 months. Good functional results may be achieved in this manner, particularly if a postsurgical stenosis is caught early. The additional use of topical steroids has no documented benefits.

Severe anal stenosis, with inability to pass the index finger through the stenosis, will always require at least some initial form of surgical intervention, if only examination under anaesthesia with graded Hagar's dilatation. The principles of surgical treatment are outlined in Box 15.4.

Four-finger manual dilatation performed under anaesthesia should be discouraged and is anyway unnecessary. It may lead to excessive damage of the anal sphincters with resultant incontinence, especially in the hands of a novice. However, a very scarred and stenotic anus, or one associated with Crohn's disease, may be self-maintained using Hagar's dilators after initial Hagar's graded dilatation under general anaesthesia.

Sphincterotomy

If the 'stenosis' is due to a hypertrophied internal anal sphincter [which is very rare – Editor], then lateral anal sphincterotomy will be indicated. Localised scars in the anal canal are not likely to cause stenosis. Circumferential mucosal scarring will usually require some form of relining of the anal canal, usually by an anoplasty. However, we believe that there

---

Box 15.4 • Principles of surgical treatment for anal stenosis

- Stool bulking
- Increase anal outlet dimensions
- Examination under anaesthesia with graded Hagar's dilatation followed by postoperative self-maintenance
- In the rare case of internal sphincter hypertrophy: internal sphincterotomy
- Removal of cutaneous scarring
- Maintain correction
- Skin advancement (inwards)
- Mucosal advancement (outwards)
- Colostomy

may also be a role for sphincterotomy in a circumferentially scarred anus. It is simple to perform and if a single sphincterotomy is insufficient to open up the stenosis, multiple sphincterotomies may be done at different positions. Open sphincterotomy has the advantage of allowing the ingrowth of anoderm to maintain the increase in diameter of the anal canal. Sphincterotomy will provide immediate relief of any pain and apprehension associated with bowel opening in these patients [Editor's comment: evidence for such an approach needs to be presented].

Flap procedures

Mucosal advancement flap

This involves the advancement of anal mucosa into the stenotic area by way of a vertical incision made in the stenotic area perpendicular to the dentate line in the lateral position. An anal sphincterotomy and excision of the scar tissue allows widening of the stenosis. The incision is then undermined for about 2 cm and closed in a transverse manner with vicryl 3/0, stitching the mucosal edge down onto the skin edge of the anoderm. This creates a minor mucosal ectropion, which will keep the stenosis open.

Y-V advancement flap

Originally described by Penn in 1948, a Y incision is made, with the vertical limb of the Y in the anal canal above the proximal level of the stenosis. The 'V' of the Y is drawn on the lateral perianal skin. The skin is incised and a V-shaped flap is raised; the length-to-breadth ratio must be less than 3. After excision of the underlying scar tissue in the anal canal with or without an additional lateral sphincterotomy, the flap can be mobilised into the anal canal and stitched into place. This may be done bilaterally with good results[69,70] and provides relief in 85–92% of cases. Tip necrosis occurs in 10–25% of cases and stenosis may then recur.

V-Y advancement flap

Unlike the Y-V advancement flap, the V-Y flap has the advantage of bringing a wider piece of skin into the stenosis to keep it open. The V is drawn with the wide base parallel to the dentate line about 2 cm long. A similar length-to-base ratio as in the Y-V flap should be maintained. The scar tissue is excised. Marking out of the skin flap is followed by its mobilisation such that it may move without tension into the anal canal. Sufficient subcutaneous tissue must be mobilised with the flap, which derives its blood supply from the perforating vessels arising within the fat. The skin is then closed behind the flap to produce the limb of the Y. A treatment success rate of 96% has been reported with this flap.

Island advancement flap

First described in 1986 by Caplin and Kodner,[71] the island flap may be constructed in various shapes (e.g. diamond, house or U-shaped). The flap is mobilised from its lateral margins together with the subcutaneous fat after the scar tissue in the stenotic area has been excised. A lateral sphincterotomy may or may not be performed. A broad skin flap (up to 50% of the circumference) may be brought into the entire length of the anal canal and simultaneously allow for closure of the donor site. Improvement of symptoms may be as high as 91% at 3 years of follow-up;[72,73] 18–50% suffer minor wound separation.

S-anoplasty

This procedure mobilises bilateral gluteal skin into the entire anal canal after excision of the scar tissue up to the dentate line. The incision is designed in an S shape, hence the name of the flap. The breadth-to-length ratio must be more than 1, with the base of the S being about 7–10 cm. The skin is rotated to line the anal canal in a tension-free manner. This extensive procedure is rarely used. Prior full bowel preparation and perioperative antibiotic cover is advocated.

Conclusion

Most of the above treatments and surgical procedures will adequately deal with postsurgical anal canal stenosis, which usually involves the lower anal canal. Occasionally, a higher stenosis (above the dentate line) is encountered. In this instance, we believe a lateral sphincterotomy or division of the fibrotic band may be sufficient as the anal canal is more distensible at this level. However, in perianal Crohn's disease-related anal stenosis, we usually try to provide symptomatic relief with anal dilators, sometimes after prior examination under anaesthesia, in the hope of avoiding surgical wound problems.

Dietary fibre – more harm than good?

The discerning reader will realise by now that we have not recommended the use of dietary supplementation of fibre in the management of haemorrhoids or anal fissure despite a generally widely accepted belief that fibre is beneficial. Whilst dietary fibre is an essential part of our daily diet, its 'therapeutic' role remains controversial.

The main feature of a high-fibre diet is its poor digestibility. Although some of the ingested insoluble fibre gets fermented in the colon, the majority of it is passed unaltered in the gastrointestinal tract and excreted in the faeces. Therefore, the more fibre ingested, the more stools will have to be passed. In addition, contrary to popular belief, the moisture content in stools is not increased following an increased intake of fibre. Many doctors advocate drinking more water to improve bowel action but this does not necessarily lead to an increase in the water content of the stool; instead, it may only lead to an increase in urinary output. We believe that the frequent straining and passage of large bulky stools as a result of an increased ingestion of fibre will lead to further damage to the supensory ligaments of Parks at the anal cushions and thus may aggravate already prolapsed haemorrhoids.[74] Also, passage of such bulky stools through the anus may cause more trauma or tearing of the anal mucosa of patients with chronic anal fissure and thus potentially worsen the anal spasm.[74] Therefore we believe that although dietary fibre and fibre supplementation may have some merits, their beneficial role in haemorrhidal disease and chronic anal fissure should be re-evaluated and should not be recommended routinely for every patient with these conditions.[75]

Key points

- Haemorrhoidal disease is common but other life-threatening diseases must first be excluded. Treatment by submucosal injection, rubber band ligation or micronised flavonoids allow for symptomatic relief but we believe consideration should be given to stapled in favour of excisional haemorrhoidectomy for prolapsing piles.
- Anal fissures are common and their aetiology multifactorial. Although chemical sphincterotomies have been performed with good results, lateral sphincterotomy remains the gold standard for chronic anal fissures.
- Pruritis ani may result from many anorectal or dermatological conditions and remains a difficult problem to manage and treat. Reduction of anal leakage and good personal hygiene remain important aspects of treatment.
- Anal stenosis has many aetiologies but the commonest is a result of anal surgery. Treatments range from anal dilatation to flap procedures.

References

1. Shanmugam V, Thaha MA, Rabindranath KS et al. Rubber band ligation versus excisional haemorrhoidectomy for haemorrhoids. Cochrane Database Syst Rev 2005; Issue 1.

   Grade 2 haemorrhoids should be treated with rubber band ligation while surgery is reserved for grade 3 haemorrhoids or recurrent haemorrhoids after rubber band ligation.

2. Ho YH, Tan M, Seow-Choen F. Micronized purified flavonidic fraction compared favourably with rubber band ligation and fiber alone in the management of bleeding haemorrhoids. Dis Colon Rectum 2000; 43:66–9.

3. Wadworth AN, Faulds D. Hydroxyethylrutosides. A review of its pharmacology and therapeutic efficacy in venous insufficiency and related disorders. Drugs 1992; 44:1013–32.

4. Duhalt J. Mecanism d'action de Daflon 500mg sur le tonus veineux noradrenergique. Arteres Veines 1992; 11:217–18.

5. Galley P. A double-blind, placebo-controlled trial of a new venoactive flavonoid fraction (S5682) in the treatment of symptomatic fragility. Int Angiol 1993; 12:69–71.

6. Damon M. Effect of chronic treatment with purified flavonoid fraction on inflammatory granuloma in the rat. Study of prostaglandin E2 and F2 and thromboxane B2 release and histological changes. Arzneimittelforschung 1987; 37:1149–53.

7. Cospite M. Double-blind versus placebo evaluation of clinical activity and safety of Daflon 500mg in the treatment of acute haemorrhoids. Angiology 1994; 6:566–73.

8. Ho YH, Foo CL, Seow-Choen F et al. Prospective randomized controlled trial of micronized flavonidic fraction to reduce bleeding after haemorrhoidectomy. Br J Surg 1995; 82:1034–5.

9. Ho YH, Goh HS. Unilateral anal electrosensation: modified technique to improve quantifications of anal sensory loss. Dis Colon Rectum 1995; 38:239–44.

10. Ho YH, Seow-Choen F, Tan M et al. Randomised trial of open and closed haemorrhoidectomy. Br J Surg 1997; 84:1729–30.

11. Seow-Choen F, Ho YH, Ang HG et al. Prospective, randomized trial comparing pain and clinical function after conventional scissor excision/ligation vs. diathermy excision without ligation of symptomatic prolapsed haemorrhoids. Dis Colon Rectum 1992; 35:1165–9.

12. Ho KS, Eu KW, Heah SM et al. Randomized clinical trial of haemorrhoidectomy under a mixture of local anaesthesia versus general anaesthesia. Br J Surg 2000; 87(4):410–3.

13. Jane Tan JY, Seow-Choen F. Prospective randomised trial comparing diathermy and harmonic scalpel haemorrhoidectomy. Dis Colon Rectum 2001; 44:677–9.

14. Ibrahim S, Tsang C, Lee YL et al. Prospective, randomized trial comparing pain and complications between diathermy and scissors for closed hemorrhoidectomy. Dis Colon Rectum 1998; 41:1418–20.

15. Ho YH, Tan M. Ambulatory anorectal manometric findings in patients before and after haemorrhoidectomy. Int J Colorectal Dis 1997; 12(5):296–7.

16. Seow-Choen F, Low HC. Prospective randomized study of radical versus four piles haemorrhoidectomy for symptomatic large circumferential prolapsed piles. Br J Surg 1995; 82:188–9.

17. Kraemer M, Seow-Choen F. Whitehead haemorrhoidectomy in older patients. Tech Coloproct 2000; 4:79–82.

18. Seow-Choen F. Stapled haemorrhoidectomy: pain or gain. Br J Surg 2000; 88:1–3.

19. Seow-Choen F. Surgery for haemorrhoids: ablation or correction. Asian J Surg 2002; 25:265–6.

20. Lloyd D, Ho KS, Seow-Choen F. Modified Longo's haemorrhoidectomy. Dis Colon Rectum 2002; 45:416–17.

21. Cheetham MJ, Mortensen NJ, Nystrom PO et al. Persistent pain and faecal urgency after stapled haemorrhoidectomy. Lancet 2000; 356:730–3.

22. Jayaraman S, Colquhoun PHD, Malthaner RA. Stapled versus conventional surgery for haemorrhoids. Cochrane Database Syst Rev 2006; Issue 4.

Stapled haemorrhoidectomy is associated with higher risk of recurrence or symptoms of prolapse than excisional haemorrhoidectomy.

23. Jayne D, Seow-Choen F. Modified stapled haemorrhoi-dectomy for treatment of massive circumferentially prolapsing piles. Tech octol 2002; 6:191–3.

24. Brown SR, Ballan K, Ho E et al. Stapled mucosectomy for acute thrombosed circumferentially prolapsed piles: a prospective randomized comparison with conventional haemorrhoidectomy. Colorectal Dis 2001; 3:175–8.

25. Milligan ETC, Morgan CN, Jones LE et al. Surgical anatomy of the anal canal and the operative treatment of haemorrhoids. Lancet 1937; ii:1119–24.

26. Morinaga K, Hacuda K, Ikeada T. A novel therapy for internal haemorrhoids: ligation of the haemorrhoidal artery with a new devised instrument in conjunction with Doppler flow meter. Am J Gastroenterol 1995; 90(4):610–13.

27. Sohn N, Aronoff JS, Cohen FS et al. Transanal haemorrhoidal dearterialization is an alternative to operative haemorrhoidectomy. Am J Surg 2001; 182:515–19.

28. Dal Monte PP, Tagariello C, Giordano P et al. Transanal haemorrhoidal dearterialization: nonexcisional surgery for the treatment of haemorrhoidal disease. Tech Coloproctol 2007; 11:333–9.

29. Ho YH, Lee J, Salleh I et al. Randomized controlled trial comparing same-day discharge with hospital stay following haemorrhoidectomy. Aust NZ J Surg 1998; 68:334–6.

30. Guy RJ, Ng CE, Eu KW. Stapled anoplasty for haemorrhoids: a comparison of ambulatory vs. inpatient procedures. Colorectal Dis 2003; 5:29–32.

31. Ho YH, Cheong WK, Tsang C et al. Stapled hemorrhoidectomy: cost and effectiveness. Randomized, controlled trial including incontinence scoring, anorectal manometry, and endoanal ultrasound assessments at up to three months. Dis Colon Rectum 2000; 43:1666–75.

32. Davies J, Duffy D, Boyt N et al. Botulinum toxin (Botox) reduces pain after haemorrhoidectomy: results of a double-blind, randomized study. Dis Colon Rectum 2003; 46:1097–102.

33. Hwang do Y, Toon SG, Kim HS et al. Effect of 0.2 percent glyceryl trinitrate ointment on wound healing after a haemorrhoidectomy: results of a randomized, prospective, double-blind, placebo-controlled trial. Dis Colon Rectum 2003; 46:950–4.

34. Mathai V, Ong BC, Ho YH. Randomized controlled trial of lateral internal sphincterotomy with haemorrhoidectomy. Br J Surg 1996; 83:380–2.

35. Nyam DCNK, Seow-Choen F, Ho YH. Submucosal adrenaline injection for post-haemorrhoidectomy haemorrhage. Dis Colon Rectum 1995; 38:776–7.

36. Eu KW, Teoh TA, Seow-Choen F et al. Anal stricture following haemorrhoidectomy: early diagnosis and treatment. Aust NZ J Surg 1995; 65:101–3.

37. Ho YH, Seow-Choen F, Tsang C et al. Randomized trial assessing anal sphincter injuries after stapled haemorrhoidectomy. Br J Surg 2001; 88:1449–55.

38. Maw A, Concepcion R, Eu KW et al. Prospective randomized study of bacteremia in diathermy

and stapled haemorrhoidectomy. Br J Surg 2003; 90:222–6.

39. Guy RJ, Seow-Choen F. Septic complications after treatment of haemorrhoids. Br J Surg 2003; 90:147–56.

40. Carapeti EA, Kamm MA, McDonald PJ et al. Double-blind randomized controlled trial of effect of metronidazole on pain after daycase haemorrhoidectomy. Lancet 1998; 351:169–72.

41. Leong AFPK, Seow-Choen F. Lateral sphincterotomy compared with anal advancement flap for chronic anal fissure. Dis Colon Rectum 1995; 38:69–71.

42. Keck JO, Staniunas RJ, Coller JA et al. Computer-generated profiles of the anal canal in patients with anal fissure. Dis Colon Rectum 1995; 38:72–9.

43. Lund JN, Parsons JL, Scholefield JH. Spasm of the internal anal sphincter in anal fissure: cause or effect? Gastroenterology 1996; 110:A711.

44. Minguez M, Tomas-Ridocci M, Garcia A et al. Pressure of the anal canal in patients with haemorrhoids or anal fissure: effect of the topical application of an anaesthetic gel. Rev Esp Enfirm Dig 1992; 81:103–7.

45. Klosterhalfen B, Vogel P, Rixen H et al. Topography of the inferior rectal artery: a possible cause of chronic, primary anal fissure. Dis Colon Rectum 1989; 32:43–52.

46. Brown AC, Sumfest JM, Rozwadowski JV. Histopathology of the internal anal sphincter in chronic anal fissure. Dis Colon Rectum 1989; 32:680.

47. Schouten WR, Briel JW, Auwerda JJ et al. Ischaemic nature of anal fissure. Br J Surg 1996; 83:63–5.

48. Smith LE. Anal fissure. Neth J Med 1990; 37:S33.

49. Colins EE, Lund JN. A review of chronic anal fissure management. Tech Coloproctol 2007; 11:209–23.

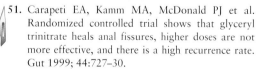

50. Lund JN, Scholefield JH. A randomized, prospective, double-blind, placebo-controlled trial of glycerin trinitrate ointment in the treatment of anal fissure. Lancet 1997; 349:11–14.

Sustained relief of pain in patients with anal fissure was demonstrated. Over two-thirds of patients treated with topical GTN avoided surgery.

51. Carapeti EA, Kamm MA, McDonald PJ et al. Randomized controlled trial shows that glyceryl trinitrate heals anal fissures, higher doses are not more effective, and there is a high recurrence rate. Gut 1999; 44:727–30.

52. Richard CS, Gregorie R, Plewes EA et al. Internal sphincterotomy is superior to topical nitroglycerin in the treatment of chronic anal fissure: results of a randomized trial by the Canadian Colorectal Surgical Trials Group. Dis Colon Rectum 2000; 43:1048–57.

Internal sphincterotomy is the treatment of choice for chronic anal fissure as it has a higher healing rate and fewer side-effects when compared with topical nitroglycerin.

53. Sajid MS, Rimple J, Cheek E et al. The efficacy of diltiazem and glyceryltrinitrate for the medical management of chronic anal fissure: a meta-analysis. Int J Colorectal Dis 2008; 23:1–6.

Diltiazem and GTN are effective in the treatment of anal fissures.

54. Cook TA, Humphreys MMS, Mortensen NJMcC. Oral nifedipine reduces resting anal pressure and heals chronic anal fissure. Br J Surg 1999; 86:1269–73.

55. Maria G, Sganga G, Civello IM et al. Botulinum neurotoxin and other treatments for fissure-in-ano and pelvic floor disorders. Br J Surg 2002; 89:950–61.

56. Brisinda G, Cadeddu F, Brandara F et al. Randomized clinical trial comparing botulinum toxin injections with 0.2 per cent nitroglycerin ointment for chronic anal fissure. Br J Surg 2007; 94:162–7.

In the medical treatment of chronic anal fissure, botulinum toxin is more effective than nitroglycerin ointment. Adverse effects in both treatments have been reported but are mild and self-limiting.

57. Brisinda G, Maria G, Bentivoglio AR et al. A comparison of injections of botulinum toxin and topical nitroglycerin ointment for the treatment of chronic anal fissures. N Engl J Med 1999; 341:65–9.

58. Nelson R. Non surgical therapy for anal fissure. Cochrane Database Syst Rev 2006; Issue 4.

Medical therapy can be used to treat anal fissure but is not as efffective as surgery. The former is also associated with a higher rate of recurrence.

59. Nelson R. Operative procedures for fissure in ano (meta-analysis). Cochrane Library 2003; Vol. 3.

60. Khubchandani IT, Reed JF. Sequelae of internal sphincterotomy for chronic fissure-in-ano. Br J Surg 1989; 76:431.

61. Littlejohn DR, Newstead GL. Tailored lateral sphincterotomy for anal fissure. Dis Colon Rectum 1997; 40:1439–42.

62. Garcia-Aguilar J, Belmonte C, Wong WD et al. Open vs closed sphincterotomy for chronic anal fissure: long-term results. Dis Colon Rectum 1996; 39:440–3.

63. Engel AF, Eijsbouts QAJ, Balk AG. Fissurectomy and isosorbide dinitrate for chronic fissure-in-ano not responding to conservative treatment. Br J Surg 2002; 89:79–83.

64. Scholz TH, Hetzer FH, Dindo D et al. Long-term follow-up after combined fissurectomy and Botox injection for chronic anal fissures. Int J Colorectal Dis 2007; 22:1077–81.

65. Fleschner PR, Schoetz DJ Jr, Roberts PL et al. Anal fissure in Crohn's disease: a plea for aggressive management. Dis Colon Rectum 1995; 38:1137–43.

66. Cundall JD, Gardiner A, Laden G et al. Use of hyperbaric oxygen to treat chronic anal fissure. Br J Surg 2003; 90:452–3.

67. Nyam DCNK, Wilson RG, Stewart KJ et al. Island advancement flaps in the management of anal fissures. Br J Surg 1995; 82:326–8.

68. Lysy J, Sistiery-Ittah M, Israelit Y et al. Topical capsaicin: a novel and effective treatment for idiopathic intractable pruritus ani. A randomised, placebo controlled, crossover study. Gut 2003; 52:1323–6.

69. Angelchik PD, Harms BA, Stanley JR. Repair of anal stricture and mucosal ectropion with YV or pedicle flap anoplasty. Am J Surg 1993; 166:55–9.

70. Ramanujam PS, Venkatesh KS, Cohen M. YV anoplasty for severe anal stenosis. Contemp Surg 1998; 3:62–8.

71. Caplin DA, Kodner IJ. Repair of anal stricture and mucosal ectropion by single flap procedures. Dis Colon Rectum 1986; 29:92.

72. Pidala MJ, Slezak FA, Porter JA. Island advancement anoplasty for anal canal stenosis and mucosal ectropion. Am Surg 1994; 60:194–6.

73. Sentovich SM, Falk PM, Christensen MA et al. Operative results of house advancement anoplasty. Br J Surg 1996; 83:1242–4.

74. Tan KY, Seow-Choen F. Fibre and colorectal disease: separating fact from friction. World J Gastroenterol 2007; 13(31):4161–7.

75. Chuwa EWL, Seow-Choen F. Dietary fibre. Br J Surg 2006; 93:3–4.

16

Sexually transmitted diseases and the anorectum

Charles B. Whitlow
David E. Beck

Introduction

Sexually transmitted diseases (STDs) are important but uncommon indications for evaluation by a colorectal surgeon. Presenting symptoms range from gastrointestinal (diarrhoea, rectal bleeding) to visible lesions in the anus and perineum. The increased prevalence and variety of STD seen in the UK and USA have been attributed to greater promiscuity, homosexuality and the use of the anorectum for sexual gratification. The incidence of any homosexual activity among British males is between 4% and 6%, but only about 1.5–2.5% of this group report homosexual activity in the preceding 5 years.[1] Unprotected anoreceptive sex and multiple partners are two common behaviours among homosexual males that put them at increased risk for anorectal STDs. Females are also affected by anorectal STDs, with more than 10% of American women and their male consorts engaging in anorectal sexual activity.[2]

The incidence of STDs (estimated at 15 million cases a year in the USA) and the non-specific gastrointestinal symptoms or cutaneous lesions associated with these infections mandate a high index of suspicion in order to make an accurate diagnosis. The presence of more than one offending organism is common. The diseases presented in Table 16.1 are categorised by aetiological agent. Medications and dosages are suggested, but clinicians are reminded

to consult the full prescribing information before using any medication mentioned in this chapter.

The more typically regarded organisms that cause STDs of the anorectum present with two main symptom complexes: proctitis or perianal ulceration. Other pathogens, less commonly listed among STDs and which can be spread by sexual practices other than anal intercourse, present with gastrointestinal symptoms such as diarrhoea or haematochezia. Paramount to the diagnosis of these diseases is a thorough history about sexual practices. These discussions may be uncomfortable for the patient and practitioner, but without them the proper diagnosis is likely to be missed.

Viral

Cytomegalovirus

Cytomegalovirus (CMV) is a common DNA virus with positive cultures or serology found in over 90% of human immunodeficiency virus (HIV)-positive homosexual men.[3] It is not always associated with pathological changes and it is often found in association with other infectious pathogens. In the context of this chapter, CMV gastrointestinal infections are included because they are most associated with immunocompromised individuals (acquired immunodeficiency syndrome (AIDS), transplant recipients). It is a common viral cause of diarrhoea in

Table 16.1 • Sexually transmitted organisms that affect the anorectum

Organism	Symptoms	Anoscopy/ proctoscopy	Laboratory	Treatment
Viral				
Cytomegalovirus	Rectal bleeding	Multiple small white ulcers	Biopsy, viral culture, antigen assay of ulcers	Intravenous ganciclovir, foscarnet
Herpes simplex virus (HSV)	Anorectal pain, pruritis, rectal bleeding	Perianal erythema, vesicles, ulcers Diffusely inflamed, friable rectal mucosa	Cytological examination of scrapings or viral culture of vesicle fluid PCR	See Box 16.1
HIV/AIDS	See text	See text	Serology	Nucleoside analogues, non-nucleoside reverse transcriptase inhibitors, protease inhibitors
Human papillomavirus (condylomata acuminatum)	Pruritis, bleeding, discharge, pain	Perianal warts	Excisional biopsy	Excision or destruction Topical agents (see text)
Molluscum contagiosum	Painless skin lesions	Flattened, round, umbilicated lesion	Excisional biopsy	Excision or destruction
Bacterial				
Campylobacter jejuni	Diarrhoea, cramps, bloating	Eythema, oedema, greyish-white ulcerations of rectal mucosa	Culture stool on selective media	Oral erythromycin 500 mg q.i.d. for 7 days
Chlamydia trachomatis	Tenesmus, perianal pain	Friable, often ulcerated mucosa	Tissue culture Nucleic acid amplification Serological antibody titres	Oral doxycycline 100 mg b.i.d. for 7 days, oral azithromycin 1 g as a single dose
Lymphogranuloma venereum	Systemic symptoms, inguinal adenopathy, anogenital ulceration	Friable ulcerated rectal mucosa	LGV serotyping with nucleic acid amplification, confirmation at specialty laboratories	Oral doxycline 100 mg b.i.d. for 14–21 days, oral erythromycin 500 mg q.i.d. for 14–21 days
Haemphilus ducreyi (chancroid)	Anal pain	Anorectal abscesses and ulcers	Culture PCR	Oral azithromycin 1 g as a single dose, oral ciprofloxacin 500 mg b.i.d. for 3 days, oral erythromycyin 500 mg q.i.d. for 7 days, i.m. ceftriaxone 250 mg as a single dose
Neisseria gonorrhoeae (gonorrhoea)	Rectal discharge	Proctitis Mucopurulent discharge	Thayer–Martin culture of discharge	Ceftriaxone 125 mg i.m. single dose plus oral doxycycline 100 mg b.i.d. for 7 days See text about quinolones
Calymmatobacterium granulomatis (granuloma inguinale)	Perianal mass, ulceration	Hard, shiny perianal masses	Smear or biopsy of mass or ulceration	Oral azithromycin, 1 g first day, then 500 mg daily until healed Oral doxycyline 100 mg b.i.d. until healed
Treponema pallidum (syphilis)	Rectal pain	Painful anal ulcer	Dark-field microscopy of ulcer scrapings Immunostaining from biopsy Serology	Benzathine benzylpenicillin 2.4 million units i.m. as a single dose

AIDS patients and is one of the more common gastrointestinal manifestations of AIDS.

CMV colitis may present with fever, abdominal pain and explosive diarrhoea with or without blood. In severe cases it may present with massive haemorrhage or intestinal perforation. Endoscopically, CMV lesions in the colon range from erythematous patches with no ulceration to wide, deep, coalescing ulcerations. Typically the edges are smooth and a whitish membrane may be present. Diagnosis is made from histopathology and immunohistochemistry of biopsies from gross lesions. The characteristic microscopic appearance includes large, basophilic, intranuclear CMV inclusions in the setting of viral cytopathic changes. Viral culture can also be performed on biopsy samples. Isolated CMV proctitis is uncommon and presents with non-specific symptoms like tenesmus, diarrhoea and haematochezia. Endoscopic and histological abnormalities are as described above but limited to the rectum.

Medical treatment of CMV requires either intravenous ganciclovir or intravenous foscarnet, lasting 3–6 weeks depending on clinical response. Relapses are not uncommon and may require maintenance therapy with oral ganciclovir.[4] Surgery is rarely required and is limited to patients with refractory haemorrhage or perforation. Subtotal colectomy with end ileostomy is the preferred approach but postoperative mortality is high.[5]

Herpes simplex virus

Herpes simplex virus (HSV) is a DNA virus endemic to the USA and the UK. The overall seroprevalence rate for HSV Type 2 (HSV-2) is 10% in the UK and it is estimated that at least 50 million patients in the USA have genital herpes infection.[6] Two serotypes cause clinical problems. Type 1 (HSV-1) is usually associated with oral–labial lesions, but with increasing oral–genital contact the rate of HSV-1 genital infections has increased.[7] HSV-1 also accounts for up to 13% of anorectal herpes infections. HSV-2 is more typically responsible for anogenital infections from direct anogenital contact. A substantial percentage of homosexual males are HSV-2 seropositive and up to one-third of homosexual males with rectal symptoms are HSV-2 culture positive.[8] HSV infection increases the risk of acquiring and transmitting HIV.

HSV is transmitted by direct contact to the skin or mucosa and infection is most commonly manifest by

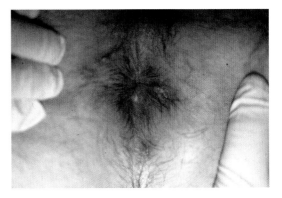

Figure 16.1 • Perianal HSV.

small painful vesicles affecting the perianal skin and the anus (**Fig. 16.1**). These lesions last for 1–2 weeks and patients are highly contagious until re-epithelialisation has completed. With secondary infection erythematous edges develop. Rectal involvement results in a painful proctitis that on sigmoidoscopy demonstrates friable mucosa, diffuse ulcerations and occasionally intact vesicles. Symptomatic infection can include systemic complaints of fevers, chills and malaise, and/or local symptoms of anal pain, tenesmus and rectal bleeding. Tender lymphadenopathy occurs in some patients. Diagnosis is confirmed by viral culture or polymerase chain reaction (PCR) of swabs from ulcerations. Type-specific serology may also be useful.

Symptomatic resolution of the acute infection is frequently followed by a chronic relapsing course. Prodromal symptoms of itching, burning or tingling may be noted, followed by the appearance of lesions which are usually in the same dermatome distribution as the initial infection.

A sacral radiculitis (Elsberg syndrome) can develop. The symptoms include urinary retention, constipation, erectile dysfunctions, paraesthesias and lower extremity weakness. Magnetic resonance imaging (MRI) reveals oedema of the spinal cord or roots and PCR of cerebrospinal fluid may aid diagnosis.[9]

Treatment is directed at two areas. The first is to provide symptomatic relief with measures such as analgesics, cool compresses, lidocaine (lignocaine) ointment or patches, sitz baths, etc. Hygiene is important to prevent bacterial superinfection. The second concern is direct treatment of severe active infections of patients with frequent reinfections. Pharmacotherapy of the initial presentation and of episodic recurrences of herpes proctitis or herpetic perianal ulcerations is with oral acyclovir, famciclovir or valacyclovir for

7–10 days (see Box 16.1).[10] While this treatment reduces the duration and severity of symptoms, it does not eradicate HSV, cure the disease or prevent recurrence or asymptomatic viral shedding.

Following initial infection and resolution most patients will experience recurrences. These recurrences tend to be shorter and less severe than the initial episode and decrease in frequency with time. Viral shedding may occur during the prodrome period, with active lesions or in the completely asymptomatic.[11]

Treatment of recurrences can be episodic or with suppressive daily treatment.

 Daily suppressive therapy is safe and reduces viral shedding, transmission of HSV and symptomatic recurrence.[12]

Part of complete treatment of HSV includes patient counselling on the risks of transmission in the absence of symptoms and despite the use of suppressive therapy and condoms. An HSV-2 vaccine is being studied.

Human immunodeficiency virus

HIV is an RNA retrovirus that infects human T lymphocytes. It is transmitted by contaminated body fluids and, after a variable latent period of up to 2 years, it produces diminished immunological function which is manifest as AIDS. As of 2004 there have been an estimated 40 million persons worldwide infected with HIV and 25 million have died of AIDS.[13] There are approximately 58 000 HIV/AIDS patients in the UK.[14] The incidence of HIV infection has apparently levelled in the USA and western Europe and the mortality from these infections has decreased as highly active antiretroviral therapy (HAART) has become widely available.

This is not meant to be an exhaustive treatise on HIV/AIDS. However, an understanding of HIV/AIDS is important to the practice of colon and rectal surgery as these patients frequently present with proctological diseases. These diseases can be divided into three categories:

1. Proctological complaints common to the population at large (e.g. haemorrhoids, fissures, pruritis) are frequently seen in HIV/AIDS patients and in the absence of routine screening may be the primary reason for seeking medical help.
2. Diseases associated with high-risk behaviours such as anoreceptive intercourse. Included in this group are the STDs which cause proctitis and anogenital ulcerations discussed later in this chapter.
3. Those illnesses associated with HIV infection such as HIV anal ulceration, unusual opportunistic infections, Kaposi's sarcoma and lymphoma.

The distribution of the most common anorectal pathologies reported in HIV patients include anal ulcer (29–32%), anal condyloma (32–43%), anal fissure (6–33%), anal fistula (6–33%), perirectal abscess (3–25%) and haemorrhoids (4–14%).[15]

Box 16.1 • Treatment of anorectal HSV*

First episode (treat 7–10 days, continue 7–10 more days if lesions persist)

Acyclovir

200 mg 5 times a day
400 mg 3 times a day

Valacyclovir

1 g 2 times a day

Famciclovir

250 mg 3 times a day

Recurrent episodes

Acylovir

200 mg 5 times a day for 5 days
800 mg 2 times a day for 5 days
800 mg 3 times a day for 2 days

Valacyclovir

500 mg 2 times a day for 3 days
1 g once a day for 5 days

Famciclovir

125 mg 2 times a day for 5 days
1 g 2 times a day for 1 day

Suppressive therapy

Acyclovir

400 mg 2 times a day

Valacylovir

500 mg once daily
1 g once daily

Famcilovir

250 mg 2 times a day

Data from Centers for Disease Control. Sexually transmitted diseases treatment guidelines 2006. MMWR 2006; 55(RR-11): 1–94.
* All doses given are oral.

The general approach to the HIV-infected patient with proctological complaints starts with a thorough history, which includes presenting symptoms, bowel and sphincter function, sexual practices and prior anorectal surgery. The current antiretroviral treatment the patient is taking as well as CD4+ counts and viral load are determined. Box 16.2 gives the most current classification system for HIV/AIDS.[16] Examiners should observe universal precautions. Most patients require only visual inspection and anoscopic or proctoscopic examination. We use disposable instruments for convenience but traditional sterilisation measures are adequate for non-disposable instruments. Abnormal lesions of the rectal mucosa or anal/perirectal region are biopsied.

Operations for anorectal pathology represent one of the most common indications for surgery in HIV-positive patients. One concern in taking care of these patients is how their disease affects wound healing. It appears that patients who are HIV positive without AIDS have no increased risk of wound problems, while those with AIDS are more likely to have delayed wound healing. Symptomatic improvement of the underlying anorectal pathology may make delayed wound healing an acceptable complication in many instances.

Patients with acute anorectal abscesses are treated by incision and drainage of the abscess. Our practice is to make a small incision and place a mushroom catheter (Pezzar, Malecot) for 5–7 days. Broad-spectrum antibiotics are prescribed, especially if there is any associated cellulitis. Fistula treatment in patients with AIDS and decreased CD4+ or leucocytes is similar to that of Crohn's patients with draining setons placed to control sepsis. Fibrin glue and the collagen fistula plug are as yet unproven, but they are low-risk treatment options to consider in this patient group. Fistulas in HIV/AIDS with normal counts are treated with the same treatment algorithm as HIV-negative patients.

Internal haemorrhoids most commonly present with symptoms of bleeding or prolapse. HIV-positive patients are treated along the same treatment schedule as HIV-negative patients. Initial management is with increased dietary fibre, bulking agents and topical preparations. Those that remain symptomatic

Box 16.2 • Revised classification system for HIV and AIDS

CD4+ T-lymphocyte categories

Category 1

≥500 cells/μL

Category 2

200–499 cells/μL

Category 3

<200 cells/μL

Clinical categories

Category A

HIV positive; asymptomatic; persistent generalised adenopathy

Category B

Symptomatic conditions not listed in clinical category C; are conditions that are attributed to HIV infection; or conditions that have a clinical course or require management that is complicated by HIV infection. Examples include: bacillary angiomatosis, oropharyngeal or vulvovaginal candidiasis, cervical dysplasia, diarrhoea (more than 1 month in duration), more than one episode of herpes zoster, pelvic inflammatory disease, peripheral neuropathy

Category C

Diagnoses included in the AIDS surveillance case definition: candidiasis (pulmonary or oesophageal), invasive cervical cancer, coccidiomycosis, extrapulmonary cryptococcosis, chronic intestinal cryptosporidiosis, cytomegalovirus disease (other than liver, spleen, nodes) or retinitis, HIV-encephalopathy, HSV (chronic ulcers, pulmonary, or oesophageal), histoplasmosis (disseminated or extrapulmonary), isosporiasis (chronic intestinal), Kaposi's sarcoma, Burkitt's lymphoma, immunoblastic lymphoma, primary brain lymphoma, *Mycobacterium avium* complex or any *Mycobacterium* species other than *M. tuberculosis* (extrapulmonary or disseminated), *M. tuberculosis, Pneumocystis carinii* pneumonia, progressive focal leucoencephalopathy, recurrent *Salmonella* septicaemia, toxoplasmosis of the brain, and HIV wasting syndrome

are treated with local measures such as rubber band ligation, infrared coagulation or sclerotherapy. The safety of rubber band ligation in HIV-positive patients without AIDS was demonstrated by Moore and Fleshner in a study of 11 patients with CD4+ counts ranging from 200 to 1000 cells/microlitre (median 450).[17] The authors typically banded one column per session and did not give prophylactic antibiotics. There were no complications related to banding and 91% of patients had at least some improvement of their presenting symptoms.

Haemorrhoidectomy is indicated in patients who fail conservative treatments. The results of haemorrhoidectomy in HIV-positive patients have been conflicting, most likely because of a difference in the severity of AIDS. Hewitt et al. compared wound healing times in HIV-negative vs. HIV-positive patients undergoing haemorrhoidectomy.[18] They found no difference in wound healing in HIV negative vs. HIV positive, HIV positive vs. HIV/AIDS, or CD4+ >200 vs. CD4+ <200. The authors point out that their patients were otherwise healthy and specifically mention that the HIV-positive patients were not malnourished or considered end-stage AIDS. While Hewitt et al. concluded that HIV status should not alter indications for surgical haemorrhoidectomy, Morandi et al. concluded that the high incidence of delayed wound healing suggested that the indication for haemorrhoidectomy in patients with AIDS needed to be considered carefully.[19] They found 50% of patients with AIDS failed to heal 32 weeks after haemorrhoidectomy. The two factors most associated with poor wound healing were AIDS and Karnofsky performance score. Symptomatic improvement was not addressed in this article. Taking these studies into account, it is our practice to offer haemorrhoidectomy to HIV-positive patients without AIDS based on standard indications just as for HIV-negative patients. AIDS patients with more advanced disease, low CD4+ counts (<100) or poor performance status are at increased risk for poor wound healing. The benefits of resolution of symptoms must be balanced against this risk.

Idiopathic anal fissures in HIV-positive patients must be distinguished from HIV-associated ulcers and STDs that cause anogenital ulcers. Treatment is similar to that of the HIV-negative population, starting with conservative measures such as warm soaks, stool softeners and topical ointments. Anoreceptive intercourse is discouraged. Two percent diltiazem ointment applied two to three times daily to the anus or botulinum toxin injected into the internal anal sphincter are alternative treatments to surgery in patients who do not respond to initial conservative measures. Lateral internal anal sphincterotomy is appropriate for patients who fail conservative measures but do not have chronic diarrhoea or pre-existing incontinence. Alternatively, a cutaneous advancement flap is preferred in those with a contraindication to sphincterotomy.

There is a paucity of data on the incidence of AIDS-associated anal ulcers. It appears that with HAART it is a less common clinical problem because these ulcers are most commonly associated with patients with clinical AIDS and lower CD4+ counts. There is one published series which reported no change in the prevalence and distribution of anal pathology (including AIDS ulcers) since the introduction of HAART.[15] These ulcers are a distinct disease process from typical anal fissures. Clinically they both result in pain with defecation, but AIDS ulcers are more likely to result in disabling pain unrelated to bowel movements. On examination AIDS ulcers are differentiated by their location proximal to the dentate line with a broad-based ulcer which may dissect between tissue plains (**Fig. 16.2**). The presence of a cavity contributes to stool and pus trapping, which may explain the severity of pain. Biopsy identifies treatable aetiologies of these ulcers, including HSV, CMV, *Treponemia pallidum*, mycobacterium, cryptococcus, *Haemophilus ducreyi*, *Chlamydia trachomatis* and cancer.

 Surgical treatment consists of debridement, unroofing cavities (to eliminate trapping) and intralesional steroid injection (80–160 mg methylprednisolone acetate in 1 mL of 0.25% bupivicaine). Repeat steroid injection is performed on patients who develop recurrent pain. The goal of this treatment is pain relief as ulcer healing is not common.[20,21]

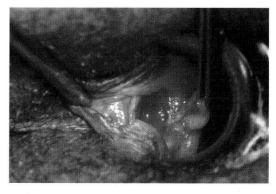

Figure 16.2 • HIV ulcer.

Human papillomavirus

Human papillomavirus (HPV) is a DNA virus that is the cause of viral warts on the skin and genitalia. There are over 118 types of HPV and about 60 of them are capable of anogenital infection. It is the most common sexually transmitted disease in the USA, with an estimated incidence of 6 million new cases per year and a prevalence of 27% for females aged 14–59 years.[22,23] HPV infection is spread by direct contact with infected skin or fluid and is frequently clinically silent. Anal intercourse is not required for anal infection to occur.[24,25] Low-risk (non-oncogenic) HPV serotypes such as HPV 6 and 11 account for the majority of anogenital warts. High-risk (oncogenic) serotypes, HPV 16 and 18, are strongly associated with anal cancer.

Patients with anal condylomata frequently present with complaints of 'haemorrhoids'. Symptoms include bleeding, pruritis, perianal wetness, bleeding and the feeling of a lump or mass. Morphologically the lesions can range in appearance from a single, pinkish-white, cauliflower-like, pinhead-sized lesion to multiple vast clusters that may obliterate the anus from view (**Fig. 16.3**). Because associated genital lesions are common, patients with anal condylomata should undergo thorough physical examination. In women this includes vaginal speculum exam and a Pap smear. Anal canal lesions that are missed on simple visual inspection of the anus can be found on anoscopy. Lesions that may be confused with anal condylomata include condyloma lata, molluscum contagiousum and hypertrophied anal papillae. Histopathology confirms the clinical diagnosis. Characteristic findings on microscopic examination include acanthosis, parakeratosis and the presence of koilocytes (large keratinocytes with an eccentric, pyknotic nucleus and perinuclear halo).

Treatment of perianal and anal condylomata is aimed at destroying gross lesions while minimising morbidity. Numerous options for treatment are available to the clinician, and the choice of treatment depends on the number, size and distribution of lesions, prior therapy, patient preference and surgeon experience, among other things. Because only gross lesions are treated, virus remains in adjacent skin and can lead to recurrence.

The most commonly used topical treatments for anal condylomata have all shown substantial failure and high recurrence rates; they include podophyllin, podophyllotoxin and trichloroacetic acid. Podophyllin resin is a non-standardised resin from the may-apple plant (*Podophyllum peltatum*) that acts as a cytotoxic agent. A 15–25% solution is applied once or twice weekly and then washed off about 4 hours later. It is not intended for use in the anal canal. Concerns about systemic side-effects when applied to larger lesions and inferior efficacy compared to podophyllotoxin have led experts, including the authors, to no longer recommend its use.[26]

Podophyllotoxin is the purified active antiwart compound from *Podophyllum* spp. which is available as a 0.5% solution or 0.15% cream. Both formulations have demonstrated clinical superiority to podophyllin in several studies.[26,27] Podophyllotoxin can be self-administered twice daily for 3 days, followed by a 4-day 'off' period. This is repeated for four cycles. Resolution of warts occurs in 60–80% of patients. Ulceration occurs in 10–20% but other local side-effects are minimal.

Trichloracetic acid as a 60–90% solution can be applied directly to perianal condylomata and lesions in the anal canal. Destruction of the lesion is by protein coagulation, so adjacent normal skin should be protected or cleaned immediately. It is applied weekly and numerous treatments are usually required. It is best reserved for small lesions that are few in number.

Imiquimod differs from the above-listed topical agents in that it acts as a local immunomodulator that induces α-interferon, tumour necrosis factor-α and other cytokines. As such it has the potential to eradicate HPV from the mucocutaneous surfaces adjacent to gross lesions, which could decrease recurrences and treatment failures. A 5% cream is applied nightly three times a week and washed off after 8 hours. This regimen can be continued for up to 16 weeks. Local skin reactions, such as erythema or excoriation, are common but only about 5% of patients cease treatment because of them. Complete resolution of lesions occurs in >50% of cases and additional patients experience a substantial

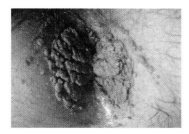

Figure 16.3 • Anal condylomata.

reduction of wart volume.[28,29] Recurrences occur in 10–20%. Imiquimod is not approved for intra-anal use, yet the use of an imiquimod suppository in 10 patients has been described with no adverse effects.[30] These authors have used imiquimod in several manners: as solitary therapy; as initial treatment followed by surgical treatment of residual disease, in effect 'debulking' large condylomata in order to minimise pain and fibrosis caused by fulguration/excision; and to treat early recurrences after surgical treatment, or as 'adjuvant' treatment after surgical treatment in patients who have demonstrated a tendency for recurrence.

Cryotherapy causes thermal-induced cytolysis and is listed in the Centers for Disease Control (CDC) treatment guideline for anal warts.[10] Proponents of this method report that anaesthesia is unnecessary. However, larger areas and more numerous lesions may require local anaesthetic. Freeze–thaw cycles can be produced with a commercially available cryoprobe, application of liquid nitrogen with a cotton-tipped applicator or with aerosolised liquid nitrogen. The procedure is inexact and it is difficult to gauge the depth of tissue destruction. Painful local tissue reaction is common, and some may experience tissue slough, ulceration and foul-smelling discharge. Liquid nitrogen is cumbersome to store and has a limited shelf-life. The authors feel the other options available are as effective and convenient to use as cryotherapy and therefore do not employ this technique in their practice.

Intralesional interferon injection has been studied, with schedules ranging from twice weekly to daily. The efficacy as primary treatment is no better than other modalities and systemic side-effects such as fever, chills, myalgias, headache and leucopenia occur. Its current use is limited to recurrences and lesions refractory to other treatments.

Immunotherapy with an autologous vaccine was described by Abcarian and Sharon.[31,32] They described weekly injections of 0.5 mL of the vaccine with no adverse reactions. Disappearance of warts occurred in 84% of patients. Similar results were reported by Eftaiha et al. on patients who had failed other treatments.[33] Vaccine preparation, the need for proper storage and treatment time prevented this from more widespread use. These issues and the lack of subsequent reports relegate autologous vaccine for condylomata to historical interest only.

A quadrivalent HPV vaccine against HPV 6, 11, 16 and 18 is now available. Its use is prophylactic

and it therefore plays no role in the treatment of visible anal condyloma. Current recommendations are to vaccinate females before exposure to HPV. No data are available on the efficacy of this vaccine for preventing anogenital HPV in males.[34]

Surgical excision can be performed in the outpatient clinic with local anaesthetic or in the operating room with local, regional or general anaesthesia. Excision has the benefit of providing tissue for histopathology. This is especially important in recurrent or atypical appearing lesions or in HIV-positive patients. Small lesions that are few in number are injected at their base with local anaesthetic and then tangential excision with scissors, a scalpel or electrocautery is performed. Haemostasis is ensured with silver nitrate or electrocautery. Postoperative care involves only daily cleansing with soap and water.

Larger lesions or patients with numerous lesions may benefit from regional anaesthesia. Broad-based lesions which would require excision of a substantial portion of perianal skin are more appropriately treated by fulguration and curettage than excision. The patient is positioned as suits the surgeon and anaesthetist. Using needle-tipped electrocautery, the most superficial layer of the condylomata is fulgurated to a grey–white appearance. This layer is then removed by curettage or by wiping it with gauze. This process is repeated until the condylomata are removed but taking care not to burn into the deep dermis or subcutaneous fat. Patients are given adequate oral narcotic analgesics and 5% topical lidocaine ointment postoperatively. Daily wound care with soap and water is adequate in most cases; however, in the USA mupirocin or sulfadiazine are given if any evidence of infection develops.

Laser destruction of warts has been advocated as being less painful and associated with fewer recurrences than other destructive techniques. No prospective, randomised data support these claims. A risk of using the laser is the problem of aerosolised active viral particles in the laser plume. Viable viral particles have been recovered from this smoke and cases of medical providers developing condylomata in their respiratory tract after using a laser to treat warts has been reported. Filter masks and smoke evacuators are recommended when lasers are used. Transmission of viral particles appears to be less of a problem with the larger-particle smoke from electrocautery. Finally, the laser is vastly more expensive than electrocautery and requires special training by both physician and ancillary staff. For these reasons many colorectal surgeons have been reluctant to abandon the less expensive and equally effective electrocautery in favour of the laser.

HPV and anal cancer

Just as HPV is linked to cervical cancer, a large body of literature has established the link between HPV and anal carcinoma. The annual incidence of new cases of anal cancer in the USA is estimated at about 4000. The incidence in HIV-negative homosexual males is roughly 35 times that rate and in HIV-positive males that rate is further doubled. It appears that in the HAART era this rate has not been decreased.[35,36]

The cervix and anal canal are similar in histology in that each has a junction of squamous epithelium with columnar epithelium. This has led some to suggest that anal HPV may progress through grades of dysplasia to invasive cancer and is the basis for screening and treatment strategies aimed at identifying these premalignant changes. Anal Pap smears are one screening test that has been suggested for homosexual men, especially those that are HIV positive. Current guidelines do not recommend routine screening as there are no randomised trials demonstrating benefit. The technique involves blind swabbing of the anal canal followed by fixing the cells on slides or in fluid. Cytological examination is performed and cells classified by a system revised from cervical cytology which includes normal, atypical squamous cells of uncertain significance (ASCUC), low-grade squamous intraepithelial lesions (LSIL) or high-grade squamous intraepithelial lesions (HSIL). The natural history and optimal evaluation and treatment of abnormal anal Pap smears is still being defined. High-resolution anoscopy has been recommended as part of an algorithm for abnormal cytology.[37] Similar to colposcopy, acetowhitening and staining with Lugol's solution is used to identify suspicious areas under an operating microscope. Gross and microscopic lesions are excised or biopsied and fulgurated. In some cases, due to burden of disease, staged treatment must be performed to reduce the risk of anal stenosis. Follow-up is frequent, with repeat examination every 6 months. No randomised study has demonstrated a decrease in anal cancer using this strategy. A less aggressive approach is to excise or biopsy/destroy only gross lesions and submit the remainder to close observation.

Molluscum contagiosum

Molluscum contagiosum is caused by a virus of the pox family and is transmitted by direct contact. It is a common cause of skin lesions anywhere in children but can be spread to the anogenital region by intercourse, skin-to-skin contact or autoinoculation. The typical lesions are papules 1–5 mm in diameter with central umbilication. Multiple lesions are common but lesions greater than 1 cm (giant molloscum contagiosum) are rare. Diagnosis is made by recognition of the typical lesions, biopsy with histopathology, or KOH preparation. While it is generally a self-limited disease, treatment is used to prevent spread and for cosmetic purposes. A variety of treatments have been described but none has proven superior in clinical trials. Curettage, cryotherapy, trichloroacetic acid and electrocautery are all discussed in the section on HPV. Topical agents such as cantharidin, tretinoin, podophyllotoxin and imiquimod have been reported in small case series but are not approved for use in the USA for this indication.[38]

Bacterial

Campylobacter jejuni

Campylobacter jejuni is a common cause of enterocolitis and infectious diarrhoea. Transmission of these curved, motile, non-spore-forming, Gram-negative rods is by ingestion of infected milk or meat. The role of sexual transmission is unclear, although it has been isolated in homosexual males, especially those with anorectal or intestinal symptoms.[39] Clinical features include crampy abdominal pain, diarrhoea with or without blood, systemic symptoms, arthritis, pericarditis or even Guillain–Barré syndrome. Most *Campylobacter* infections are self-limited and supportive treatment is all that is required. Antibiotics (erythromycin, quinolones) are used for treatment in severe or prolonged cases. Some resistant strains have been reported.[40]

Chlamydia and *Lymphogranuloma venereum* (LGV)

Chlamydia trachomatis is the most commonly reported bacterial sexually transmitted infection in western countries. Clinical syndromes resulting from chlamydial infection include cervicitis, pelvic inflammatory disease, urethritis and proctitis. Over 1 million *Chlamydia* infections were reported in the USA in 2006, but when unreported cases are included the total estimated annual incidence is about 3 million.[41]

Chlamydia are broadly divided into two groups based on serotyping. Rectal infection with non-LGV serotypes (serotyped D–K) may result in a proctitis, but lack of symptoms is common. Non-specific symptoms of proctitis include tenesmus, rectal urgency, bloody discharge and anorectal pain. More proximal involvement of the colon may produce bloody diarrhoea. The endoscopic appearance of chlamydial proctitis is diffuse inflammation, small ulcerations and nodular lymphoid follicle hyperplasia.[42] Diagnosis is by culture, microimmunofluorescent antibody titres or PCR. The technique for transport of biopsies for culture is important and involves placing the biopsy in sucrose phosphate media on ice for immediate tissue culture inoculation. Nucleic acid amplification tests are currently not FDA approved. There are data supporting their accuracy in rectal specimens and they have been recommended in cases where culturing *Chlamydia* is not available.[43] The treatment for non-LGV anorectal *Chlamydia* is supplied in Table 16.1.

Infection with LGV serotypes (L1, L2, L3) has been endemic to some tropical countries, but in the past 5 years an increasing number of cases of LGV proctitis has been seen in western countries almost exclusively in HIV-positive homosexual males.[44] Before these reports, LGV was more commonly associated with anogenital ulceration. Small vesicles that become ulcerated are the initial signs of infection that occur at the site of inoculation. After resolution of these lesions, an anogenitorectal syndrome occurs, which comprises signs of systemic infection (fevers, chills, myalgias) and a proctitis that is more severe than that seen with non-LGV strains. Mucosal ulceration and regional adenopathy may make the proctitis indistinguishable from Crohn's disease. Long-term chronic inflammation from LGV results in stricture, fistulas and lymphoedema. Diagnosis of LGV is made by serotyping in patients determined to have *Chlamydia* by the methods listed above. Unfortunately, serotyping is not rapid nor is it widely available. This has led to the recommendation to treat patients with anorectal *Chlamydia* who are at high risk of LGV (those with proctitis on proctoscopy, >10 white blood cells/high-power field on anorectal smear, or those who are HIV positive)

presumptively.[45] Treatment for LGV is doxycycline 100 mg twice daily for 3 weeks.

Chancroid

Haemophilus ducreyi is a Gram-negative coccobacillus which is a frequent cause of painful anogenital ulcerations in underdeveloped countries but is uncommon in the USA and western Europe.[46] Transmission is via sexual intercourse, although some perianal ulcerations have been seen in females without anal intercourse. The ulcerations are frequently multiple. In addition to ulceration, regional lymphadenopathy and bubo formation may be noted. The lymphadenopathy is frequently unilateral and is more common in males. A health concern that extends beyond the clinical effects described is the understanding that genital ulcerations facilitate HIV transmission.

Culture of *H. ducreyi* from ulcer material requires special laboratory techniques and at best is 80% sensitive. Gram stain is unreliable and non-specific. PCR detection of *H. ducreyi* is more sensitive than culture and although not commercially available is becoming more widely used at specialised labs.[47] Fluctuant bubos are aspirated or incised and drained. Antibiotic treatment regimens include erythromycin, azithromycin, ceftriaxone or ciprofloxacin[48] (see Table 16.1).

Gonorrhoea

Gonorrhoea is an extremely common STD with rates of over 1000 per 100 000 reported for homosexual men in the UK in 2000–2002.[49] In the USA it is the second most commonly reported STD, with about 600 000 new cases annually.[10] The causative organism, *Neisseria gonorrhoeae* (a Gram-negative intracellular diplococcus), can infect the mucous lining of all body orifices. The clinical syndromes associated with gonorrhoeal infection include urethritis, cervicitis, PID, pharyngitis, conjunctivitis and proctitis.

Up to 55% of homosexual men seen in screening clinics harbour gonorrhoea. The rectum is the only site of infection in 40–50% of these and the majority are asymptomatic. Transmission is by anal receptive intercourse and, after an incubation period of 3 days to 2 weeks, proctitis or cryptitis results. In women, the majority of cases with anorectal involvement are caused by autoinoculation from vaginal infection. Stansfield reported that only 6% of women have rectal involvement in the absence of cervical or urethral involvement.[50]

Symptoms of anorectal involvement include pruritis ani, bloody or mucoid discharge, tenesmus, and anorectal pain. Untreated gonococcal infection leads to disseminated disease which manifests as perihepatitis, meningitis, endocarditis, pericarditis or a migratory arthritis. Mucopurulent discharge in combination with proctitis is the characteristic physical finding in gonocoocal proctitis. This thick, viscid mucopus can be expressed from anal crypts with pressure applied to the anus. The proctitis is non-specific and consists of oedema, friability and mucus.

Culture of the mucopus is diagnostic, but the yield may be decreased if lubricants other than water are used on the anoscope. The diagnostic yield is highest when the discharge is swabbed under direct vision and immediately plated onto an enriched medium, such as Thayer–Martin or GC agar base. Gram stain from rectal samples has low sensitivity but is rapid, inexpensive and highly specific.[51] Nucleic acid amplification tests are not currently in use for rectal gonorrhoea.[52]

Treatment of anorectal gonorrhoea is listed in Table 16.1. Penicillin G was the treatment of choice until the 1970s, when penicillinase-producing N. gonorrhoeae emerged. More recently, quinolone-resistant N. gonorrhoeae (QRNG) has been reported and increased in Asia, the Pacific, the west coast of the USA and parts of Europe.[10] Fenton et al. reported an increase in the rate of QRNG to 9.8% in England and Wales in 2002.[53]

These reports have led to the recommendation that quinolones no longer be used as treatment for N. gonorrhoeae in areas where resistant strains are reported. USA guidelines no longer include quinolones for homosexual males with N. gonorrhoeae.[10]

Obviously, local surveillance data will play an important role in these therapeutic decisions. In addition to the treatments in Table 16.1, UK national guidelines include ampicillin/probenicid for N. gonorrhoeae.[53] Antibiotic susceptibility testing should be performed in patients who fail to respond to appropriate treatment or who are infected from an area known to have resistant strains. Additionally, because of the high rate of concomitant infection with Chlamydia,

all patients treated for N. gonorrhoeae infections should be treated for Chlamydia if infection is not ruled out.

As with all bacterial STDs, management of sexual partners is an integral part of decreasing disease spread and reinfection. Sexual partners from the past 60 days should be evaluated and treated, and patients should abstain from sexual activity until treatment is completed and symptoms resolved. Routine testing after treatment is not indicated. Patients who remain symptomatic after treatment should undergo culture and antibiotic sensitivity testing for persistent infection, such as urethritis, cervicitis or proctitis.[10]

Granuloma inguinale (Donovanosis)

Calymmatobacterium granulomatis (also known as Donovania granulomatis, and in the future may be reclassified as Klebsiella granulomatis) is a rare cause of genital ulceration in western countries but is common in parts of Africa and South America. Efforts to eradicate this disease in Australia appear to have been successful. Transmission is felt to be mostly via sexual means but autoinoculation and faecal contamination may also play a role.[54]

Initially a firm papule appears and then subsequently ulcerates. Four morphological manifestations have been described, the most common being ulcerogranulomatous. These are non-tender, beefy-red ulcers. Less common types are hypertrophic or verrucous ulcers, necrotic ulcers or the cicatricial type. While genital involvement is the most common location, anal involvement either alone or contiguous with the genitalia is seen (**Fig. 16.4**).

In endemic areas diagnosis may be made on clinical grounds alone. Examination of stained tissue

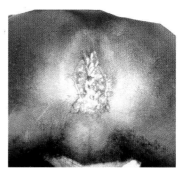

Figure 16.4 • Perianal granuloma inguinale.

from ulcers showing Donovan bodies is diagnostic. Staining of biopsy specimens may also be useful. PCR is not widely available.[55] Recommended antibiotic regimens are listed in Table 16.1.

Syphilis

Syphilis is a mucocutaneous STD caused by the spirochaete *Treponema pallidum*. Recent surveillance suggests rates in the USA and UK are increasing again, especially among homosexual males.[41,56] The disease manifests itself in several stages and as it progresses from a local to systemic infection the sites of infection and symptoms become protean. Like the section on HIV, this discussion will be, for the most part, limited to anorectal infections from *T. pallidum*.

Anorectal syphilis is largely a disease of homosexual males, with the first stage presenting with a chancre at the site of contact (**Fig. 16.5**). This is a raised, 1–2 cm, indurated, ulcerated lesion occurring at the anal margin or canal. Chancres may be eccentrically located, multiple or irregular, and two ulcers may be opposite each other in a 'kissing' configuration. The ulcers may be painless or painful and are associated with discharge and inguinal adenopathy. Untreated they resolve in 2–4 weeks. Rectal mucosal involvement results in tenesmus, rectal discharge or rectal bleeding.[57,58]

Secondary syphilis presents with systemic symptoms and as a non-pruritic macular rash on the trunk, limbs, palms and/or soles. Condylomata lata

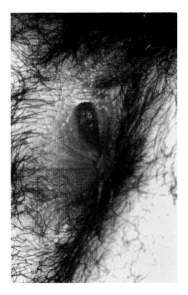

Figure 16.5 • Anal chancre.

may be found near the initial chancre and are spirochaete-laden, wart-like lesions. Mucosal patches or ulcerations may appear in the rectum.[58–60] As with primary infection, this stage resolves spontaneously after 3–12 weeks. About one-quarter of untreated patients relapse in the first year – this is termed early latent syphilis. It should be noted that concomitant HIV infection may lead to more severe symptoms that take longer to resolve. Untreated for years, the tertiary stage of syphilis develops with involvement of the nervous and vascular system and formation of gummas.

Treponema pallidum cannot be cultured. Darkfield microscopy of scrapings from chancres or lymph nodes is useful for diagnosis. Because of the presence of commensal spirochaetes in the rectum, it is less accurate in this location. Specific immunofluorescent staining, or silver staining of biopsy specimens, can also diagnose *T. pallidum*. Serology is useful in the diagnosis of syphilis and typically a two-stage process is followed. The initial test is a non-treponemal test which if positive is followed by a treponemal test. Non-treponemal tests are not specific for *T. pallidum* and include Venereal Disease Research Laboratory (VDRL) and rapid plasma regain (RPR). Treponemal tests include *T. pallidum* enzyme immunoassay (EIA), *T. pallidum* particle assay (TPPA) and the fluorescent antibody absorbed test (FTA-abs). EIA and TPPA can be used jointly as confirmatory tests. Qualitative VDRL/RPR are used to assess an appropriate response to treatment. PCR is available in some speciality labs.[60–63]

Treatment of syphilis is with benzathine penicillin G, 2.4 million units as a single intramuscular injection. The most commonly used alternative regimen is doxycycline 100 mg orally given twice a day for 1 week. Recommendations for managing sex partners depend on the stage of diagnosis of the index case. In general, any sexual contact within the 90 days before diagnosis is treated presumptively. Any sexual partners for the past 6 months are considered at risk for patients with secondary syphilis and those for the past year for early latent syphilis.[10]

Syndromic treatment

Several factors have led some authors to recommend treatment of STDs based on the clinical presenting syndrome: (1) point of care testing is not widely available for the pathogens discussed above;

(2) the two common presenting complaints (proctitis or genital ulceration) are not specific to a particular organism; and (3) infection with multiple organisms is not uncommon.

 Patients with proctitis or anogenital ulcers in whom an STD is suspected should undergo thorough physical examination to include inspection and palpation for inguinal lymphadenopathy. For those with proctitis, specimen collection should be performed for all the common pathogens that produce this symptom: HSV, gonorrhoea, Chlamydia/LGV and *T. pallidum*. It is rational to treat empirically for gonorrhoea and Chlamydia (e.g. ceftriaxone and doxycline) in these patients if anorectal exudate is noted or if polymorphonuclear leucocytes are seen on Gram stain. Additional treatment is determined by the results of testing for specific organisms.[10,60]

Likewise, syndromic management of anogenital ulcers, even in the presence of HIV, can be successful.[64] Again, thorough physical examination and appropriate testing for the most common causative organisms are performed: HSV, *T. pallidum*, *C. trachomatis* (LGV serovars), *H. ducreyi* and *C. granulomatis*. Empirical therapy for syphilis is initiated. Patients with vesicles or other indications of HSV should be started on appropriate therapy for HSV. Additionally patients can be started on empirical treatment for LGV,

chancroid or granuloma inguinale based on the local prevalence of these diseases. If not treated empirically, treatment is based on the laboratory results.[65]

Prevention

While this chapter has focused on the recognition, diagnosis and treatment of STDs of the anorectum, a brief word about prevention is necessary. As was mentioned in the introduction, a thorough sexual practices history should be obtained in any patient suspected of having an STD. This history should include the number and gender of sexual partners from the past 12 months, sexual practices, use of protection, past history of STDs and past HIV testing. Part of the complete treatment of STDs includes educating the patient as to the mode of transmission and ways to avoid subsequent reinfection. This frequently includes treatment and counselling of sexual partners.

 Resources for appropriate treatment of sexual partners and guidance for counselling and education are available through several organisations, including the Centers for Disease Control and the World Health Organisation.[10,65]

Key points

- Sexually transmitted diseases are common and increasing in frequency.
- A high index of suspicion and knowledge of lesions is required.
- An appropriate sexual history is important in diagnosing these conditions.
- Patients and their partners must be treated.
- Excision has produced the best results for anal condylomata but imiquimod has shown promise.
- Quinolone-resistant *N. gonorrhoeae* is becoming more common.
- Review of current testing and treatment recommendations is suggested when managing uncommon sexually transmitted infections.

References

1. Johnson A, Wadsworth J, Wellings K et al. Sexual attitudes and lifestyles (Wellcome Trust). Oxford: Blackwell Scientific, 1994; pp. 463–5.

2. Voeller B. AIDS and heterosexual anal intercourse. Arch Sex Behav 1991; 20:233–76.

3. Collier AC, Meyers JD, Cory L et al. Cytomegalovirus infection in homosexual men. Am J Med 1987; 82:593–601.

4. Whitley RJ, Jacobson MA, Friedberg DN et al. Guidelines for the treatment of cytomegalovirus diseases in patients with AIDS in the era of potent antiretroviral therapy: recommendations of an international panel. Arch Intern Med 1998; 158:957–69.

5. Wexner SD, Smithy WB, Trillo C et al. Emergency colectomy for cytomegalovirus ileocolitis in patients with the acquired immune deficiency syndrome. Dis Colon Rectum 1988; 31:755–61.

6. Morris-Cunnington M, Brown D, Pimenta J et al. New estimates of herpes simplex virus type 2 seroprevalance in England. Sex Transm Dis 2004; 31:243–6.

7. Edwards S, Carne C. Oral sex and the transmission of viral STIs. Sex Transm Inf 1998; 74:6–10.

8. Krone MR, Wald A, Tabet SR. Herpes simplex virus type 2 shedding in human immunodeficiency virus-negative men who have sex with men: frequency, patterns, and risk factors. Clin Infect Dis 2000; 30:261–7.

9. Eberhardt O, Kuber W, Dichgans J et al. HSV-2 sacral radiculitis (Elsberg syndrome). Neurology 2004; 63:758–9.

10. Centers for Disease Control. Sexually transmitted diseases treatment guidelines 2006. MMWR 2006; 55(RR-11):1–94.

11. Kimberlin DW, Rouse DJ. Genital herpes. N Engl J Med 2004; 350:1970–7.

12. Corey L, Wald A, Patel R. Once-daily valacyclovir to reduce the risk of transmission of genital herpes. N Engl J Med 2004; 350:11–20.

13. Jayasurlya A, Robertson C, Allan PS. Twenty-five years of HIV management. J R Soc Med 2007; 100:363–6.

14. Dua RS, Wajed SA, Winslet MC. Impact of HIV and AIDS on surgical practice. Ann R Coll Surg Engl 2007; 89:354–8.

15. Gonzalez-Ruth C, Heartfield W, Briggs B et al. Anorectal pathology in HIV/AIDS-infected patients has not been impacted by highly active antiretroviral therapy. Dis Colon Rectum 2004; 47:1483–6.

16. Centers for Disease Control. 1993 revised classification system for HIV infection and expanded surveillance case definition for AIDS among adolescents and adults. MMWR 1992; 41(RR-17):1–19.

17. Moore BA, Fleshner PR. Rubber band ligation for hemorrhoidal disease can be safely performed in select HIV-positive patients. Dis Colon Rectum 2001; 44:1079–82.

18. Hewitt WR, Sokol TP, Fleshner PR. Should HIV status alter indications for hemorrhoidectomy? Dis Colon Rectum 1996; 39:615–18.

19. Morandi E, Merlini D, Savaggio A et al. Prospective study of healing time after hemorrhoidectomy. Dis Colon Rectum 1999; 42:1140–4.

20. Brar HS, Gottesman L, Surawicz C. Anorectal pathology in AIDS. Gastrointest Endosc Clin North Am 1998; 8:913–31.

21. Modesto VL, Gottesman L. Surgical debridement and intralesional steroid injection in the treatment of idiopathic AIDS-related anal ulcerations. Am J Surg 1997; 174:439–41.

22. Nielson CM, Harris RB, Dunne EF et al. Risk factors for anogenital human papillomavirus infection in men. J Infect Dis 2007; 196:1137–45.

23. Dunne EF, Unger ER, Sternberg M et al. Prevalence of HPV infection among females in the United States. JAMA 2007; 297:813–19.

24. Hernandez BY, McDuffe K, Zhu X et al. Anal human papillomavirus infection in women and

its relationship with cervical infection. Cancer Epidemiol Biomarkers Prev 2005; 14:2550–6.

25. Guiliano AR, Neilson CM, Flores R et al. The optimal anatomic sites for sampling heterosexual men for human papillomavirus (HPV) detection: the HPV detection in men study. J Infect Dis 2007; 196:1146–52.

26. von Krogh G, Longstaff E. Podophyllin office therapy against condyloma should be abandoned. Sex Transm Inf 2001; 77:409–12.

27. Lacey CJN, Goodall RL, Tennvall GR et al. Randomised controlled trial and economic evaluation of podophyllotoxin solution, podophyllotoxin cream, and podophyllin in the treatment of genital warts. Sex Transm Infect 2003; 79:270–5.

28. Beutner KR, Tyring SK, Tofatter KF et al. Imiquimod, a patient-applied immune-response modifier for treatment of genital warts. Antimicrob Agents Chemother 1998; 42:789–94.

29. Maitland JE, Maw R. An audit of patients who have received imiquimod cream 5% for the treatment of anogenital warts. Int J STD AIDS 2000; 11:268–70.

30. Kaspari M, Gutzmer R, Kaspari T et al. Application of imiquimod by suppositories (anal tampons) efficiently prevents recurrences after ablation of anal canal condyloma. Br J Derm 2002; 147:757–9.

31. Abcarian H, Sharon N. The effectiveness of immunotherapy in the treatment of anal condyloma. J Surg Res 1977; 22:231–6.

32. Abcarian H, Sharon N. Long-term effectiveness of the immunotherapy of anal condyloma acuminatum. Dis Colon Rectum 1982; 25:648–51.

33. Eftaiha MS, Amshel AL, Shonberg IL et al. Giant and recurrent condyloma acuminatum: appraisal of immunotherapy. Dis Colon Rectum 1982; 25:136–8.

34. Palefsky J. Human papillomavirus in HIV-infected persons. Top HIV Med 2007; 15:130–3.

35. Palefsky JM, Holly EA, Efirdc JT et al. Anal intraepithelial neoplasia in the highly active antiretroviral therapy era among HIV-positive men who have sex with men. AIDS 2005; 19:1407–14.

36. Gervaz P, Hirshel B, Morel P. Molecular biology of squamous cell carcinoma of the anus. Br J Surg 2006; 93:531–8.

37. Whitlow C, Gottesman L. Sexually transmitted diseases. In: Wolf BG, Fleshman JW, Beck DE et al. (eds) The ASCRS textbook of colon and rectal surgery. New York: Springer, 2007; pp. 256–68.

38. Trager JDK. Sexually transmitted diseases causing genital lesions in adolescents. Adol Med Clin 2004; 15:323–52.

39. Quinn TC, Stamm WE, Goodell SE. The polymicrobial origin of intestinal infections in homosexual men. N Engl J Med 1983; 309:576–82.

40. Gaudreau C, Michaud S. Cluster of erythromycin- and ciprofloxacin-resistant *Campylobacter jejuni* subsp. *Jejuni* from 1999 to 2001 in men who have sex with men, Quebec, Canada. Clin Infect Dis 2003; 37:131–6.

41. Centers for Disease Control. Trends in reportable sexually transmitted diseases in the United States, 2006. National surveillance data for Chlamydia, gonorrhoea, and syphilis. CDC, 2007; pp. 1–7.

42. Ootani A, Mizuguchi M, Tsunada S et al. *Chlamydia trachomatis* proctitis. Gastrointest Endosc 2004; 60:161–2.

43. Carder C, Mercey D, Benn P. *Chlamydia trachomatis*. Sex Transm Infect 2006; 82(S4):S10–12.

44. Stark D, van Hal S, Hillman R et al. Lymphogranuloma venereum in Australia: anorectal *Chlamydia trachomatis* serovar L2b in men who have sex with men. J Clin Microbiol 2007; 45:1029–31.

45. Van der Bij AK, Spaargearn J, Morre SA et al. Diagnostic and clinical implications of anorectal lymphogranuloma venereum in men who have sex with men: a retrospective case–control study. Clin Infect Dis 2006; 42:186–94.

46. Spinola SM, Bauer ME, Munson RS. Immunopathogenesis of *Haemophilus ducreyi* infection (chancroid). Infect Immun 2002; 70:1667–76.

47. Alfa M. The laboratory diagnosis of *Haemophilus ducreyi*. Can J Infect Dis Med Microbiol 2005; 16:31–4.

48. Lewis DA. Chancroid: clinical manifestations, diagnosis, and management. Sex Transm Infect 2003; 79:68–71.

49. Brown AE, Sadler KE, Tomkins SE et al. Recent trends in HIV and other STIs in the United Kingdom: data to the end of 2002. Sex Transm Infect 2004; 80:159–66.

50. Stansfield VA. Diagnosis and management of anorectal gonorrhoea in women. Br J Venereal Dis 1980; 56:319–21.

51. Grover D, Prime KP, Prince MV et al. Rectal gonorrhoea in men – is microscopy still a useful tool? Int J STD AIDS 2006; 17:277–9.

52. Bignell C, Ison CA, Jungmann E. Gonorrhoea. Sex Transm Infect 2006; 82(S4):S6–9.

53. Fenton KA, Ison C, Johnson AP et al. Ciprofloxacin resistence in *Neiserria gonorrhoeae* in England and Wales in 2002. Lancet 2003; 361:1867–9.

54. O'Farrell N. Donovanosis. Sex Transm Infect 2002; 78:452–7.

55. Richens J. Donovanosis (granuloma inguinale). Sex Transm Infect 2006; 82(S4):S21–22.

56. Chakraborty R, Luck S. Syphilis is on the increase: the implications for child health. Arch Dis Chile 2008; 93:105–9.

57. Mindel A, Tovey SJ, Timmins DJ et al. Primary and secondary syphilis, 20 years' experience. Clinical features. Genitourinary Med 1989; 65:1–3.

58. Smith D. Infectious syphilis of the anal canal. Dis Colon Rectum 1963; 6:7–10.

59. Marino AWM. Proctologic lesions observed in male homosexuals. Dis Colon Rectum 1964; 7:121.

60. Rampalo AM. Diagnosis and treatment of sexually acquired proctitis and proctocolitis: an update. Clin Infect Dis 1999; 28(Suppl 1):S84–90.

61. Zetola NM, Engelmen J, Jensen TP et al. Syphilis in the United States: an update for clinicians with an emphasis on HIV coinfection. Mayo Clin Proc 2007; 82:1091–102.

62. Hamlyn E, Taylor C. Sexually transmitted proctitis. Postgrad Med J 2006; 82:733–6.

63. Lewis DA, Young H. Syphilis. Sex Transm Infect 2006; 82(Suppl 4):S13–15.

64. Moodley P, Sturm P, Vanmali T et al. Association between HIV-1 infection, the etiology of genital ulcer disease, and response to syndromic management. Sex Transm Dis 2003; 30:241–5.

65. World Health Organisation. Guidelines for the management of sexually transmitted infections, 2003; pp. 11–15.

17

Laparoscopic surgery and enhanced recovery programmes in colorectal disease

Ian Jenkins
Robin Kennedy

Introduction

Despite the introduction of laparoscopic colorectal surgery in the early 1990s, its adoption has been slow due to a difficult learning curve, the requirement for significant local service reconfiguration, and a number of concerns. Inadequate oncological clearance of colorectal cancer and the specific complication of port-site recurrence are concerns that have been resolved. The technique's general applicability in colorectal surgery is also clearer and there is more understanding regarding cost issues and when to convert to traditional open surgery.

When performed by surgeons with adequate experience and training, it is clear that laparoscopic colorectal surgery dramatically improves the functional outcome following bowel resection. In early 2000, Henrik Kehlet transformed the surgical landscape introducing a multimodal approach to improve functional recovery after conventional surgery – the enhanced recovery programme (ERP) was born. The use of an ERP combined with laparoscopic colorectal surgery further improves results. We therefore anticipate that this combined approach in colorectal surgery will become the gold standard: after elective segmental colectomy, postoperative hospital stays of 3–4 days, with commensurate improvements in functional recovery, will become routine.

This chapter will discuss the main issues relevant to laparoscopic colorectal surgery and introduce the important areas in enhanced recovery (ER) care.

Because of the considerable benefits to patients, we are at the threshold of transition from utilisation of these approaches by a small minority of enthusiasts, to them becoming the preferred approach in the vast majority of elective resections.

Outcomes of laparoscopic colorectal surgery

The safety and advantages of laparoscopic colectomy for cancer have been much debated and several randomised controlled trials (RCTs) have clarified these issues. The published large RCTs comparing late cancer outcomes following open or laparoscopic resection of colonic cancer are from Spain,[1] North America[2] (COST trial – Comparison of Laparoscopically-assisted and Open Colectomy for Colon Cancer), Hong Kong,[3] the UK[4] (MRC-CLASICC trial – Conventional versus Laparoscopic-Assisted Surgery In Colorectal Cancer) and Europe (CoLOR trial – Colon cancer Laparoscopic or Open Resection).[5] It is important to note that the only trial specifically addressing rectal cancer was the CLASICC trial.

Oncological outcomes

Initial fears regarding poor results for laparoscopic colorectal cancer resection, particularly port-site recurrences, resulted in its suspension outside trials in some countries. Concerns regarding port-site recurrence have now been dispelled and major RCTs report abdominal wall recurrence to be the same following either type of surgery, and <1%. Short- and medium-term oncological outcomes are at least equivalent between open and laparoscopic groups, and in the highly cited study by Lacy et al., an improved cancer-specific survival for stage III disease was identified.[1] This improvement for the laparoscopic patients may be explained by an improved host response to malignancy or earlier initiation of adjuvant therapy. Critics have, however, attributed the difference to poor results in the open group.

Although oncological outcome is equivalent in the large multicentre studies, this is despite conversion rates of 17–29%, which probably reflect the relative inexperience of participating surgeons. In contrast, Lacy et al. reported a conversion rate of 11% and the largest reduction in hospital stay after laparoscopy, suggesting a smaller effect from the learning curve. If a difference in oncological outcome is not detected with conversion rates around 20%, then it is a tantalising prospect that once conversion rates decrease to single figures, due to increased expertise and appropriate case selection, an oncological benefit might be confirmed.

The CLASICC trial recently reported results at 3 years which showed no difference in overall survival between laparoscopic and open surgery.[6] Reports on the equivalence in oncological outcomes and the improvements in postoperative recovery prompted the National Institute for Health and Clinical Excellence (NICE) in 2006 to endorse the use of laparoscopic surgery for colorectal cancer (www.nice.org.uk). NICE have provided the following guidance:

- Laparoscopic resection is recommended as an alternative to open resection for individuals with colorectal cancer in whom both laparoscopic and open surgery are considered suitable.
- It should only be performed by surgeons who have completed appropriate training in the technique and who perform this procedure often enough to maintain competence.
- The decision about which of the procedures (open or laparoscopic) is undertaken should be made after informed discussion between the patient and the surgeon.

Hospital stay and complications

The results of both RCTs and observational studies assessing laparoscopic colorectal surgery have been submitted to meta-analysis and have produced similar results.

 Following laparoscopic resection, operation times are longer, but benefits are a reduced wound infection rate, less pain and narcotic use, less overall morbidity and a shorter hospital stay.[7–9]

Compared to conventional surgery, minimal access surgery may reduce the necessity for re-operation caused by adhesions or incisional hernias, although this has not yet been reported in prospective studies. A retrospective study of 716 patients by Duepree et al. identified a decreased rate in the laparoscopic group for both incisional hernia and small-bowel obstruction.[10] The overall re-operation rate in the open group was double that of the laparoscopic group (7.7% vs. 3.8%); however, further studies are required for confirmation.

Blood loss

A case–control study by Kiran et al. of 147 patients confirmed that the laparoscopic approach for colorectal surgery led to significantly less blood loss and blood usage than after open colectomy.[11]

Mortality

The major RCTs report no difference in the 30-day mortality, possibly reflecting their size and that they were not powered to detect differences in mortality, particularly when the surgeons had conversion rates of >20%. If laparoscopy reduces complications then it is likely to have a similar effect on mortality. Recently, Law et al. reported a reduced mortality with laparoscopic resection in a non-randomised study of 1134 colon and upper rectal resections (401 laparoscopic procedures) and in a meta-analysis of 17 RCTs assessing 4013 procedures by Tjandra and Chan, laparoscopic resection of colonic and rectosigmoid cancer had a significantly lower perioperative mortality (odds ratio 0.33, $P = 0.005$).[12,13]

Economic considerations

Although laparoscopic colectomy has demonstrated a variety of advantages, it has been unclear whether reduced hospital stay and morbidity offset the potential cost increases resulting from increased operating time and the use of extra disposable instruments. Braga et al. assessed 517 patients undergoing laparoscopic colonic and rectal cancer resection, finding a slight increase in hospital costs.[14] Similarly Murray et al. found laparoscopic techniques to be more costly overall.[15,16] This analysis informed the NICE assessment, estimating the difference in cost to be £265. This is a modest additional cost, considering the short-term benefits associated with a more rapid recovery. Conversely, King et al. found no cost difference and a systematic review by Dowson et al. reported cost equivalence between open and laparoscopic groups.[17,18] For resection of diverticular disease, Senagore et al. found laparoscopic surgery to be less costly.[19]

The length of hospital stay is an important element of the total cost and with laparoscopic surgery hospital stay is known to decrease. Although current evidence is limited, it seems likely that as operative times and conversion rates decrease, the total cost of laparoscopic surgery will reduce.

Conversion to open surgery

The possibility of conversion is inherent in laparoscopic surgery. Reported conversion rates vary considerably in laparoscopic colorectal surgery, but it is important to emphasise that conversion to open surgery should not be regarded as a failure of the technique: it may be entirely appropriate. Problems arise as definitions of conversion are unclear and, when quoting rates, authors do not define the percentage of their population undergoing open surgery. The sum of three numbers – open interventions, operations attempted laparoscopically and converted, and those completed laparoscopically – will be the denominator. Without defining this, quoted conversion rates are virtually impossible to interpret. Based upon appropriate experience and a suitable clinical workload, we believe laparoscopic resection can be attempted in over 90% of elective colorectal cancer patients, with a conversion rate of <10%.[20] In support of this, the laparoscopic unit in Brisbane reports a low conversion rate of 6.6%[21] and the authors' conversion rate in a recent RCT was 7.3%.[22]

The definition of conversion

To ensure an unambiguous definition, we regard conversion as the inability to complete specimen mobilisation laparoscopically, including vascular division, usually but not always resulting in a larger incision than would otherwise have been required for specimen removal. The emphasis on vascular division is because after bowel transection retrieval is possible through a very small incision such as 4–5 cm – provided vascular and mesenteric division has occurred – maximising the benefit from laparoscopic surgery. Attempting to ligate vessels through the incision will invariably produce a larger incision than the anticipated 4–5 cm, or problematic ligation. Using this definition there will be patients in whom much of the mobilisation will have been undertaken laparoscopically and who will derive considerable benefit from this, even though conversion is required.

Predicting the risk of conversion

Defining the patient group most likely to be converted would be beneficial, yet this has proved difficult. A recent European Association of Endoscopic Surgeons (EAES) consensus statement on laparoscopic surgery for colonic cancer indicated the most common cause for conversion is the presence of a bulky or locally advanced tumour.[23] Obesity and previous abdominal operations were not considered absolute contraindications for laparoscopic colon cancer surgery, though most studies cite these factors as being risk factors for conversion.

Obese patients carry a higher risk of wound and cardiopulmonary complications in addition to a greater incidence of comorbidity, which has the potential adversely to affect outcome after surgery. This group may therefore achieve the greatest benefit from laparoscopic resection. Schwandner et al. assessed obesity (body mass index (BMI) $>30\,kg/m^2$) in 589 laparoscopic colorectal patients, finding no difference in conversion rates (7.3% vs. 9.5%) in 95 obese patients and 494 'non-obese' patients.[24] Overall complication rates were similar (23.3% in the obese group vs. 24.5% in the non-obese group). These results are perhaps a testament to the level of expertise exhibited by the surgeons treating these patients. Senagore et al. compared 59 obese (BMI $>30\,kg/m^2$) and 201 non-obese patients, identifying differences between the two groups: in the obese group significantly more conversions (23.7% vs. 10.9%), longer operations (109 vs. 94 minutes), a higher morbidity rate (22% vs. 13%) and more anastomotic leakage (5.1% vs. 1.2%).[25] Buchanan et al. reported that a BMI $\geq 28\,kg/m^2$ increased conversions from 3% to 22% in colorectal cancer resection.[20] The results from these last two groups are perhaps more recognisable for most surgeons and reflect the degree of difficulty in obese patients.

Previous abdominal surgery has been considered a risk factor for conversion. Arteaga Gonzalez et al. found a higher conversion rate following previous abdominal surgery (26.1% vs. 5.1%),[26] but with increasing experience this effect seems to disappear.[20]

Tumour location also affects the likelihood of conversion. Buchanan et al. identified rectal cancer resections to have an increased conversion rate over colonic resections, but this decreased with experience. The difficulty undertaking laparoscopic rectal resection derives from the location of the rectum within a confined space and the concern that the technique may compromise tumour clearance. In addition, the rectal dissection follows vascular ligation and bowel mobilisation, often involving splenic flexure mobilisation, so the novice surgeon may be challenged by a subsequent complex rectal mobilisation. Law et al. assessed the outcomes of 265 patients with upper and mid rectal cancers, of which 37% were performed laparoscopically, the latter goup having less advanced disease. Cancer-specific survival and local recurrences rates, stratified by disease stage, were not compromised by the laparoscopic approach.[27] The CLASICC study did not demonstrate a significant worsening of oncological outcome following laparoscopic rectal cancer resection; however, it specifically noted that positive margin rates were non-significantly higher in laparoscopic resections (16/129 (12%) vs. 4/64 (6%), $P = 0.19$),[4] probably reflecting the learning curve.

Disease extent may also influence conversion rates and Buchanan et al. report that a magnetic resonance imaging (MRI)-predicted threatened resection margin in rectal cancer is associated with higher conversion rates.[20] Moloo et al. compared laparoscopic resection between stage IV colorectal cancer and stage I–III disease. Thirteen percent of the 375 laparoscopic resections were with palliative intent yet no significant differences were found between the groups for intraoperative (4% vs. 9%) or postoperative complications (14% vs. 12%),

perioperative mortality (8% vs. 4%), or length of hospital stay.[28] However, the conversion rate was increased in the palliative group (22% v 11%) owing to tumour fixation or bulk. These results support the view of many experienced surgeons that laparoscopic resection of contiguous involvement is technically possible and not contraindicated in certain patients.

High hospital case volume has been associated with improved outcome after open operation for colorectal malignancy and it is likely that the volume of laparoscopic surgery performed will impact upon outcomes such as conversion. Kuhry et al. assessed data from the CoLOR trial and stratified outcomes by low, medium and high case volumes: a high colorectal case load resulting in decreased conversions and improved short-term outcomes.[29]

 Tekkis et al. have developed a regression analysis model to predict the likelihood of conversion.[30] Predictors of conversion were BMI, ASA grade, type of resection, presence of intraoperative abscess or fistula, and surgeon seniority. Marusch et al. assessed results in a total of 1658 patients from the Laparoscopic Colorectal Surgery Study Group.[31] This group reported a low conversion rate of 5.2% and identified elevated BMI, rectal resection and intraoperative complications as predictors for conversion.

Outcome after conversion

Concerns remain that conversion is associated with increased morbidity and greater hospital costs. A case–control study by Casillas et al. with a conversion rate of 12% found conversion did not significantly increase operation time, morbidity, length of stay, cost or unplanned readmissions, compared with similar complex open surgery.[32] Marusch et al. found the opposite: after conversion, operation time increased and postoperative morbidity (47.7% vs. 26.1%), mortality (3.5% vs. 1.5%) and hospital stay were all negatively influenced.[31] Buchanan et al. observed similar outcomes and cautions that although technically challenging resections may be attempted laparoscopically, when surgeons are sufficiently experienced, patients with a high chance of conversion represent the most challenging procedures and probably occur in a subset of people with the greatest comorbidity.

The likelihood of conversion is greatest in patients undergoing rectal surgery, when there is an increased BMI, following previous major abdominal surgery, and in inflammatory bowel disease. Earlier rather than delayed conversion, especially when progress is not being made, is the authors' current policy. This will minimise errors due to tiredness or technical difficulties that might have been handled best by open resection.

Benign colorectal conditions suitable for laparoscopic surgery

The role of laparoscopic surgery for patients with ileocaecal Crohn's disease has been a contentious issue as adhesions secondary to inflammation or previous surgery increase technical difficulty. A key technical aspect of ileocolonic Crohn's resection is to mobilise fully the right colon, in order that when performing the anastomosis there is no restriction on the colon. A comparative study by Bemelman et al. found that laparoscopic resection for Crohn's disease was associated with similar morbidity rates to open surgery but a shorter hospital stay and improved cosmetic results.[33] The cosmetic aspect is relatively important as many Crohn's patients are young adults and also likely to require re-operation. Further studies confirm improvements in outcome with laparoscopic resection for this disease and some suggest that initial minimal access surgery increases the chance that future resections will be possible laparoscopically.[34,35] The first RCT assessing this subject demonstrated a benefit to laparoscopy with a decrease in complications and hospital stay.[36] Maartense et al. later randomised 60 patients with a conversion rate of 10%, demonstrating similar results but also a significant reduction in hospital costs.[37]

Schwandner et al. assessed the outcomes of laparoscopic resection for diverticulitis compared to non-diverticular disease and found a low conversion rate of ≈7% in both groups, with similarly low and comparable morbidity.[38] Purkayastha et al. performed a meta-analysis on 12 non-randomised studies finding equivalent results for laparoscopic and open surgery in diverticular disease, with possible reductions in complications and hospital stay. However, significant study heterogeneity was identified, indicating likely bias.

To clarify the most appropriate technique for resection, the outcomes of open and laparoscopic total colectomy and ileoanal pouch surgery have been compared in several studies. The laparoscopic approach should only be recommended when an experienced team is available. Studies confirm similar benefits to those reported for other indications.[39,40] Study heterogeneity in the meta-analyses assessing these procedures underlines the fact that total colectomy and proctocolectomy are demanding procedures unsuitable for surgeons early in their experience of laparoscopic colorectal surgery. We would suggest that when experienced laparoscopic teams are available patients are likely to derive as much, if not more, benefit from this technique as patients undergoing laparoscopic segmental colectomy.

Laparoscopic colorectal technique

All patients considered for elective laparoscopic colorectal cancer resection will undergo preoperative staging by computed tomography (CT) of the abdomen, chest and pelvis, with MRI in addition for rectal cancer. This confirms tumour location, defines adjacent organ involvement that may pose technical problems, and excludes both synchronous pathology and widespread disease. Patients will undergo colonoscopy or virtual colonoscopy to evaluate the whole colon before surgery. Endoscopic India Ink marking techniques are used for the intraoperative identification of colonic polyps and early neoplasms in order to avoid on-table colonoscopy. Tumours are tattooed based on their location in the colon by an agreed protocol (**Fig. 17.1**), but rectal lesions below 12 cm from the anal verge are not tattooed to avoid discolouring the fascia of Denonvillier. This approach has been found to be safe and effective in aiding lesion identification at laparoscopy.[41]

Patients undergoing laparoscopic colorectal resection are positioned using a modified Lloyd–Davies position, with shoulder restraints owing to the steep Trendelenburg and lateral tilt required for left-sided and rectal resections: care should be exercised in the morbidly obese as bilateral brachial plexus injury has been reported.

For elective laparoscopic left colonic, sigmoid or rectal cancer resection, our approach is similar. Our favoured technique uses a four-port approach with an additional port added for low rectal dissection in laparoscopic total mesorectal excision

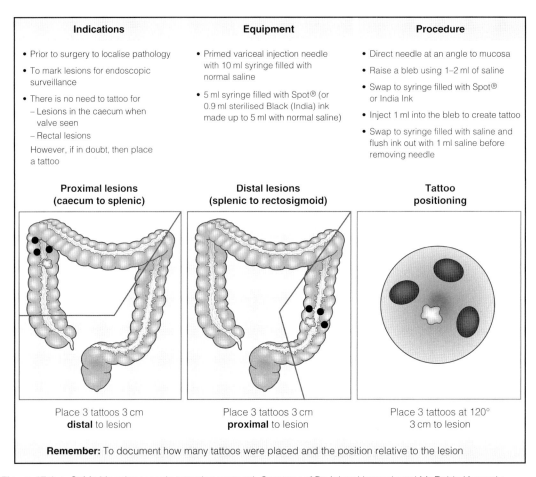

Indications	Equipment	Procedure

• Prior to surgery to localise pathology
 	
• To mark lesions for endoscopic surveillance
 	
• There is no need to tattoo for
  – Lesions in the caecum when valve seen
  – Rectal lesions
  However, if in doubt, then place a tattoo
	• Primed variceal injection needle with 10 ml syringe filled with normal saline
	
	• 5 ml syringe filled with Spot® (or 0.9 ml sterilised Black (India) ink made up to 5 ml with normal saline)
		• Direct needle at an angle to mucosa
		
		• Raise a bleb using 1–2 ml of saline
		
		• Swap to syringe filled with Spot® or India Ink
		
		• Inject 1 ml into the bleb to create tattoo
		
		• Swap to syringe filled with saline and flush ink out with 1 ml saline before removing needle

Proximal lesions (caecum to splenic) — Place 3 tattoos 3 cm **distal** to lesion

Distal lesions (splenic to rectosigmoid) — Place 3 tattoos 3 cm **proximal** to lesion

Tattoo positioning — Place 3 tattoos at 120° 3 cm to lesion

Remember: To document how many tattoos were placed and the position relative to the lesion

Figure 17.1 • St Mark's colonoscopic tattooing protocol. Courtesy of Dr Adam Haycock and Mr Robin Kennedy, St Mark's Hospital.

(TME) (**Fig. 17.2**). A zero-degree telescope is used for all resections. Following identification of the relevant anatomy, an operative strategy is planned, skeletonising the vessels and proceeding to early vascular ligation using single clips or sutures. We generally mobilise the colon from medial to lateral using a harmonic scalpel, identifying the left ureter and gonadal vessels before the lateral peritoneal attachments are divided. The splenic flexure mobilisation is performed as required, and when it is mobilised a medial to lateral approach is again favoured. The distal end of the specimen is cross-stapled, divided intracorporeally and the specimen extracted via a muscle-separating incision near the left groin. A stapled intracorporeal transanal anastomosis is then fashioned laparoscopically and leak-tested.

For resection of malignant right and right transverse colonic lesions we use a five-port technique (**Fig. 17.3**). Following an assessment of the anatomy and formulation of an operative strategy, we perform early vascular ligation of the ileocolic vessels near their origin, after identification of the superior mesenteric vein. Medial to lateral mobilisation is then performed before the middle colic vessels are identified and the right branch divided. Not only must surgeons be aware of the considerable variation in the vascular anatomy of this region, but also that the right gastroepiploic vessels consistently lie intimately opposed to the posterior aspect of the middle colic vessel. The 'right colic' artery is usually a branch of the middle colic vessel and its division allows further dissection of the transverse mesocolon from the pancreas. Having divided all vessels, the transverse

Sigmoid colectomy; TME;
Rectopexy; Left hemicolectomy

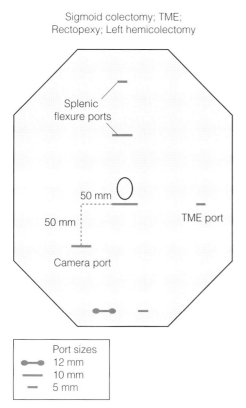

Figure 17.2 • Port positions for sigmoid colectomy, TME, rectopexy and left hemicolectomy.

Right hemicolectomy

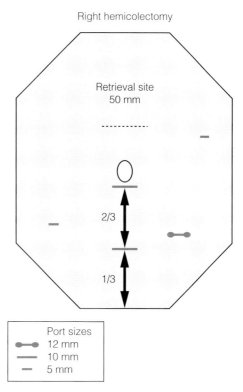

Figure 17.3 • Port positions for right hemicolectomy.

colon and hepatic flexure are mobilised from medial to lateral, ensuring adequate clearance of the transverse colon distal to the proposed anastomosis. This allows the colon to be delivered via a 4–5 cm incision unimpeded by attached omentum. The operative site then moves to the pelvic brim, where the right ureter and gonadal vessels are identified. The peritoneum overlying these structures is incised, with dissection proceeding in the avascular plane anterior to the fascia of Toldt, to join the previous dissection. The resection and anastomosis is via a transverse, supraumbilical, muscle-separating incision and the mesenteric defect is closed laparoscopically.

Difficult aspects of laparoscopic resection

Laparoscopic colorectal resection can be made more difficult by the patient factors described above; however, certain technical aspects of laparoscopic resection require caution depending on the surgeon's experience.

Though a right hemicolectomy may be regarded as an initial stepping stone in open surgery, this is not always comparable for laparoscopic resection. In Crohn's disease, one should not hesitate to convert when there is extensive mesenteric thickening or difficult inflammatory adhesions. There is still likely to be benefit from bowel mobilisation even if conversion – using the strict definition provided above – occurs. Vascular control and dissection of the transverse colon can also be problematic for the novice.

Further technical issues relate to splenic flexure mobilisation and rectal dissection. Laparoscopic splenic flexure mobilisation by any approach can prove difficult. We would normally recommend a medial to lateral approach using dissection along the anterior surface of the pancreas, after division of the inferior mesenteric vein (IMV). We would then separate the greater omentum from the superior surface of the transverse colon in a medial to lateral direction. This flexure can be challenging and the surgeon should be familiar with all approaches. Rectal dissection and particularly TME will continue to prove difficult in males with a narrow pelvis, irrespective of whether the procedure is open or laparoscopic. It is, however, a step too far for novices, even in women. The views obtained of the rectum at laparoscopy are unrivalled and with increasing experience laparoscopic TME is a satisfying procedure.

Specific contraindications to laparoscopic resection are gross peritonitis, toxic megacolon and obstructing carcinoma. However, with the advent and improvement in colonic stenting it is not unusual for obstructed patients to undergo elective laparoscopic resection following successful stenting.[42] Contiguous organ involvement may also be resected laparoscopically without conversion, when appropriate. For some large tumours, vascular ligation and the majority of mobilisation can be undertaken laparoscopically, in order to allow completion of the dissection through a smaller targeted incision than would otherwise have been possible using an open technique. This is often appropriate in TME when the rectal dissection may be completed through a much smaller incision than would otherwise have been possible. Some laparoscopic enthusiasts report small series when laparoscopic re-intervention has been feasible in the setting of clinical anastomotic leakage, with improved subsequent outcomes compared to open re-operation.[43,44] However, such small studies have inherent biases and in the setting of gross peritonitis from a leak we would not advocate laparoscopy. We have employed laparoscopy with benefit when doubt remains regarding situations such as an internal hernia, a small leak or unexplained postoperative pain.

The learning curve and training in laparoscopic colorectal surgery

The laparoscopic learning curve is known to vary between surgeons and will be influenced by patient selection and operative complexity, with comparisons requiring appropriate case-mix adjustment. Several authors have attempted to define a learning curve for laparoscopic colorectal resection. In one of the largest assessments to date, Tekkis et al. reported that more than 50 cases of each type of segmental colectomy were necessary to see a reduction in conversion rates.[45] Having adjusted for case-mix, a learning curve of 55 cases for right-sided colonic resections versus 62 cases for left-sided resections was found. The reader should be aware that as experience builds surgeons will often attempt more

complex cases, with inherently higher chances of conversion. This explains Tekkis et al.'s finding that a greater number of cases are necessary than was previously thought to be the case.

In an excellent study, MacRae et al. reviewed conversion and outcome in ileocolonic resection for Crohn's, reporting that despite increasing case complexity outcome improved over time. This, like Buchanan et al.'s study on colorectal cancer, is one of the few that includes the totality of practice – thus conversion rates can be interpreted with respect to the proportion of patients undergoing open surgery.[46]

The appropriate method of imparting laparoscopic colorectal skills remains an area of debate and a full exploration is beyond the scope of this chapter. It is likely that the combination of teaching adjuncts and simultaneous clinical training will add value for trainees. Favourable reports have come from the use of virtual reality training[48,49] or videotaping and playback[50] for skills assessment. Video production by trainees may also prove useful in training. Our own approach is to separate components of each laparoscopic procedure into modules so that each module can be learned before the entire operation is attempted. In addition each procedure is broken down into logical sequential steps, which are presented on a teaching video. The teaching video and recorded footage of the trainee are then used for regular review to optimise technique in training. This standardised, didactic approach is taught along with the identification of predicted operative difficulty so that the surgeon can proceed to independent practice without the necessity to relearn unnecessary lessons.

The most appropriate methods to optimise training in laparoscopic colorectal surgery remain unclear, although various systems have been initiated in the UK. These can be broadly categorised as preceptorship programmes for consultant surgeons, laparoscopic fellowships for senior trainees, animal and cadaver training courses, and more recently the set-up of a National Training Programme for consultant surgeons.

Summary

The multiple benefits of laparoscopic colorectal surgery have been repeatedly proven in large studies. Consequently the laparoscopic approach has changed from being the preserve of a few enthusiasts, in a limited number of patients, to becoming the preferred approach. We anticipate a dramatic increase in the number of laparoscopic colorectal procedures performed in the UK, which will be fuelled by increasing patient awareness and demand. As NICE highlighted, further information is required on cost-effectiveness, late oncological results, postoperative incisional hernias, neuralgia and small-bowel obstruction.

Enhanced recovery programmes

Surgical injury induces a series of complex responses in endocrine/metabolic and humoral cascade systems that may subsequently pose a risk to the surgical patient, resulting in organ dysfunction and delayed recovery. By making many modifications to traditional perioperative care, enhanced recovery or 'fast-track' programmes (ERPs) are designed to reduce this surgical stress response and its consequences (**Fig. 17.4**). ERPs have evolved as a result of evidence-based advances and important aspects include patient education, physiological optimisation, improved anaesthetic and analgesic techniques, modifications in surgical technique, and an improved understanding of early feeding and mobilisation.

Traditional perioperative care

A hospital stay of 10–14 days following colorectal resection has been accepted as normal when accompanied by traditional perioperative care. Despite this a postoperative stay of 2–3 days was first reported by Kehlet in Copenhagen and similar results have subsequently been achieved by other groups.[51–55] An understanding of what 'traditional' care means comes from Lassen et al.'s survey of colorectal surgeons in five Northern European countries.[56] This study highlighted the marked variation in practice between countries, suggesting that most surgeons have ignored evidence-based advances in perioperative care. Nygren et al. subsequently assessed these same five countries as part of the Enhanced Recovery After Surgery (ERAS) Group, comparing results in four centres with those from patients within an established ERP in Denmark.[57] This study was used to develop a consensus and a formal core protocol for ER care.[58] The core protocol was published by Fearon in 2005 and the key elements are summarised in **Fig. 17.5**.

Perioperative interventions in enhanced recovery programmes

Reducing metabolic stress

To prevent aspiration, starvation for solids and fat is required for 6 hours before elective surgery, but for only 2 hours when considering liquids (unless there has been previous gastric surgery or there is a known hiatus hernia). Evidence came initially from Ljungqvist's group in Stockholm that surgery is best conducted when the patient is in the fed state.[59–61] This can be achieved by the use of a 'complex carbohydrate' drink, which when taken 2 hours preoperatively decreases postoperative insulin resistance. Traditional starvation increases insulin resistance and patients thus behave more like type II diabetics, with a consequent increase in postoperative complications.

 Small detailed RCTs have also shown that protein balance is better maintained following preoperative carbohydrate loading.[62,63] Postoperative oral nutritional supplements significantly decrease postoperative complications and fatigue, maintaining nitrogen balance; hence early postoperative nutrition using supplements is encouraged.[63–65]

Preoperative bowel preparation

Systematic reviews and meta-analyses have assessed the role of preoperative bowel preparation in colorectal surgery and derived similar conclusions. A

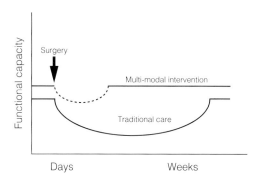

Figure 17.4 • Enhanced recovery and traditional care. Courtesy of Professor Henrik Kehlet.

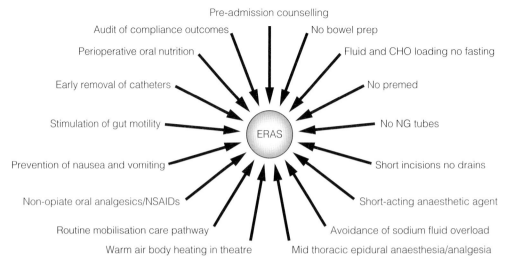

Figure 17.5 • Key elements of enhanced recovery care. ERAS, enhanced recovery after surgery. Courtesy of Professor Ken Fearon.

Cochrane Review by Guenaga et al. and at least two further meta-analyses confirm that mechanical bowel preparation does not reduce anastomotic leakage and may even increase wound infections.[66–68] Two recent large RCTs assessing the role of mechanical bowel preparation have provided conflicting results.[69,70] Based on the existing evidence we now only use mechanical bowel preparation in patients undergoing TME. For other people who require left-sided colonic or other forms of rectal resection we merely employ a preoperative enema in order to allow the anastomosis to be performed without gross faecal loading. A recent study from Sweden reported that a defunctioning stoma decreases symptomatic anastomotic leakage following rectal surgery and has recommended it for all low anterior resections.[71] Our TME patients therefore receive bowel preparation, as it seems illogical to defunction them and leave faeces between the stoma and the defunctioned anastomosis.

Perioperative fluid balance

Perioperative fluid therapy is the subject of much controversy and clinical trials investigating the effect of fluid therapy on the outcome of surgery are contradictory. Areas of debate in current surgical practice are that evaporative loss from the abdominal cavity is likely to be overestimated and assumptions regarding any third space loss may be based on methodologically flawed studies. The fluid volume that actually accumulates in traumatised tissue is likely to be minimal and volume preloading

following neuroaxial blockade causes postoperative overload.[72,73]

 Strong evidence from RCTs exists indicating that gut function, tissue healing, postoperative morbidity and hospital stay are adversely affected by the excessive prescription of perioperative fluid and sodium in elective surgery.[73,74]

Lobo et al. investigated the effect of fluid therapy on gastric emptying after colorectal surgery. The patients 'restricted' to <2 litres of crystalloid and 77 mmol of sodium per day had significantly improved gastric emptying, compared to those with standard fluids of >3 litres and 154 mmol of sodium per day.[74] Bowel function and hospital stay were also significantly improved. Fluid and sodium restriction was examined further by Brandstrup in a multicentre RCT which compared a traditional fluid replacement regimen with a restricted one. The latter aimed to maintain preoperative body weight and euvolaemia,[72] and it significantly reduced cardiopulmonary (7% vs. 24%), improved tissue healing (16% vs. 31%) and reduced overall complications (33% vs. 51%). Mortality was higher in the traditional group though this was not significant (0% vs. 4.7%, $P = 0.12$).

Perioperative fluid administration also influences cardiac function, fluid overload producing a suboptimal right-shifted position on the Starling curve, and fluid deficit does the opposite. Both situations increase the risk of perioperative cardiac morbidity. Intraoperative 'goal-directed' fluid therapy aims to optimise cardiac function addressing these risks.[75] The timing of intraoperative fluid administration may also be important. Noblett et al. investigated the administration of colloid boluses, guided by oesophageal Doppler monitoring of cardiac function, in a double-blind RCT. The intervention group experienced a reduction in complications and hospital stay, largely resulting from the administration of relatively small amounts of colloid early in the intervention.[76]

Surgical technique and wound drainage

Transverse and smaller incisions have been encouraged within ERPs.[77] There is evidence that smaller incisions improve outcome and that is likely to be one of the mechanisms of benefit in laparoscopic surgery. The direction of the incision is more contentious. A recent Cochrane Review found that although both analgesia use and pulmonary complications may be reduced with a transverse or oblique incision, this does not seem to be significant clinically as complication rates and recovery times are the same as with a midline incision.[78] Owing to heterogeneity in these studies the conclusions should be interpreted with caution.

The laparoscopic technique has been shown to decrease the stress response, with lower levels of interleukin-6 and C-reactive protein observed than after traditional open surgery; however, not all authors have identified this.[79–81]

The use of drains in elective colorectal surgery has been extensively studied in many RCTs. A Cochrane Review of 1140 patients from six such trials reported that 573 were allocated to drainage and 567 to no drainage.[82] No benefit was found for routine anastomotic drainage and we would regard drainage as unnecessary in most situations; in addition it impairs patient mobility. In order to minimise pelvic haematoma formation after low rectal surgery, drainage for 12–18 hours may be appropriate. This is our current practice but it is unsupported by objective data.

Mobilisation

One of the central tenets of ER care is early mobilisation, with patients sitting out of bed on the day of surgery and walking regularly thereafter. This is made much less feasible if there are multiple attachments restricting mobilisation. It would be normal for us to remove all tubes, excluding the epidural catheter and with capping of the intravenous cannula, on day one following colonic surgery in order to allow patients to mobilise. Should patients fail to mobilise on day one then the urinary catheter is retained. Similarly, following low rectal surgery we would delay removal of the urinary catheter for 2–3 days in case bladder denervation has occurred.

Pain control

There is consistent evidence from meta-analysis that epidural local anaesthetic, usually mixed with a low concentration of opiate, hastens return of postoperative gastrointestinal function after abdominal surgery by 24–37 hours and improves pain control.[83] It is not clear, however, that this technique reduces postoperative complications, other than pulmonary morbidity, largely as studies have been underpowered.[84] The epidural should be thoracic rather than lumbar to avoid lower limb motor paralysis and urinary retention. Compared to patient-controlled intravenous opiate analgesia (PCA), epidurals seem to provide better analgesia, particularly during exercise, without the nausea and ileus incurred with opiates.[83] In addition, it has become routine to supplement analgesia with paracetamol and administer non-steroidal anti-inflammatory drugs (NSAIDs) just before the epidural is stopped. Contrary views exist and Delaney et al. have routinely used PCA followed by multimodal oral analgesics with good results.[55] The debate on optimal postoperative analgesia therefore continues, particularly as the laparoscopic technique reduces postoperative pain. Evidence is contradictory as publications are frequently heterogeneous, mixing outcomes from different age groups and different comorbidities. Hence we have continued to use a thoracic epidural analgesic technique postoperatively as, to date, the only studies achieving a postoperative stay of less than 4 days in an elderly population have used it.[22,51]

Enhanced recovery trials

The principles of ER care have been applied in several RCTs with favourable outcomes. Anderson et al. randomised 25 patients and reported that optimisation was associated with maintained grip strength, earlier mobilisation, lower pain and fatigue scores, and reduced hospital stay (median 3 vs. 7 days, $P = 0.002$).[53] These results were supported by Delaney et al. in an RCT of 64 patients and a later study by Gatt et al. reiterated the benefits, even when epidural analgesia was used postoperatively in both ERP and traditional groups.[54]

Compared to traditional perioperative care, hospital stay and morbidity are significantly reduced in ERPs without significantly increasing readmission rates or mortality.[85]

One of the initial concerns regarding ERPs was related to an increased readmission rate. Proponents addressed this by changing the planned discharge date from 2 to 3 days, significantly reducing the readmission rate.[86] Setting up further RCTs to examine individual components that contribute to an ERP is problematic, since it is difficult to randomise patients to traditional care in an institution that has spent 1–2 years developing ER care, particularly when the developments are evidence based and should be regarded as best practice.

The issue of whether ER care results in a transfer of cost to the community has been analysed in a carefully controlled study. Detailed cost and quality-of-life analyses were performed and did not demonstrate an increase in cost or deterioration in quality of life resulting from this change in care.[17] We anticipate that larger trials will confirm an improvement in these outcomes in the future.

ERPs applied to laparoscopic surgery

It is clear that with appropriate training the use of the laparoscopic technique can considerably improve functional results after colorectal resection. The debate has therefore shifted to whether optimisation of the perioperative care associated with open surgery can produce similar outcomes. To date, two RCTs have assessed this question and have produced conflicting results.[22,86]

Basse et al. randomised 60 patients to open or laparoscopic surgery and observed no difference in outcome, with both groups having a median stay of 2 days after surgery. There were high readmission rates of 20% and 29% and 0 vs. 4 deaths for laparoscopic and open patients respectively. Neither of these outcomes were, however, significantly different between the groups. King et al. assessed 62 patients with a 2:1 randomisation, the format used in the CLASICC trial. The length of hospital stay after laparoscopic resection was 32% shorter than for open resection ($P = 0.018$). Combined hospital, convalescent and readmission stay was 37% shorter ($P = 0.012$) and the chance of readmission significantly less (5% vs. 26%).

The EnROL trial (Enhanced Recovery Open versus Laparoscopic) in the UK and the LAFA trial (LAparoscopy and/or FAst-track multimodal management versus standard care) in the Netherlands have been devised to re-examine this question in a multicentre setting.

Who should ERPs be applied to?

As yet, it is unclear whether this multimodal approach to perioperative optimisation can be broadly applied to all patients or whether modification is required in certain subgroups. Further, more conclusive data will hopefully clarify the place of epidural analgesia in patients treated by experienced laparoscopic surgeons who have low conversion rates. We do not use NSAIDs in people with known impairment of renal function or when the creatinine is rising postoperatively. Despite these issues, we currently use an ERP for all our patients undergoing elective colorectal surgery and it would seem logical that the more unfit a patient is, the greater the potential benefit in perioperative optimisation from an ERP.

Starting an ERP

This development requires a multidisciplinary approach to perioperative care and requires extensive retraining of staff. Modest resource requirements are necessary, but a large change in the healthcare culture is essential. We use multidisciplinary courses directed at all key team members in order to start the training. A nurse facilitator to lead, teach and audit outcomes is also necessary to manage the process of change. The change requires many months to reach maximal effectiveness and will be aided by regular audit of compliance with the different interventions (Fig. 17.5). As the percentage compliance achieved for each intervention increases, patient recovery improves.[87]

Summary

ERPs represent an evidence-based approach to perioperative care that aims to reduce the stress response to surgery. Until recently, this evidence base has largely been ignored by the surgical community. Interest is now increasing in the benefits of this approach that have been confirmed in RCTs.

Fluid management in the perioperative period remains an area of debate but euvolaemic fluid replacement should be encouraged. The importance of opioid-sparing analgesia has been recognised and the use of peripheral opioid antagonists to reduce postoperative ileus is an area for development. Carbohydrate loading and early feeding contribute to a reduction in the stress response but other agents such as glucocorticoids may also have

a role. We anticipate that further research will clarify the place of epidural anaesthesia in laparoscopic surgery and the relative contributions of other components within the programme.

In conclusion, colorectal surgeons should not restrict enhancement of recovery to unimodal interventions, such as laparoscopic surgery, but should offer it within the context of multimodal optimisation to obtain the best outcomes following colorectal surgery.

Key points

Laparoscopic colorectal surgery

- Though operation times are currently slightly longer, laparoscopic colorectal surgery reduces wound infection rates, blood loss and postoperative pain, and results in a shorter hospital stay.
- Laparoscopic resection for colorectal cancer yields similar overall and cancer-specific survival. Future studies with potentially lower conversion rates may identify improved cancer outcomes.
- Although most authors report an increased cost associated with minimal access surgery, increased experience and future decreases in instrument costs are likely to result in an economic benefit.
- Increased conversion rates are observed in rectal surgery, the obese patient and following previous major surgery. It is important to recognise the technical challenges associated with this procedure in order to minimise potential adverse outcomes.
- The most effective method of training in laparoscopic colorectal surgery is unclear but a structured, repetitive approach paying attention to operative complexity is essential.

Enhanced recovery programmes

- Key components of an ERP include preoperative conditioning of expectation, modifications of surgical and anaesthetic technique, improved postoperative analgesia allowing early mobilisation and reduction of ileus, reduction of metabolic stress and the avoidance of fluid overload.
- This mutimodal approach to rehabilitation improves recovery, reducing complications and hospital stay.
- Further research is necessary to demonstrate the extra benefit derived from the addition of laparoscopic surgery to an ERP.
- The establishment of an ERP requires extensive multidisciplinary training but the benefits are likely to be equally applicable to other surgical disciplines.

References

1. Lacy AM, Garcia-Valdecasas JC, Delgado S et al. Laparoscopy-assisted colectomy versus open colectomy for treatment of non-metastatic colon cancer: a randomised trial. Lancet 2002; 359(9325):2224–9.

2. A comparison of laparoscopically assisted and open colectomy for colon cancer. N Engl J Med 2004; 350(20):2050–9.

3. Leung KL, Kwok SP, Lam SC et al. Laparoscopic resection of rectosigmoid carcinoma: prospective randomised trial. Lancet 2004; 363(9416):1187–92.

4. Guillou PJ, Quirke P, Thorpe H et al. Short-term endpoints of conventional versus laparoscopic-assisted surgery in patients with colorectal cancer (MRC CLASICC trial): multicentre, randomised controlled trial. Lancet 2005; 365(9472):1718–26.

5. Veldkamp R, Kuhry E, Hop WC et al. Laparoscopic surgery versus open surgery for colon cancer: short-term outcomes of a randomised trial. Lancet Oncol 2005; 6(7):477–84.

6. Jayne DG, Guillou PJ, Thorpe H et al. Randomized trial of laparoscopic-assisted resection of colorectal carcinoma: 3 year results of the UK MRC CLASSIC Trial Group. J Clin Oncol 2007; 25(21):3061–8.

7. Abraham NS, Young JM, Solomon MJ. Meta-analysis of short-term outcomes after laparoscopic resection for colorectal cancer. Br J Surg 2004; 91(9):1111–24.

 8. Schwenk W, Haase O, Neudecker J et al. Short term benefits for laparoscopic colorectal resection. Cochrane Database Syst Rev 2005; 3:CD003145.

 9. Abraham NS, Byrne CM, Young JM et al. Meta-analysis of non-randomized comparative studies of the short-term outcomes of laparoscopic resection for colorectal cancer. Aust NZ J Surg 2007; 77(7):508–16.

These meta-analyses assess the outcomes of randomised clinical trials and observational studies and highlight the short-term benefits of laparoscopic resection of colorectal cancer over open surgery.

10. Duepree HJ, Senagore AJ, Delaney CP et al. Does means of access affect the incidence of small bowel obstruction and ventral hernia after bowel resection? Laparoscopy versus laparotomy. J Am Coll Surg 2003; 197(2):177–81.

11. Kiran RP, Delaney CP, Senagore AJ et al. Operative blood loss and use of blood products after laparoscopic and conventional open colorectal operations. Arch Surg 2004; 139(1):39–42.

12. Law WL, Lee YM, Choi HK et al. Impact of laparoscopic resection for colorectal cancer on operative outcomes and survival. Ann Surg 2007; 245(1):1–7.

13. Tjandra JJ, Chan MK. Systematic review on the short-term outcome of laparoscopic resection for colon and rectosigmoid cancer. Colorectal Dis 2006; 8(5):375–88.

14. Braga M, Vignali A, Gianotti L et al. Laparoscopic resection in rectal cancer patients: outcome and cost–benefit analysis. Dis Colon Rectum 2007; 50:464–71.

15. Lourenco T, Murray A, Grant A et al. Laparoscopic surgery for colorectal cancer: safe and effective? – A systematic review. Surg Endosc 2007 (Epub ahead of print).

16. Murray A, Lourenco T, de Verteuil R et al. Clinical effectiveness and cost-effectiveness of laparoscopic surgery for colorectal cancer: systematic reviews and economic evaluation. Health Technol Assess 2006; 10(45):1–141, iii–iv.

17. King PM, Blazeby JM, Ewings P et al. The influence of an enhanced recovery programme on clinical outcomes, costs and quality of life after surgery for colorectal cancer. Colorectal Dis 2006; 8(6):506–13.

18. Dowson HM, Huang A, Soon Y et al. Systematic review of the costs of laparoscopic colorectal surgery. Dis Colon Rectum 2007; 50(6):908–19.

19. Senagore AJ, Duepree HJ, Delaney CP et al. Cost structure of laparoscopic and open sigmoid colectomy for diverticular disease: similarities and differences. Dis Colon Rectum 2002; 45(4):485–90.

20. Buchanan GN, Malik A, Parvaiz A et al. Laparoscopic resection for colorectal cancer. Br J Surg 2008; 95(7):893-902.

21. Lumley J, Stitz R, Stevenson A et al. Laparoscopic colorectal surgery for cancer: intermediate to long-term outcomes. Dis Colon Rectum 2002; 45(7):867–72; discussion 872–5.

22. King PM, Blazeby JM, Ewings P et al. Randomized clinical trial comparing laparoscopic and open surgery for colorectal cancer within an enhanced recovery programme. Br J Surg 2006; 93(3):300–8.

23. Veldkamp R, Gholghesaei M, Bonjer HJ et al. Laparoscopic resection of colon cancer: consensus of the European Association of Endoscopic Surgery (EAES). Surg Endosc 2004; 18(8):1163–85.

24. Schwandner O, Farke S, Schiedeck TH et al. Laparoscopic colorectal surgery in obese and nonobese patients: do differences in body mass indices lead to different outcomes? Surg Endosc 2004; 18(10):1452–6.

25. Senagore AJ, Delaney CP, Madboulay K et al. Laparoscopic colectomy in obese and nonobese patients. J Gastrointest Surg 2003; 7(4):558–61.

26. Arteaga Gonzalez I, Martin Malagon A, Lopez-Tomassetti Fernandez EM et al. Impact of previous abdominal surgery on colorectal laparoscopy results: a comparative clinical study. Surg Laparosc Endosc Percutan Tech 2006; 16(1):8–11.

27. Law WL, Choi HK, Ho JW et al. Outcomes of surgery for mid and distal rectal cancer in the elderly. World J Surg 2006; 30(4):598–604.

28. Moloo H, Bedard EL, Poulin EC et al. Palliative laparoscopic resections for Stage IV colorectal cancer. Dis Colon Rectum 2006; 49(2):213–18.

29. Kuhry E, Bonjer HJ, Haglind E et al. Impact of hospital case volume on short-term outcome after laparoscopic operation for colonic cancer. Surg Endosc 2005; 19(5):687–92.

30. Tekkis PP, Senagore AJ, Delaney CP. Conversion rates in laparoscopic colorectal surgery: a predictive model with 1253 patients. Surg Endosc 2005; 19(1):47–54.

31. Marusch F, Gastinger I, Schneider C et al. Importance of conversion for results obtained with laparoscopic colorectal surgery. Dis Colon Rectum 2001; 44(2):207–14; discussion 214–16.

32. Casillas S, Delaney CP, Senagore AJ et al. Does conversion of a laparoscopic colectomy adversely affect patient outcome? Dis Colon Rectum 2004; 47(10):1680–5.

33. Bemelman WA, Slors JF, Dunker MS et al. Laparoscopic-assisted vs. open ileocolic resection for Crohn's disease. A comparative study. Surg Endosc 2000; 14(8):721–5.

34. Duepree HJ, Senagore AJ, Delaney CP et al. Advantages of laparoscopic resection for ileocecal Crohn's disease. Dis Colon Rectum 2002; 45(5):605–10.

35. Lawes DA, Motson RW. Avoidance of laparotomy for recurrent disease is a long-term benefit of laparoscopic resection for Crohn's disease. Br J Surg 2006; 93(5):607–8.

36. Milsom JW, Hammerhofer KA, Bohm B et al. Prospective, randomized trial comparing laparoscopic vs. conventional surgery for refractory ileocolic Crohn's disease. Dis Colon Rectum 2001; 44(1):1–8; discussion 8–9.

37. Maartense S, Dunker MS, Slors JF et al. Laparoscopic-assisted versus open ileocolic resection for Crohn's disease: a randomized trial. Ann Surg 2006; 243(2):143–9; discussion 150–3.

38. Schwandner O, Farke S, Bruch HP. Laparoscopic colectomy for diverticulitis is not associated with increased morbidity when compared with non-diverticular disease. Int J Colorectal Dis 2005; 20(2):165–72.

39. Pokala N, Delaney CP, Senagore AJ et al. Laparoscopic vs open total colectomy: a case-matched comparative study. Surg Endosc 2005; 19(4):531–5.

40. Tilney HS, Lovegrove RE, Heriot AG et al. Comparison of short-term outcomes of laparoscopic vs open approaches to ileal pouch surgery. Int J Colorectal Dis 2007; 22(5):531–42.

41. Arteaga-Gonzalez I, Martin-Malagon A, Fernandez EM et al. The use of preoperative endoscopic tattooing in laparoscopic colorectal cancer surgery for endoscopically advanced tumors: a prospective comparative clinical study. World J Surg 2006; 30(4):605–11.

42. Law WL, Choi HK, Lee YM et al. Laparoscopic colectomy for obstructing sigmoid cancer with prior insertion of an expandable metallic stent. Surg Laparosc Endosc Percutan Tech 2004; 14(1):29–32.

43. Pera M, Delgado S, Garcia-Valdecasas JC et al. The management of leaking rectal anastomoses by minimally invasive techniques. Surg Endosc 2002; 16(4):603–6.

44. Wind J, Koopman AG, van Berge Henegouwen MI et al. Laparoscopic reintervention for anastomotic leakage after primary laparoscopic colorectal surgery. Br J Surg 2007; 94(12):1562–6.

45. Tekkis PP, Senagore AJ, Delaney CP et al. Evaluation of the learning curve in laparoscopic colorectal surgery: comparison of right-sided and left-sided resections. Ann Surg 2005; 242(1):83–91.

46. Evans J, Poritz L, MacRae H. Influence of experience on laparoscopic ileocolic resection for Crohn's disease. Dis Colon Rectum 2002; 45(12):1595–1600.

47. Braga M, Vignali A, Zuliani W et al. Training period in laparoscopic colorectal surgery. Surg Endosc 2002; 16(1):31–5.

48. Aggarwal R, Grantcharov T, Moorthy K et al. A competency-based virtual reality training curriculum for the acquisition of laparoscopic psychomotor skill. Am J Surg 2006; 191(1):128–33.

49. Aggarwal R, Ward J, Balasundaram I et al. Proving the effectiveness of virtual reality simulation for training in laparoscopic surgery. Ann Surg 2007; 246(5):771–9.

50. Dath D, Regehr G, Birch D et al. Toward reliable operative assessment: the reliability and feasibility of videotaped assessment of laparoscopic technical skills. Surg Endosc 2004; 18(12):1800–4.

51. Basse L, Hjort Jakobsen D, Billesbolle P et al. A clinical pathway to accelerate recovery after colonic resection. Ann Surg 2000; 232(1):51–7.

52. Basse L, Raskov HH, Hjort Jakobsen D et al. Accelerated postoperative recovery programme after colonic resection improves physical performance, pulmonary function and body composition. Br J Surg 2002; 89(4):446–53.

53. Anderson AD, McNaught CE, MacFie J et al. Randomized clinical trial of multimodal optimization and standard perioperative surgical care. Br J Surg 2003; 90(12):1497–1504.

54. Gatt M, Anderson AD, Reddy BS et al. Randomized clinical trial of multimodal optimization of surgical care in patients undergoing major colonic resection. Br J Surg 2005; 92(11):1354–62.

55. Delaney CP, Zutshi M, Senagore AJ et al. Prospective, randomized, controlled trial between a pathway of controlled rehabilitation with early ambulation and diet and traditional postoperative care after laparotomy and intestinal resection. Dis Colon Rectum 2003; 46(7):851–9.

56. Lassen K, Hannemann P, Ljungqvist O et al. Patterns in current perioperative practice: survey of colorectal surgeons in five northern European countries. BMJ 2005; 330(7505):1420–1.

57. Nygren J, Hausel J, Kehlet H et al. A comparison in five European Centres of case mix, clinical management and outcomes following either conventional or fast-track perioperative care in colorectal surgery. Clin Nutr 2005; 24(3):455–61.

58. Fearon KC, Ljungqvist O, Von Meyenfeldt M et al. Enhanced recovery after surgery: a consensus review of clinical care for patients undergoing colonic resection. Clin Nutr 2005; 24(3):466–77.

59. Ljungqvist O, Soreide E. Preoperative fasting. Br J Surg 2003; 90(4):400–6.

60. Soreide E, Ljungqvist O. Modern preoperative fasting guidelines: a summary of the present recommendations and remaining questions. Best Pract Res Clin Anaesthesiol 2006; 20(3):483–91.

61. Soreide E, Ljungqvist O. Preoperative fasting. Can J Surg 2006; 49(3):218–19; author reply 219.

62. Svanfeldt M, Thorell A, Hausel J et al. Randomized clinical trial of the effect of preoperative oral carbohydrate treatment on postoperative whole-body protein and glucose kinetics. Br J Surg 2007; 94(11):1342–50.

291

63. Soop M, Carlson GL, Hopkinson J et al. Randomized clinical trial of the effects of immediate enteral nutrition on metabolic responses to major colorectal surgery in an enhanced recovery protocol. Br J Surg 2004; 91(9):1138–45.

These elegant small RCTs assess the effect of perioperative feeding in attenuating the metabolic response. This group have identified benefits with this approach in maintaining whole-body protein balance and that the suppressive effects of endogenous glucose release are better maintained with pre-op carbohydrate loading and post-op feeding.

64. Keele AM, Bray MJ, Emery PW et al. Two phase randomised controlled clinical trial of postoperative oral dietary supplements in surgical patients. Gut 1997; 40(3):393–9.

65. Rana SK, Bray J, Menzies-Gow N et al. Short term benefits of post-operative oral dietary supplements in surgical patients. Clin Nutr 1992; 11(6):337–44.

66. Guenaga KF, Matos D, Castro AA et al. Mechanical bowel preparation for elective colorectal surgery. Cochrane Database Syst Rev 2005; 1:CD001544.

67. Bucher P, Mermillod B, Gervaz P et al. Mechanical bowel preparation for elective colorectal surgery: a meta-analysis. Arch Surg 2004; 139(12):1359–64; discussion 1365.

68. Slim K, Vicaut E, Panis Y et al. Meta-analysis of randomized clinical trials of colorectal surgery with or without mechanical bowel preparation. Br J Surg 2004; 91(9):1125–30.

69. Contant CM, Hop WC, van't Sant HP et al. Mechanical bowel preparation for elective colorectal surgery: a multicentre randomised trial. Lancet 2007; 370(9605):2112–17.

70. Platell C, Barwood N, Makin G. Randomized clinical trial of bowel preparation with a single phosphate enema or polyethylene glycol before elective colorectal surgery. Br J Surg 2006; 93(4):427–33.

71. Matthiessen P, Hallbook O, Rutegard J et al. Defunctioning stoma reduces symptomatic anastomotic leakage after low anterior resection of the rectum for cancer: a randomized multicenter trial. Ann Surg 2007; 246(2):207–14.

72. Brandstrup B, Svensen C, Engquist A. Hemorrhage and operation cause a contraction of the extracellular space needing replacement – evidence and implications? A systematic review. Surgery 2006; 139(3):419–32.

73. Brandstrup B, Tonnesen H, Beier-Holgersen R et al. Effects of intravenous fluid restriction on postoperative complications: comparison of two perioperative fluid regimens: a randomized assessor-blinded multicenter trial. Ann Surg 2003; 238(5):641–8.

74. Lobo DN, Bostock KA, Neal KR et al. Effect of salt and water balance on recovery of gastrointestinal function after elective colonic resection: a randomised controlled trial. Lancet 2002; 359(9320):1812–18.

These studies have had a potent effect on our renewed interest in perioperative fluid management. Brandstrup et al.'s paper shows clear benefits to fluid restriction compared to traditional practice, with significantly elevated morbidity levels in the traditional group who received large fluid volumes in the perioperative period. Lobo et al.'s study on a small number of patients confirms the important effects of fluid management on gut function and recovery.

75. Pearse R, Dawson D, Fawcett J et al. Early goal-directed therapy after major surgery reduces complications and duration of hospital stay. A randomised, controlled trial (ISRCTN38797445). Crit Care 2005; 9(6):R687–93.

76. Noblett SE, Snowden CP, Shenton BK et al. Randomized clinical trial assessing the effect of Doppler-optimized fluid management on outcome after elective colorectal resection. Br J Surg 2006; 93(9):1069–76.

77. O'Dwyer PJ, McGregor JR, McDermott EW et al. Patient recovery following cholecystectomy through a 6 cm or 15 cm transverse subcostal incision: a prospective randomized clinical trial. Postgrad Med J 1992; 68(804):817–19.

78. Brown SR, Goodfellow PB. Transverse versus midline incisions for abdominal surgery. Cochrane Database Syst Rev 2005; 4:CD005199.

79. Delgado S, Lacy AM, Filella X et al. Acute phase response in laparoscopic and open colectomy in colon cancer: randomized study. Dis Colon Rectum 2001; 44(5):638–46.

80. Braga M, Vignali A, Zuliani W et al. Metabolic and functional results after laparoscopic colorectal surgery: a randomized, controlled trial. Dis Colon Rectum 2002; 45(8):1070–7.

81. Dunker MS, Ten Hove T, Bemelman WA et al. Interleukin-6, C-reactive protein, and expression of human leukocyte antigen-DR on peripheral blood mononuclear cells in patients after laparoscopic vs. conventional bowel resection: a randomized study. Dis Colon Rectum 2003; 46(9):1238–44.

82. Jesus EC, Karliczek A, Matos D et al. Prophylactic anastomotic drainage for colorectal surgery. Cochrane Database Syst Rev 2004; 4:CD002100.

83. Gendall KA, Kennedy RR, Watson AJ et al. The effect of epidural analgesia on postoperative outcome after colorectal surgery. Colorectal Dis 2007; 9(7):584–98; discussion 598–600.

84. Liu SS, Wu CL. Effect of postoperative analgesia on major postoperative complications: a systematic update of the evidence. Anesth Analg 2007; 104(3):689–702.

85. Wind J, Polle SW, Fung Kon Jin PH et al. Systematic review of enhanced recovery programmes in colonic surgery. Br J Surg 2006; 93(7):800–9.

86. Basse L, Jakobsen DH, Bardram L et al. Functional recovery after open versus laparoscopic colonic resection: a randomized, blinded study. Ann Surg 2005; 241(3):416–23.

87. Maessen J, Dejong CH, Hausel J et al. A protocol is not enough to implement an enhanced recovery programme for colorectal resection. Br J Surg 2007; 94(2):224–31.

18

Intestinal failure

Carolynne Vaizey
Janindra Warusavitarne

Introduction

The term intestinal failure encompasses a spectrum of conditions that manifests itself as an inability to maintain adequate nutritional, fluid and electrolyte homeostasis without supportive therapy.[1] The vast majority of cases are transient, without significant gut pathology, and are routinely managed in general surgical units. They frequently occur secondary to postoperative ileus. However, there is a group of cases distinguished by loss of functional gut that results in prolonged intestinal failure lasting from months to years, some patients requiring permanent parenteral nutrition. These cases may be due to massive gut loss secondary to surgery, or loss of functioning intestine available for absorption, as occurs after enterocutaneous fistula formation.

Management of these cases may be complex, prolonged and expensive, in terms of both financial cost and clinical input. Care may be optimised by involvement of a multidisciplinary unit devoted to the management of intestinal failure. This unit will include a nutrition support team with the capacity to facilitate the transition of the patient's care from a hospital environment to a home environment. The care of patients with intestinal failure is prolonged and involves specialist gastroenterological, surgical and nursing input. Surgical treatment is generally the last of many steps in the management but accounts for an important part of the workload of specialised intestinal failure units.[1]

The nursing staff on the ward and in clinic, specialist nutrition nurses and the home parenteral nutrition (HPN) team are the backbone of delivery of care to these patients and their families. The different functions of each of these groups and their separate physical locations make it imperative that all are coordinated in their approach to each patient. Failure to achieve this results in confusion and demoralisation of this psychologically vulnerable group of patients, who have been faced with prolonged hospital admission, a debilitating illness, the prospect of no longer being able to eat normally or at all and the likelihood of less than fully functional recovery. Those who do survive find it difficult to accept the major limitations to their opportunities in life, especially in the case of young adults who constitute a significant proportion of these patients. A high level of technical training in the carers is required, which necessitates a specialist centre to maintain the technical base to these skills.

In addition, congenial working conditions will help prevent high staff turnover and consequent loss of skills. Coordination is achieved by a sense of team purpose and familiarity, consultant-led weekly multidisciplinary rounds, and a consensus approach to patient management that is explicitly stated in a protocol, but which allows flexibility for medical and social demands.

The British Government has set up and funded two supraregional units in England through the National Specialist Commissioning Advisory Body. One is at St Mark's Hospital in London (Northwick Park,

Watford Road, Harrow, Middlesex HA1 3UJ), the other is at Hope Hospital in Salford (Hope Hospital, Stott Lane, Salford, Manchester M6 8HD).

Intestinal failure: criteria for referral

The following criteria[2] are an indication of the type of cases that warrant referral to a nationally designated intestinal failure unit:

1. Persistence of intestinal failure beyond 6 weeks, without any evidence of resolution and/or complicated by venous access problems.
2. Multiple intestinal fistulation in a totally dehisced abdominal wound.
3. An intestinal fistula outside the expertise of the referring unit (e.g. recurrent in a non-specialist unit) or second and third recurrences in a colorectal centre.
4. Total or near-total small-bowel enterectomy, resulting in less than 30 cm of residual small bowel.
5. Recurrent venous access problems in patients needing sustained parenteral nutrition. This definition includes recurrent severe infections and recurrent venous thrombosis, where all upper limb and cervical venous access routes have become obliterated.
6. Persistent intra-abdominal sepsis, complicated by severe metabolic derangement (characterised by hypoalbuminaemia), that is not responding to radiological/surgical drainage of sepsis and provision of nutritional support.
7. Metabolic complications relating to high-output fistulas and stomas and to prolonged intravenous feeding, not responsive to medication and adjustment of the feeding regimen. Disorders of hepatic and renal function associated with intravenous nutrition that are resistant to metabolic and nutritional supplementation.
8. Chronic intestinal failure (from whatever cause) in a hospital without adequate experience/expertise to manage the medical/surgical and nutritional requirements of such patients.

Epidemiology

The prevalence of intestinal failure is unknown, but estimates can be made by considering those who require home parenteral nutrition (HPN). The incidence of HPN in Europe is estimated to be 3 per million population and the prevalence at 4 per million population, of whom 35% have short-bowel syndrome (SBS).[3] In the USA the use of HPN is estimated to be 120 per million population, of whom approximately 25% have SBS.[4] Such data do not include the patients who have not required HPN or those who have been successfully weaned off HPN. In the UK the estimated incidence of intestinal failure requiring treatment at a specialised unit is 5.5 per million population.[1]

As SBS is an uncommon condition, specialised centres with expertise in SBS have been created.[1,5,6] A recent study showed an overall survival rate of 86% in patients undergoing autologous surgical reconstruction at a median follow-up period of 2 years in a specialised unit.[7] Similar results have been achieved in other units and highlight the importance of multidisciplinary care.[1,8]

Causes

The causes of intestinal failure are multifactorial but can be categorised into four broad areas:

1. loss of intestinal length;
2. loss of functional intestinal length;
3. loss of intestinal absorptive capacity;
4. loss of intestinal functional ability.

Loss of intestinal length

In the adult population the aetiology of intestinal failure is most commonly related to a loss of intestinal length as a result of multiple intestinal resections or one massive intestinal resection.[9,10] Multiple resections are most common in recurrent Crohn's disease; an isolated massive enterectomy usually follows a vascular catastrophe, such as mesenteric arterial thrombosis or embolism, or a venous thrombosis. Massive resection can also be necessary in cases of volvulus, trauma or, in the case of children, necrotising enterocolitis or gastroschisis.

The relation between the amount of bowel removed and the degree of intestinal failure is variable, influenced by the age of the patient, the site of resection and the presence or absence of colon. The normal small bowel is around 600 cm in length but may range between 300 and 800 cm. The important figure is not how much small bowel is removed but how much remains. An approximate figure of less than 100 cm in the presence of an ileostomy or less than 50 cm with colon present is likely to result in dependence on parenteral nutrition (PN) at 3 months. Children may function with less bowel as small-bowel adaptation (see below) may be very dramatic. The function of the remaining bowel may also be influenced by the presence of active Crohn's disease as well as the aforementioned presence or absence of colon, as this may have a significant absorptive function.

Loss of functional absorptive capacity

Enterocutaneous fistula is the commonest cause of intestinal failure where the mechanism is loss of functional absorptive capacity. Fistulous disease commonly bypasses otherwise normal functional small intestine. This is usually the result of an enterocutaneous fistula, but hidden internal fistulas may also be responsible.

At a specialised intestinal failure unit, 42% of patients had Crohn's disease and the commonest complication necessitating admission was formation of enterocutaneous fistulas.[1] The second most common cause of fistulas is abdominal surgery. The majority of fistulas occurring in postoperative patients[11,12] are the consequence of anastomotic breakdown. Risks for this include the age of the patient, the state of the bowel undergoing anastomosis, preoperative nutritional status and the site of anastomosis.[11] When associated with malignancy, factors including tumour fixity, presence of obstruction, previous radiotherapy, associated abscess and surgical technique all affect the risk. Non-absorbable mesh can erode into the bowel and cause fistulas, particularly where there is fragile postoperative or diseased bowel. The use of vacuum-assisted closure (VAC) systems in the open abdomen can result in fistula when applied next to the bowel wall. In patients with intestinal or peritoneal inflammation and/or multiorgan failure there is a 20% rate of intestinal fistulisation associated with the use of a VAC system.[13]

Other causes of fistulas include colorectal cancer, diverticular disease and radiation. Fistulas resulting from radiation damage are usually complex and carry a high mortality. Rarer conditions include trauma and congenital fistulas, such as a patent vitello-intestinal tract. Tuberculosis may fistulate

as a complication of an ileal mass, and actinomycosis is an alternative possibility. Ulcerative colitis may fistulate, but this is more commonly postoperational, and occasionally the diagnosis needs reviewing as to the possibility of Crohn's disease.

Loss of intestinal absorptive capacity

Inflammatory conditions of the small bowel can result in non-functioning enterocytes that reduce absorptive capacity. Such conditions include inflammatory bowel disease, sprue, scleroderma, amyloid, coeliac disease and radiation enteritis.

Loss of intestinal functional ability

In the acute setting, postoperative ileus is the commonest reason for a loss of intestinal function, but this is usually self-remitting and does not require more than short-term supportive treatment. More chronic conditions such as pseudo-obstruction, visceral myopathy or autonomic neuropathy can result in functional disability and present a significant challenge for management.

Pathophysiology

The three stages of intestinal failure

Following the initiating event, intestinal 'recovery' results in three recognisable phases that have implications for management.

Stage I: hypersecretory phase

Of the 7 litres secreted daily by the duodenum, stomach, small intestine, pancreas and liver, about 6 litres are reabsorbed proximal to the ileocaecal valve. A further 800 mL are reabsorbed in the colon, leaving just 200 mL of water in the faeces.

Lack of absorption results in large volume losses. This phase can last 1–2 months and is characterised by copious diarrhoea and/or high stoma or fistula outputs. The main focus of treatment is on fluid and electrolyte replacement while PN may be required to maintain nutrition.

Stage II: adaptation phase

The process of intestinal adaptation involves a series of histological changes in the intestinal mucosa that allow for enhanced mucosal absorption within the residual intestine. The triggers for adaptation are the maintenance of fluid and electrolyte balance and the gradual introduction of enteral feeding. The process of adaptation takes 3–12 months and the degree of adaptation varies with patient age (more adaptation occurs in the paediatric population), underlying disease extent and the site of resection (ileum has better capacity for adaptation than jejunum).

Stage III: stabilisation phase

Maximum intestinal adaptation may take up to 1–2 years and the extent and route of nutritional support will vary. The overall goal for the patient is to achieve as normal a lifestyle as possible, which means achieving stability at home.

Normal physiological functioning of the intestine involves complex fluid, electrolyte and nutrient exchanges to maintain homeostasis. Interruption of this arrangement can result in gross imbalances which require supplementation enterally or parenterally. The normal physiology of the intestine is discussed below.

Fluid and electrolytes

Sodium absorption in the small bowel is actively linked to the absorption of glucose and certain amino acids. Water absorption is passive and follows the sodium. The jejunum is freely permeable to water, so the contents remain isotonic.

> Movement of sodium into the lumen occurs if sodium concentration is low, but absorption of sodium, and hence water, occurs only when the concentration is greater than 100 mmol/L.[14]

Sodium reabsorption normally occurs in the ileum and colon. In the absence of the absorptive capacity of the ileum and colon the net sodium losses are expectedly high. This occurs in the presence of a high fistula or jejunostomy. If there is a high fistula or jejunostomy, the daily net loss of sodium and net loss of water from the body will be approximately 300–400 mmol and 3–4 L respectively. This highlights the importance of sodium replacement when there is a high jejunostomy or fistula. Oral fluid con-

centrated in sodium will help reduce enteric fluid losses. The minimum required daily oral sodium replacement is 100 mmol. The sodium concentration that is absorbable is limited by palatability.[15]

The colon has a significant absorptive capacity, amounting to 6–7 L of water, up to 700 mmol of sodium and 40 mmol of potassium per day. Connection of colon in continuity with the residual small bowel will significantly reduce water and sodium losses.

Potassium absorption is usually adequate unless there is less than 60 cm of small bowel. In this scenario, standard daily intravenous requirements of 60–100 mmol of potassium are required. Magnesium is usually absorbed in the distal jejunum and ileum. Loss of these will result in significant magnesium loss and deficiency. Magnesium deficiency may precipitate calcium deficiency because hypomagnesaemia impairs the release of parathyroid hormone.

Nutrients

Carbohydrates, proteins and water-soluble vitamins

The upper 200 cm of jejunum absorbs most carbohydrates, protein and water-soluble vitamins. Nitrogen is the macronutrient least affected by a decrease in the absorptive surface, and utilisation of peptide-based diets rather than protein-based ones has demonstrated no benefit.[15] Water-soluble vitamin deficiencies are rare in patients with SBS, although thiamine deficiency has been reported.[16]

Fat, bile salts and fat-soluble vitamins

Fat and the fat-soluble vitamins (A, D, E and K) are absorbed over the length of the small intestine.[17] Hence loss of ileum will impair absorption. Bile salts are also reabsorbed in the ileum and bile salt deficiency will contribute to reduced fat absorption. However, bile salt supplements such as cholestyramine have shown no benefit and may worsen steatorrhoea due to binding of dietary lipid[18] and may also worsen fat-soluble vitamin deficiency. In view of multifactorial metabolic bone disease, vitamin D_2 supplements are often given empirically along with calcium supplements. Vitamin A and E deficiencies have been reported, but usually an awareness that visual or neurological symptoms may indicate deficiency combined with infrequent monitoring of serum levels are all that is necessary. If the patient is wholly dependent on PN, then replacement along with vitamin K injections is required. Most patients have lost their terminal ileum and so require vitamin B_{12} replacement. Trace elements appear not to be a problem, with normal levels being found in patients on long-term PN.

Loss of bowel results in not only decreased absorptive capacity but also rapid transit. Reduced time for absorption will exacerbate nutritional deficiencies.

Adaptation

Following massive small-bowel resection there are changes in the mucosal surface of the remaining small intestine. Most experimental work has been in small animals such as rats. It appears that adaptation will occur only if there is enteral feeding. Patients who are wholly dependent on PN have mucosal atrophy, which is reversed on refeeding enterally. The mechanism for this is at present unknown, but various trophic factors have been proposed. Current theory is that increased crypt cell proliferation leads to lengthening of villi and deepening of crypts, so resulting in increased surface area. Because the ileum has shorter villi it is able to adapt further, but is unfortunately more frequently resected. The stimulation to adapt appears to be threefold: (i) direct absorption of enteral nutrients leading to local mucosal hyperplasia; (ii) enteral nutrition resulting in the release of trophic hormones and a paracrine effect; and (iii) increased fluid and protein secretion with subsequent resorption, leading to increased enterocyte workload and adaptation.[17]

Another form of adaptation occurs in neonates, infants and young children, where continued developmental growth of the small intestine may make the difference between dependence on PN and managing with an enteral diet.[18]

Role of the colon in SBS

The colon has significant absorptive capacity, not only for fluid and electrolytes as described above, but also for short-chain fatty acids.[19,20] These are an energy substrate and in the region of 500 kcal may be derived in this way. It is estimated that having a colon is the equivalent of approximately 50 cm of small bowel for energy purposes.[21] The colon will also slow intestinal transit, particularly if the ileocaecal valve is present, which will improve absorption.

Having overcome the immediate problems of fluid balance and nutritional replacement, a frequent problem for those patients who still have their large bowel in continuity is diarrhoea. Excessive carbohydrate entry into the colon may result in osmotic diarrhoea.[22,23] Alternatively, choleric diarrhoea may be brought on by failure to reabsorb bile salts completely. Colonic bacteria deconjugate and dehydroxylate these into bile acids, which stimulate water and electrolyte secretion. In the more extreme cases of SBS, bile salt depletion may occur that will then give rise to steatorrhoea from incompletely digested long-chain fatty acids. Bile salts increase colonic permeability to oxalate. As the undigested fatty acids bind calcium in preference to oxalate, there is a resultant increase in enteric oxalate uptake and hence increased renal stone formation.[23]

 There is also an increased frequency of mixed gallstones, possibly because of interruption of the enterohepatic circulation.[24]

Lastly, D-lactate acidosis[25] is a rare syndrome that comprises headache, drowsiness, stupor, confusion, behavioural disturbance, ataxia, blurred vision, ophthalmoplegia and/or nystagmus. The exact mechanism is unknown. It may be provoked by a carbohydrate load and is relieved by antibiotics. Whether it is a direct result of D-lactate or whether this is a marker for some other substance is unclear. There is anecdotal evidence that neomycin or vancomycin has led to improvements.

Surgical catastrophe and management

The management of intestinal failure and enterocutaneous fistulas can present a paradigm of multidisciplinary care. In those patients who fail to heal spontaneously, surgical treatment is generally one of the last of many steps in treatment. Owing to the heterogeneity of this condition, randomised placebo-controlled trials have not been performed in patients and most recommendations are based on expert opinions. The multidisciplinary approach to management involves the initial 'damage control' and medical management followed by definitive surgical management. It is vitally important to initiate wound and psychological management early in order to prevent and reduce effluent-associated excoriation and prepare the patient mentally for what may be at least a few months of therapy.

Resuscitation

As discussed above, the scenarios in which patients usually develop intestinal failure are often acute catastrophes, and the very nature of intestinal failure is such that patients are often severely fluid and electrolyte depleted. In light of this, urgent fluid and electrolyte replacement is vital. This will often have been undertaken when the patient was first admitted to hospital, before transfer to a specialist intestinal failure centre.

Restitution

The key components of restitution may be summarised by the acronym SNAPP, representing sepsis, nutrition, anatomy, protection of skin and planned surgery. Each is considered in turn.

Sepsis

Sepsis is often present in patients who have developed intestinal failure and adversely influences outcome.

In a study of patients with enterocutaneous fistulas, Reber et al.[11] reported an overall mortality of 11%, with 65% of these associated with sepsis. In patients who had their sepsis controlled within 1 month the mortality was 8%, with spontaneous closure of the fistula in 48%. In those where sepsis remained uncontrolled the mortality was 85%, with a spontaneous closure rate of 6%.

Awareness of the high probability of associated sepsis is vital, and if the suspicion arises patients should be thoroughly investigated. Currently the optimum tool to identify collections is computed tomography (CT). Management includes appropriate antibiotics and drainage of sepsis. This is usually possible and successful radiologically, and is the preferred option where possible. Surgical drainage carries a high risk of further bowel damage.

Nutrition

Sepsis and inflammatory bowel disease can add to the patient's state of malnutrition. Replacement of fluid, electolytes and nutrients, including carbohydrate, protein, fat and vitamins, is vital. Monitoring fluid and electrolyte replacement is a vital part of nutritional support and involves serum electrolyte measurements

and regular weight measurements. Hiram Studley in 1936 commented that 'Weight loss is a basic indicator of surgical risk' and this still remains true today.

Fluid and electrolytes

Following resuscitation, fluid and electrolyte requirements will depend on the patient's losses. As described above, the first stage of intestinal failure is a hypersecretory phase, with high outputs and gastric hypersecretion. Fluid and electrolyte replacement should be by the intravenous route, with the following requirements:

Water: losses + 1 L
Na^+: losses (100 mmol/L effluent) + 80 mmol
K^+: 80 mmol/day
Mg^{2+}: 10 mmol/day.

Nutritional support

Early return to enteral nutrition should be the aim as soon as the patient is haemodynamically stable and fluid and electrolyte replacement complete. Parenteral nutrition should be regarded as a support mechanism rather than the main source of calories. Overall energy requirements depend on the size and weight of the patient, activity levels and metabolic status, with sepsis increasing demand. The rule of thumb is that males require 25–30 kcal/day and females 20–25 kcal/day of non-protein energy. For research purposes, more exact estimates can be made using the Harris–Benedict equation:

$$\text{Male energy expenditure} = [66 + (13.7 + W) + (5 + H) - (6.8 + A)] + SF$$
$$\text{Female energy expenditure} = [665 + (9.6 + W) + (1.7 + H) - (4.7 + A)] + SF$$

where W represents weight (kg), H height (cm), A age (years) and SF stress factor. However, the Harris–Benedict equation is inconvenient for daily use. Replacement should also include 1.0–1.5 kg/day of protein.

Daily requirements from the American Gastroenterological Association[26] for patients with SBS are recorded in Table 18.1.

Parenteral nutrition will provide calories (carbohydrate and fat), protein (amino acids), vitamins and trace elements. The volume should also be considered as part of the daily fluid requirement, with additional fluid requirements given as normal saline.

Reduction of output

Losses from stomas, fistulas or per anus may be very substantial, making replacement and simple management difficult. A number of strategies should be

Table 18.1 • Dietary macronutrient recommendations for short-bowel syndrome

	Colon present	Colon absent
Carbohydrate	Complex carbohydrate, 30–35 kcal/kg daily Soluble fibre	Variable, 30–35 kcal/kg daily
Fat	MCT/LCT, 20–30% of caloric intake, with or without low fat/high fat	LCT, 20–30% of caloric intake, with or without low fat/high fat
Protein	Intact protein, 1.0–1.5 g/kg daily, with or without peptide-based formula	Intact protein, 1.0–1.5 g/kg daily, with or without peptide-based formula

LCT, long-chain triglyceride; MCT, medium-chain triglyceride.
From AGA technical review on short bowel syndrome and intestinal transplantation. Gastroenterology 2003; 124:1111–34. With permission from the American Gastroenterological Association.

introduced to reduce these losses. Although they should be allowed to eat solids, patients should be restricted to around 500 mL of water orally per day, as hypotonic drinks will increase output in patients with SBS as described above. They should instead be cautioned against consumption of plain water and be given electrolyte solution, which will reduce intestinal fluid and electrolyte losses. There are several commercially available formulas. The St Mark's electrolyte solution is made from 1 L of water, to which is added 20 g of glucose (six tablespoons), 3.5 g of sodium chloride (one level 5-mL teaspoon) and 2.5 g of sodium bicarbonate (one heaped 2.5-mL teaspoon). This provides 100 mmol of sodium per litre. The problem is palatability, although this may be improved by the addition of orange squash or similar flavourings. Patients at home can make up this solution themselves. The World Health Organisation recommendations are similar but also contain 20 mmol of potassium chloride.[27]

Medication is also given to reduce gastric hypersecretion. H_2 receptors can reduce gastric hypersecretion,[28] as can proton-pump inhibitors, but not always enough to obviate the need for parenteral fluid supplements.[29,30]

Patients are routinely started on omeprazole to reduce gastric output. Octreotide produces a similar action but is more expensive and has been shown to be of little benefit to patients except in the first 2 weeks.

A review of all controlled studies evaluating the effects of somatostatin or octeotride showed that no study demonstrated a significant increase in the rate of fistula closure.[31] Medication to slow intestinal transit or gastric emptying should in theory improve absorption,[28] so both codeine phosphate and loperamide[32,33] are used on an empirical basis. They are given before meals and often at higher doses than normal, frequently crushed. However, codeine runs

the risk of addiction and clinical trials are equivocal as to the benefit of both,[34] so monitoring the effluent and weighing patients daily are essential for individual assessment. Bulking agents have shown no benefit in reducing stomal effluent. Cholestyramine may be used to treat hyperoxaluria, but it has no place in those with a jejunostomy, and in those with a colon in continuity it may reduce jejunal bile salt concentration to a level below the minimal micellar concentration for absorption of fat, resulting in steatorrhoea. A review of long-term medication is always useful, paying particular heed to site of uptake. Enteric-coated tablets are unlikely to be useful.

Dietary modification

Oral feeding should be introduced gradually with additions made one at a time and assessed. Patients should remain fluid restricted and continue on oral rehydration solution, gastric antisecretory drugs and antidiarrhoeal medication, the latter taken 30–60 minutes before meals. Drinking should be avoided during meals as this increases losses. It is important to continue intravenous maintenance therapy during this time as this will reduce the pressure on the patient to drink. In the early part of the second clinical stage it may be necessary to feed the patient wholly using PN, as gastric hypersecretion in response to even the smallest volume of enteral feeding can prejudice newly stabilised fluid balance.

A change of eating pattern to one of 'grazing' or 'little and often' increases the absorption window for the small intestine. Alternatively, overnight nasogastric tube or percutaneous endoscopic gastrostomy feeding can utilise otherwise unproductive absorption time.[35]

Oral magnesium oxide capsules, 12–16 mmol daily, are started and intravenous therapy is gradually withdrawn. Magnesium replacement may need to remain intravenous, albeit intermittent.

The precise balance between oral and parenteral requirements will vary between patients. As a rule of thumb, daily stoma/fistula losses below 1500 mL may be managed with oral replacement alone; losses between 1500 and 2000 mL require sodium and water replacement, usually as subcutaneous or intravenous fluids, but no parenteral nutrition; and losses of more than 2000 mL per day require parenteral nutrition. Requirements will change over time as adaptation occurs; this can continue for up to 2 years and in the case of children can be very dramatic.

Outcome aims and monitoring

Clinically, the aim is for the patient to have no thirst or signs of dehydration, with acceptable strength, energy and appearance. Biochemical targets should include the following:

Gut loss: <2 L/day
Urine: >1 L/day
Urine Na^+: >20 mmol/L
Serum Mg^{2+}: >0.7 mmol/L
Body weight within 10% of normal.

The mainstays of monitoring in the first stage are those used in the normal postoperative patient (temperature, pulse, blood pressure, postural hypotension, urinary output, and daily urea and electrolytes), combined with random estimations of urinary sodium osmolality. If urinary sodium content falls below 20 mmol/L, then deficiency is likely. As the patient stabilises, fluid balance is monitored with daily weight estimation and the acute observations are reduced in frequency. A meticulous watch is kept on the input/output volumes, with specifically designed charts for ease and clarity of recording. With the fluid balance under control and the eradication of any associated septic foci, reassessment of the underlying trend of the patient's nutritional status is performed. This is done by calculating body mass indices, skinfold thickness and serum albumin, and by making an estimate of likely return to normal activities. As the patient moves into the third stage of maximum adaptation, the common nutrient deficiencies are assessed (Table 18.2) and the rarer complications are clinically looked for (Box 18.1).

Total parenteral nutrition (TPN)

TPN is used either as a temporary measure to maintain fluid and energy intake while the remaining small bowel undergoes adaptation or as definitive treatment in itself. It may also be used as non-TPN in the third clinical stage. The advantages of maintaining some enteral nutrition, even if unable to be totally sufficient in terms of energy needs, include maintenance of normal gut flora, increased gastrointestinal adaptation and prevention of biliary sludge accumulation. With better understanding has come a willingness to maintain patients at home on PN.

Table 18.2 • Supplementation required in patients with intestinal failure depending on whether the patient needs partly enteral or wholly parenteral feeding

Nutrient	Parenteral	Partly enteral	Route
Potassium	Yes	If <60 cm and a jejunostomy	In TPN or oral supplement
Magnesium	Common with a jejunostomy Uncommon with a colon		Magnesium oxide 12–24 mmol daily
Calcium	Uncertain	Vitamin D_2 400–900 IU daily	
Vitamin D	Uncertain		
Vitamin A	Uncommon		Watch for visual and neurological symptoms and monitor levels 3-yearly
Vitamin E	Uncommon		
Vitamin K	Yes	Normal	Monthly injections
Vitamin B complex	Yes	Normal	In TPN
Vitamin C	Yes	Normal	In TPN
Vitamin B_{12}	If terminal ileum lost (most patients)	Bimonthly hydroxycobalamin 1000 μg	
Iron	Yes	Normal	In TPN
Zinc	Yes	Normal	In TPN
Copper	Yes	Normal	In TPN

TPN, total parenteral nutrition.

Box 18.1 • Complications of intestinal failure

Early

- Dehydration
- Hyponatraemia
- Shock
- Hypokalaemia

Intermediate

- Morale
- Weight loss
- Immune compromise
- Peptic ulcers
- Gastro-oesophageal reflux disease
- Proximal small-bowel inflammation
- Diarrhoea
- Bacterial overgrowth
- Peristomal excoriation

Late

- Vitamin deficiency syndromes
- Growth retardation in children
- Depression
- Total parenteral nutrition-induced liver disease
- Recurrent sepsis
- Intravenous line-related complications
- Cholelithiasis
- D-Lactic acidosis
- Urolithiasis

This is a great advantage for those who are dependent on PN and who have not otherwise responded to medical therapy. The benefits of the home environment cannot be overestimated in terms of morale and psychological well-being in an otherwise chronically hospitalised patient.[36] Home PN depends upon a stable physiological condition, other medical pathology, a suitable social set-up and good patient education, coupled with a dedicated PN team providing technical support and advice. Even then, it is not without complications, the chief among them being catheter sepsis.[37,38] Meticulous aseptic technique on the part of the team and patient is essential if this is to be avoided. It takes about 3 weeks as an inpatient for the nursing staff to teach sufficiently rigorous self-care of the feeding line. Other complications, such as catheter occlusion, hepatic dysfunction, gallstones and bone disease, may occur.[39] Guidelines to its use are well established.[40]

Anatomy or mapping

Defining the anatomy is important in terms of both planned management and prediction of long-term outcome. This may vary from determining how much small bowel remains, which may give an indication as to the likely necessity for perma-

nent parenteral nutrition, to defining the anatomy of enterocutaneous fistulas that will enable planned surgery later. The key facts to identify therefore are small-bowel anatomy, site of origin of a fistula (if present) and the anatomy of fistulous tracts.

Radiological contrast studies are the investigations of choice for assessing remaining bowel length and may include small-bowel follow-throughs or enemas, and fistulograms. CT enteroclysis and magnetic resonance (MR) enteroclysis can also be very useful in examining pathological bowel and areas of ongoing pathology, such as areas of ongoing obstruction or septic collections.[41–43] CT scanning can also provide valuable information, such as safe sites of entry into the abdominal cavity. Active discussion between the intestinal failure team and the radiologists is essential as each case is unique and poses different questions.

Protection of skin

Protection of the skin is an essential component of management of patients with intestinal failure. Small-bowel output is caustic and excoriation of skin around a stoma or fistula is a painful, demoralising and highly visible immediate complication. The extent of the problem will vary, ranging from a standard end ileostomy, through patients with an enterocutaneous fistula, to those with a laparostomy wound and multiple open loops of small bowel visible in the wound. This requires specialist stoma care from highly skilled nurses who will use a wide variety of shaped appliances, wide-necked bags, and protective dressings and pastes to protect the skin and contain the small-bowel contents. In rare situations, emergency surgery is indicated to either refashion a stoma or construct a controlled proximal stoma in the presence of a more distal fistula. An example of the need for this may be an enterovaginal fistula where a proximal stoma is the only means of control possible.

The resolution of wounds over time may be very significant. This is usually a factor of time, nutrition and skin protection. In the case of patients with laparostomies, there is usually significant reduction in the diameter of the wound and bowel loops become indistinguishable following growth of granulation tissue over them.

Planned surgery

Surgical intervention should be planned and frequently delayed. In the case of intestinal failure associated with enterocutaneous fistulas, early operative intervention to close the fistula is contraindicated by the associated high mortality due to re-fistulisation, sepsis, malnutrition and difficulties with fluid balance.[44] Indications for early surgery may include the following:[45]

1. drainage of pus when this cannot be achieved percutaneously;
2. excision of ischaemic bowel;
3. laying open of abscess cavities in the abdominal wall;
4. construction of a controlled proximal stoma;
5. catastrophic anastomotic failure, by exteriorisation of proximal and distal bowel ends.

These are usually the most septic patients and there is an associated high mortality with these procedures. Only in life-threatening situations should surgery be undertaken early in these patients and the decision should not be taken lightly as early surgery can result directly in multiple complications.

Patients managed with an open abdomen have a higher mortality and enterocutaneous fistula rate when compared with historical case-matched controls with a closed abdomen,[46] patients with an open abdomen having a mortality rate of 25% and fistula formation rate of 14.8%.

Reconstruction

When considering reconstructive surgery, the aim is to have a well patient, with no signs of dehydration or evidence of sepsis and with a good nutritional status. The aim of the management described above is to produce this scenario, such that surgery can be undertaken as safely as possible. The decisions then concern when to operate and what to do.

The decision about when to operate is vital. In the 1960s, Edmunds et al. proposed that early intervention using a conservative approach was associated with 80% mortality compared with 6% mortality for an operative approach. Supportive care has changed significantly since that time, however, particularly the use of PN. In 1978, Reber et al.[11] proposed planned intervention following eradication of sepsis. In the case of enterocutaneous fistulas, they reported a proportion of spontaneous closures, of which 90% occurred within 1 month, 10% within the next 2 months and none thereafter.

As discussed above, early surgery is made extremely difficult by the severity of the adhesions. It is important to delay surgery until these adhesions have softened, thereby reducing the risk of iatrogenic complications.

This will often necessitate a delay of 5–6 months following the patient's previous surgical intervention. Clinically, this may be indicated by the identification of prolapse of stomas or fistulas, and by the impression, on examination, that the abdominal wall is moving separately to the underlying bowel (**Fig. 18.1**).

The second decision is what definitive reconstruction to undertake and this must be individualised. It may range from connecting an end ileostomy to the remaining colon, with the aim of bringing the colon into continuity, to closure of multiple complex fistulas in a hostile abdomen full of severe adhesions.

Surgery to increase nutrient and fluid absorption by either slowing intestinal transit or increasing intestinal surface area is not commonly undertaken in the adult population. The operations include reversed small-bowel segments,[47–49] colonic interposition, and tapering with small-bowel lengthening.[50–52] The first two attempt to slow the transit of luminal contents by antiperistaltic activity or interposition of colonic tissue. They have achieved some clinical success but run the risk of further sacrifice of small bowel, obstruction or anastomotic leakage. Tapering with small-bowel lengthening has been applied in children with some success.[53] It involves dividing the dilated adapted bowel in two longitudinally, while maintaining mesenteric blood supply via careful dissection in the axis of the mesentery, allocating vessels to either segment. The bowel is then tubularised and joined sequentially.[54–56] However, no new mucosa is formed and there are risks of multiple adhesions and leakage or stenosis from the long anastomotic line.

Artificial valves, recirculation loops, electrical pacing,[57–59] tapering and plication, growth of neomucosa and mechanical tissue expansion[60] are all

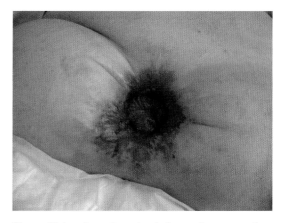

Figure 18.1 • A small, contracted wound some months after admission suitable for reconstruction surgery.

experimental techniques that are either untried in clinical practice or limited to case reports only.

Enterocutaneous fistula

High-output proximal small-bowel fistulas are associated with intestinal failure by producing functionally short bowel, and are often associated with significant problems with sepsis, malnutrition and difficulties with fluid balance.[44] Initial management is as described above.

Natural resolution of the fistula depends on the underlying pathology. Postoperative fistulas heal in around 70% of cases,[61] usually within the first 6 weeks of starting PN. Factors preventing healing may be specific to the fistula itself, as indicated in Table 18.3, or general, including ongoing sepsis, nutritional deficiency and infiltration of the tract by underlying disease, such as malignancy, Crohn's or tuberculosis.

Surgical intervention tends to be somewhat 'freestyle' as, despite detailed investigations, findings at surgery may be unexpected. General principles are well described.[62] The abdominal cavity is entered and the small bowel mobilised carefully as the adhesions are usually considerable. The fistula-bearing segment(s) of bowel is resected en bloc and the remaining ends of bowel re-anastomosed. This includes resection of any cutaneous abdominal wall component of the fistulous tract. If an anastomosis is likely to be in an area of residual sepsis, a stoma is usually advisable. Abdominal wall closure may be problematic and may necessitate a components separation abdominoplasty in order to obtain fascial closure due to tissue loss from the abdominal wall or the use of Vicryl mesh.

Rehabilitation

The goal of therapy is for the patient to resume work and a normal lifestyle, or as normal a one as possible. This can be a considerable undertaking as the patient will generally have spent a prolonged period of time in hospital, sometimes up to 6 months. Sending patients home on PN whilst they await surgery can reduce the time to long-term rehabilitation.

Rehabilitation must be multidisciplinary, involving stoma care, physiotherapy, dietetics and occupational health. There needs to be detailed stoma care for patients with high-output stomas and referral to a community continence service for patients with intestinal continuity and incontinence due to liquid stools. Referral to a medical social worker for assistance with social security benefits is important. A proportion of patients will need to remain on intravenous therapy, either saline or PN. Patients must be taught how to manage their tunnelled feeding lines appropriately in order to allow them to move from a hospital environment to home.

Considerable psychological support may be required and patients should be put in contact with supporting organisations. Long-term sequelae must also be considered. This may involve long-term HPN or recurrence of the underlying disease. Long-term care will include regular monitoring and review of therapy, vitamin B_{12} replacement if more than 1 m of terminal ileum has been resected, and review of other nutrients such as zinc, iron and folic acid and fat-soluble vitamins.

Transplantation

Around 2 patients per million commence HPN and 50% are suitable for consideration of small-bowel transplantation. In the UK this results in a possible 50 cases per year (50% children). A study of 124 consecutive adult SBS patients with non-malignant disease at two centres in France reported survival of 86% at 2 years and 75% at 5 years.[63] Dependence on PN was 49% at 2 years and 45% at 5 years. Small-bowel transplantation remains an experimental procedure. At the last update of the international

Table 18.3 • Factors influencing spontaneous fistula closure

	Unfavourable	Favourable
Anatomy	Jejunum	Ileum
	Short and wide fistula	Long and narrow fistula
	Mucocutaneous continuity	Mucocutaneous discontinuity
	Discontinuity of the bowel	Continuity of the bowel
Small bowel	Active disease	No active disease
	Distal obstruction	No distal obstruction

Box 18.2 • St Mark's intestinal failure protocol

Stage 1: Establish stability

1. Restrict oral fluids to 500 mL daily

Achieve and maintain reliable venous access

1. Administer intravenous sodium chloride 0.9% until the concentration of sodium in the urine is greater than 20 mmol/L

Maintain equilibrium by infusing

1. Fluid: calculated from the previous day's losses and daily body weight records
2. Sodium: 100 mmol/L for every litre of previous days' intestinal loss plus 80 mmol (more if the intestinal loss is excessive)
3. Potassium: 60–80 mmol daily
4. Magnesium: 8–14 mmol daily
5. Calories, protein, vitamins, trace elements: only if enteral absorption is inadequate

Stage 2: Transfer to oral intake

1. Continue intravenous maintenance therapy
2. Start low-fibre meals
3. Start antidiarrhoeal medication 30–60 minutes before meals
4. Start gastric antisecretory drugs
5. Start oral rehydration solution. Discourage drinking around meal times
6. Restrict the intake of non-electrolyte drinks to 1 L daily
7. Encourage snacks and supplementary nourishing drinks, within above limits

Consider the need for enteral tube feeding

1. Start oral magnesium oxide capsules 12–16 mmol daily
2. If intestinal losses remain high, start octreotide 50–100 mg s.c. t.d.s.
3. Gradually withdraw intravenous therapy

Stage 3: Rehabilitation

1. The patient and family should by now understand the physiological changes that have occurred and the rationale for treatment
2. There needs to be detailed stoma care for patients with high-output stomas
3. Referral to community continence service for patients with intestinal continuity and incontinence due to liquid stools
4. Referral to medical social worker for assistance with social security benefits
5. If intravenous therapy cannot be withdrawn because of continuing intestinal losses (>2 L/day), teach the patient/family to perform intravenous therapy at home

Stage 4: Long-term care

1. Regular monitoring and review of therapy
2. Vitamin B_{12} replacement if more than 1 m of terminal ileum resected
3. Review other nutrients such as zinc, iron and folic acid and also fat-soluble vitamins

registry (www.intestinaltransplant.org), 1292 intestinal transplants had been performed on 1210 patients in 64 different centres. This included intestine-only transplants (45%), combined intestine/liver transplants (40%) and multivisceral transplants (15%). The majority have been performed in patients under the age of 16 years (62%).[64]

The most recent evaluation has reported 1-year patient and graft survival of 79% and 64% respectively for intestine-only transplants, and 50% and 49% respectively for intestine/liver transplants. Long-term patient and graft survival for intestine-only transplants is 62% and 49% respectively at 3 years, and 50% and 38% at 5 years.[65] Because survival is poorer than that of patients on HPN, the indication for transplantation is SBS not maintainable on dietary supplements, and in whom PN is no longer possible due to severe complications. These usually include lack of access sites because of central venous occlusion, or cholestatic liver disease progressing to fibrosis and cirrhosis. The possibility of gut-lengthening operations must be considered first. The portal vein must be patent and should be checked by Doppler studies, as should the other great veins, in a search for vascular access for the perioperative period.

Complications are chiefly due to graft rejection and immunosuppression. Rejection leads to bacterial translocation and sepsis in an immunosuppressed patient who is often already malnourished. Current immunosuppressives such as tacrolimus have been paramount in reducing graft sepsis but have adverse effects of neurotoxicity, nephrotoxicity and glucose intolerance. The antiproliferative agents may cause bone marrow suppression. The consequences of chronic steroid use are osteoporosis, cataracts and diabetes, and growth retardation in children. Opportunistic infections are a major problem, particularly cytomegalovirus.[66]

Recently, a report of an experimental procedure in beagles described the transplantation of ileal mucosa to the colonic lumen. This raises the possibility of autogenic allotropic small-bowel mucosa transplantation.

Supporting organisations

Like most chronic conditions, a supporting structure has evolved to assist in overall management. The patient support group is Patients on Intravenous and Nasogastric Nutrition Therapy (PINNT, 258 Wennington Road, Rainham, Essex RM13 9UU). The paediatric version is called half-PINNT. Apart from the functions of providing advice and understanding from patients in a similar condition, the association also enables the borrowing of portable equipment to allow holidays away from home.

The professional supporting body is the British Association of Parenteral and Enteral Nutrition (BAPEN, PO Box 922, Maidenhead, Berkshire SL6 4SH). Keeping an overall view of intestinal failure is the British Artificial Nutritional Survey (BANS, 4 Low Moor Road, Lincoln LN 3JY), which maintains a census of patients on long-term nutritional support. Most importantly, the pharmaceutical firms that supply the various nutritional mixtures are also involved in providing and delivering the bags to patients at home; this also includes maintenance contracts that ensure continued functioning of the necessary fridges and emergency back-up in case of failure.

Summary

Recent developments in intestinal failure, including HPN and a greater understanding of the pathophysiology of massive intestinal resection, have allowed clinicians to treat and maintain such patients, resulting in long-term survival. The complex medical and surgical management is prolonged and multidisciplinary. It is summarised in Box 18.2.

Key points

- Intestinal failure is a multifactorial entity with improved long-term outcome with developments in nutritional and specialised care.
- Nutritional requirements will vary according to phase of intestinal failure. In the hypersecretory phase the aim is to maintain fluid balance and reduce stoma output and total parenteral nutrition may be required. In the adaptation and stabilisation phases enteral nutrition is encouraged and total parenteral nutrition requirements may be reduced or weaned.
- A clear understanding of normal intestinal physiology is required to understand the pathophysiology of intestinal failure.
- Prevention of intestinal failure is important and involves meticulous attention to anastomotic technique and techniques to preserve intestinal length in conditions such as Crohn's disease. The use of non-absorbable mesh and VAC dressings should be avoided in the setting of intestinal inflammation.
- A staged approach to management will ensure good long-term outcome. Nutritional management, defining the anatomy by radiological means and skin protection should be the initial steps in management. Any definitive surgery should be deferred till nutritional optimisation has been achieved, all sepsis is eradicated and maturation of adhesions has occurred.
- The multidisciplinary team approach to management of intestinal failure is the standard of care and consideration should be given to referring these patients to a centre dedicated to the management of intestinal failure.
- Intestinal transplantation is a valuable addition to the armentarium of treatments available for intestinal failure.

References

1. Scott NA, Leinhardt DJ, O'Hanrahan T et al. Spectrum of intestinal failure in a specialised unit. Lancet 1991; 337(8739):471–3.

2. Anonymous. Intestinal failure: criteria for referral. London: St Mark's Hospital, 1999 (internal).

3. Bakker H, Bozzetti F, Staun M et al. Home parenteral nutrition in adults: a European multicentre survey in 1997. ESPEN-Home Artificial Nutrition Working Group. Clin Nutr 1999; 18(3):135–40.

4. Howard L, Ament ME, Fleming CR. Current use and clinical outcome of home parenteral and enteral nutrition therapies in the United States. Gastroenterology 1995; 109:355–65.

5. Carlson GL. Surgical management of intestinal failure. Proc Nutr Soc 2003; 62(3):711–18.

6. Nightingale JM. Parenteral nutrition: multi-disciplinary management. Hosp Med 2005; 66(3): 147–51.

7. Sudan D, DiBaise J, Torres C et al. A multidisciplinary approach to the treatment of intestinal failure. J Gastrointest Surg 2005; 9(2):165–76.

8. DiBaise JK, Young RJ, Vanderhoof JA. Intestinal rehabilitation and the short bowel syndrome: part 2. Am J Gastroenterol 2004; 99(9):1823–32.

9. Buchman AL. Etiology and initial management of short bowel syndrome. Gastroenterology 2006; 130(2, Suppl 1):S5–15.

10. DiBaise JK, Young RJ, Vanderhoof JA. Intestinal rehabilitation and the short bowel syndrome: part 1. Am J Gastroenterol 2004; 99(7):1386–95.

11. Reber H, Roberts C, Way L et al. Management of external gastrointestinal fistulas. Ann Surg 1978; 188:460–7.

   Excellent paper that provides clear management strategies which still remain current.

12. McIntyre P, Ritchie J, Hawley P et al. Management of enterocutaneous fistulas: a review of 132 cases. Br J Surg 1984; 71:293–6.

13. Rao M, Burke D, Finan PJ et al. The use of vacuum-assisted closure of abdominal wounds: a word of caution. Colorectal Dis 2007; 9(3):266–8.

14. Spiller RC, Jones BJM, Silk DBA. Jejunal water and electrolyte absorption from two proprietary enteral feeds in man: importance of sodium content. Gut 1987; 28:671.

15. Lennard-Jones J. Oral rehydration solutions in short bowel syndrome. Clin Ther 1990; 12(Suppl A):129–37.

16. Allou M, Ehrinpreis M. Shortage of intravenous multivitamin solution in the United States. N Engl J Med 1997; 337:54–5.

17. Vanderhoof JA, Young RJ, Thompson JS. New and emerging therapies for short bowel syndrome in children. Paediatr Drugs 2003; 5(8):525–31.

18. Kurkchubasche A, Rowe M, Smith S. Adaptation in short-bowel syndrome: reassessing old limits. J Pediatr Surg 1997; 28:1069–71.

19. Hoffman A, Poley R. Role of bile acid malabsorption in pathogenesis of diarrhoea and steatorrhea in patients with ileal resection. Gastroenterology 1972; 62:918–34.

20. Gouttebel MC, Saint-Aubert B, Astre C et al. Total parenteral nutrition needs in different types of short bowel syndrome. Dig Dis Sci 1986; 31(7):718–23.

21. Jeppesen P, Mortensen P. Significance of a preserved colon for parenteral energy requirements in patients receiving home parenteral nutrition. Scand J Gastroenterol 1998; 33:1175–9.

22. Spiller R, Brown M, Phillips P. Decreased fluid tolerance, accelerated transit, and abnormal motility of the human colon induced by oleic acid. Gastroenterology 1986; 91:100–7.

23. Ammon H, Phillips S. Inhibition of colonic water and electrolyte absorption by fatty acids in man. Gastroenterology 1973; 65:744–9.

24. Nightingale JM, Lennard-Jones JE, Gertner DJ et al. Colonic preservation reduces need for parenteral therapy, increases incidence of renal stones, but does not change high prevalence of gall stones in patients with a short bowel. Gut 1992; 33(11):1493–7.

   Seminal paper on the role of the colon in reducing extraintestinal manifestations of intestinal failure.

25. Oh M, Phelps K, Traube M et al. d-Lactic acidosis in a man with the short bowel syndrome. N Engl J Med 1979; 301:1493–7.

26. AGA technical review on short bowel syndrome and intestinal transplantation. Gastroenterology 2003; 124:111–34.

27. WHO. Treatment and prevention of dehydration in diarrhea diseases: a guide for use at the primary level. Geneva: World Health Organisation, 1976.

28. Nightingale JM, Kamm MA, van der Sijp JR et al. Disturbed gastric emptying in the short bowel syndrome. Evidence for a 'colonic brake'. Gut 1993; 34(9):1171–6.

29. Goldman C, Rudloff M, Ternberg J. Cimetidine and neonatal small bowel adaptation: an experimental study. J Pediatr Surg 1987; 22:484–7.

30. Jacobsen O, Ladefoged K, Stage J et al. Effects of cimetidine on jejunostomy effluents in patients with severe short-bowel syndrome. Scand J Gastroenterol 1986; 824-8.

31. Hesse U, Ysebaert D, de Hemptinne B. Role of somatostatin-14 and its analogues in the management of gastrointestinal fistulae: clinical data. Gut 2001; 49(Suppl 4):iv11–21.

32. Schlemminger R, Lottermoser S, Sostmann H et al. Metabolic parameters and neurotensin liberation after resection of the small intestine, syngeneic and allogeneic segment transplantation in the rat. Langenbeck's Arch Chir 1993; 378:265–72.

33. Farthing M. Octreotide in dumping and short bowel syndromes. Digestion 1993; 54(Suppl 1):47–52.

34. Rodrigues C, Lennard-Jones J, Thompson D et al. The effects of octreotide, soy polysaccharide, codeine and loperamide on nutrient, fluid and electrolyte absorption in the short-bowel syndrome. Aliment Pharmacol Ther 1989; 3:159–69.

35. McIntyre P, Wood S, Powell-Tuck J et al. Nocturnal nasogastric tube feeding at home. Postgrad Med J 1983; 59:767–9.

36. Gulledge A, Gipson W, Steiger E et al. Home parenteral nutrition for the short bowel syndrome. Psychological issues. Gen Hosp Psychiat 1980; 2:271–81.

37. Lake A, Kleinman R, Walker W. Enteric alimentation in specialized gastrointestinal problems: an alternative to total parenteral nutrition. Adv Pediatr 1981; 28:319–39.

38. Kurkchubasche A, Smith S, Rowe M. Catheter sepsis in short-bowel syndrome. Arch Surg 1992; 127:21–4.

39. Foldes J, Rimon B, Muggia-Sullam M. Progressive bone loss during long-term home total parenteral nutrition. J Parenteral Enteral Nutr 1990; 14:139–42.

40. Anonymous. Guidelines in the use of total parenteral nutrition in hospital patients. J Parenteral Enteral Nutr 1987; 10:441–5.

41. Lappas JC. Imaging of the postsurgical small bowel. Radiol Clin North Am 2003; 41(2):305–26.

42. Umschaden HW, Gasser J. MR enteroclysis. Radiol Clin North Am 2003; 41(2):231–48.

43. Wiarda BM, Kuipers EJ, Houdijk LP et al. MR enteroclysis: imaging technique of choice in diagnosis of small bowel diseases. Dig Dis Sci 2005; 50(6):1036–40.

44. Chapman R, Foran R, Dunphrey J. Management of intestinal fistulas. Am J Surg 1964; 108:157–64.

45. Keighley MR. Intestinal fistula. In: Keighley MR, Williams N (eds) Surgery of the anus, rectum and colon. London: WB Saunders, 1993; pp. 2014–43.

46. Adkins AL, Robbins J, Villalba M et al. Open abdomen management of intra-abdominal sepsis. Am Surg 2004; 70(2):137–40.

47. Pigot F, Messing B, Chaussade S et al. Severe short bowel syndrome with a surgically reversed small bowel segment. Dig Dis Sci 1990; 35(1):137–44.

48. Panis Y, Messing B, Rivet P et al. Segmental reversal of the small bowel as an alternative to intestinal transplantation in patients with short bowel syndrome. Ann Surg 1997; 225(4):401–7.

49. Hennessy K. Nutritional support and gastrointestinal disease. Nurs Clin North Am 1989; 24:373–82.

50. Thompson J, Pinch L, Murray N et al. Experience with intestinal lengthening for the short-bowel syndrome. J Pediatr Surg 1991; 26:721–4.

51. Thompson J, Vanderhoof J, Antonson D. Intestinal tapering and lengthening for short bowel syndrome. J Pediatr Surg 1985; 4:495–7.

52. Weinberg G, Matalon T, Brunner M et al. Bleeding stomal varices: treatment with a transjugular intrahepatic portosystemic shunt in two pediatric patients. J Vasc Intervent Radiol 1995; 6:233–6.

53. Bianchi A. Longitudinal intestinal lengthening and tailoring: results in 20 children. J R Soc Med 1997; 90:429–32.

54. Pokorny WJ, Fowler CL. Isoperistaltic intestinal lengthening for short bowel syndrome. Surg Gynecol Obstet 1991; 172(1):39–43.

55. Boeckman C, Traylor R. Bowel lengthening for short gut syndrome. J Pediatr Surg 1981; 16:996–7.

56. Dionig IP, Spada M, Alessiani M. Potential small bowel transplant recipients in Italy. Italian National Register of Home Parenteral Nutrition. Transpl Proc 1994; 26:1444–5.

57. Cullen J, Kelly K. The future of intestinal pacing. Gastroenterol Clin North Am 1994; 23:391–402.

58. Gladen HE, Kelly KA. Electrical pacing for short bowel syndrome. Surg Gynecol Obstet 1981; 153(5):697–700.

59. Brousse N, Canioni D, Rambaud C. Small bowel transplant cyclosporine-related lymphoproliferative disorder: report of a case. Transpl Proc 1994; 26:1424–5.

60. Stark GB, Dorer A, Walgenbach KJ et al. The creation of a small bowel pouch by tissue expansion – an experimental study in pigs. Langenbeck's Arch Chir 1990; 375(3):145–50.

61. Levy E, Frileux P, Sandrucci S. Continuous enteral nutrition during the early adaptive stage of the short bowel syndrome. Br J Surg 1988; 75:549–53.

62. Fazio V. Intestinal fistulas. In: Keighley M, Pemberton J, Fazio V et al. (eds) Atlas of colorectal surgery. New York: Churchill Livingstone, 1996; pp. 363–71.

63. Carbonnel F, Cosnes J, Chevret S et al. The role of anatomic factors in nutritional autonomy after extensive small bowel resection. J Parenteral Enteral Nutr 1996; 20(4):275–80.

64. Grant D. Intestinal transplantation: 1997 report of the international registry. Transplantation 2000; 69:555–9.

65. US Scientific Registry of Transplant Recipients and the Organ Procurement and Transplantation Network. 2000 Annual Report. Transplant data 1990–1999. Rockville, MD: United Network of Organ Sharing. Richmond, VA: US Department of Health and Human Services, Health Resources and Services Administration, Office of Special Programs, Division of Transplantation.

66. Pirenne J. Short-bowel syndrome. Medical aspects and prospects of intestinal transplantation. Acta Chir Belg 1996; 96(4):150–4.

M